2nd edition
obstetrics and gynecology

The National Medical Series for Independent Study

2nd edition
obstetrics and gynecology

William W. Beck, Jr., M.D.

Professor
Department of Obstetrics and Gynecology
University of Pennsylvania School
  of Medicine
Pennsylvania Hospital
Philadelphia, Pennsylvania

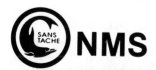 **NMS**

National Medical Series from Williams & Wilkins
Baltimore, Hong Kong, London, Sydney

Harwal Publishing Company, Malvern, Pennsylvania

**Williams
& Wilkins**

Illustrations: Wieslawa B. Langenfeld
Layout artist: Adriana Kulczycky
Composition: June Sangiorgio Mash

The author of the Introduction to the Challenge Exam, Michael
J. O'Donnell, Ph.D., holds the positions of Assistant Professor of
Psychiatry and Director of Biomedical Communications at the
University of New Mexico School of Medicine, Albuquerque,
New Mexico.

Library of Congress Cataloging-in-Publication Data

Obstetrics and gynecology/editor, William W. Beck, Jr.—
  2nd ed. p.   cm.—(The National medical series
  for independent study)
(A Williams & Wilkins medical publication)
  Includes bibliographies and index.
  ISBN 0-683-06240-9 (pbk.)
    1. Gynecology—Examinations, questions, etc.   2.
Obstetrics—Examinations, questions, etc. 3. Gynecology—Outlines, syllabi, etc.   4. Obstetrics—Outlines,
syllabi, etc.   I. Beck, William W., 1939-   . II.
Series. III. Series: A Williams & Wilkins medical
publication.
    [DNLM: 1. Gynecology—examination questions.
2. Gynecology—outlines. 3. Obstetrics—examination questions.   4. Obstetrics—outlines. WQ 18 014]
RG111.035   1988
618'.076—dc19
DNLM/DLC
for Library of Congress   88-39731
                                               CIP

10 9 8 7

Contents

Contributors

William W. Beck, Jr., M.D.
Professor
Department of Obstetrics and Gynecology
University of Pennsylvania School
   of Medicine
Pennsylvania Hospital
Philadelphia, Pennsylvania

PonJola Coney, M.D.
Assistant Professor and Director of
   Reproductive Endocrinology and Infertility
Department of Obstetrics and Gynecology
University of Nebraska Medical Center
Omaha, Nebraska

Luciano Lizzi, M.D.
Assistant Professor
Department of Obstetrics and Gynecology
University of Pennsylvania School
   of Medicine
Pennsylvania Hospital
Philadelphia, Pennsylvania

John Riva, M.D.
Attending Physician
Department of Obstetrics and Gynecology
Pennsylvania Hospital
Philadelphia, Pennsylvania

Nancy S. Roberts, M.D.
Director, Division of Perinatology
Department of Obstetrics and Gynecology
Lankenau Hospital
Philadelphia, Pennsylvania

Edward E. Wallach, M.D.
Professor and Chairman
Department of Obstetrics and Gynecology
Johns Hopkins University School
   of Medicine
Baltimore, Maryland

Preface to Second Edition

The second edition of *Obstetrics and Gynecology* is marked by the addition of two new chapters and 200 new questions and explanations. The new chapters, written by two new contributors—Drs. John Riva and Luciano Lizzi—cover sexually transmitted disease, which is of particular relevance since the AIDS epidemic, and medicolegal concerns in obstetrics and gynecology.

In addition, all of the existing chapters have been updated, and many have been expanded. Also, inaccuracies from the first edition were corrected throughout thanks to very helpful letters from readers—both students and teachers. This feedback is very much appreciated.

The intent of this book remains the same—to serve as a resource and a study guide for students and residents learning obstetrics and gynecology.

William W. Beck, Jr.

Preface to First Edition

Obstetrics and Gynecology has evolved as an extension of the core curriculum offered to students at the University of Pennsylvania School of Medicine who elect their clinical rotations at Pennsylvania Hospital, Philadelphia, Pennsylvania. A group of the faculty, some of whom have since departed for other institutions, began with the subject matter presented to the students and increased both the scope and depth of the material. The result is *Obstetrics and Gynecology*, an outline book aimed at medical students and residents in the specialty. Aspects of certain topics have been purposefully omitted as they were thought to be inappropriate or unnecessary for the basic needs of a student learning the important concepts of the specialty. This book should serve as a good study guide and resource, regardless of the curriculum taught at a specific medical center.

William W. Beck, Jr.

Acknowledgment

Once again I would like to express my appreciation for all the work done by Ms. Jane Edwards in editing the second edition of *Obstetrics and Gynecology*. She does her job very efficiently, providing a perfect balance of suggestion, encouragement, patience, urgency, and understanding. Even when the manuscript schedule fell behind, Ms. Edwards' approach was always positive, a characteristic that I find both helpful and appealing.

Introduction

Obstetrics and Gynecology is one of six clinical science review books in a series entitled *The National Medical Series for Independent Study*. This series has been designed to provide students and house officers, as well as physicians, with a concise but comprehensive instrument for self-evaluation and review within the clinical sciences. Although *Obstetrics and Gynecology* would be most useful for students preparing for the National Board of Medical Examiners examinations (Part II, Part III, FLEX, and FMGEMS), it should also be useful for students studying for course examinations. These books are not intended to replace the standard clinical science texts but, rather, to complement them.

The books in this series present the core content of each clinical science area, using an outline format and featuring 500 study questions. The questions are distributed throughout the book at the end of each chapter and in a challenge examination at the end of the text. In addition, each question is accompanied by the correct answer, a paragraph-length explanation of the correct answer, and specific reference to the outline points under which the information necessary to answer the question can be found.

We have chosen an outline format to allow maximal ease in retrieving information, assuming that the time available to the reader is limited. Considerable editorial time has been spent to ensure that the information required by all medical school curricula has been included and that the question format parallels that of the National Board examinations. We feel that the combination of the outline and board-type study questions provides a unique teaching device.

We hope you will find this series interesting, relevant, and challenging. The authors and the staff at Harwal/Wiley welcome your comments and suggestions.

Part I
Obstetrics

1
Endocrinology of Pregnancy
Edward E. Wallach

I. INTRODUCTION

A. Endocrine changes during pregnancy. The most important endocrine changes are the production of human chorionic gonadotropin (HCG), human placental lactogen (HPL), prolactin, progesterone, and estrogens by the placenta. **Maternal hormone levels**, which differ from those in the nonpregnant state, **are dependent upon**:

1. **The presence of a placenta**, a rich store of steroid and protein hormones

2. **The presence of a fetus** whose endocrine structures—the pituitary gland, thyroid, adrenal cortex, pancreas, and the gonads—function as early as the eleventh week of pregnancy
   a. In the male fetus, the testes, in response to placental gonadotropin, produce testosterone, which is necessary for normal male development.
   b. In the female fetus, although the ovaries are responsive to placental gonadotropins, fetal ovarian steroid production is not obligatory for normal development.

3. **The presence of elevated circulating estrogens**, which have the following effects:
   a. They elevate binding proteins, such as thyroid-binding globulin (TBG) and cortisol-binding globulin (CBG). These proteins bind thyroxine and cortisol and spuriously raise their levels in the maternal circulation. The free fraction, however, changes little, and thus, the metabolic processes that are dependent on these hormones are usually unaltered.
   b. They partially inhibit the enzyme 3-β-hydroxysteroid dehydrogenase. This enzyme is necessary to convert steroid precursors with a Δ-5,3-hydroxyl configuration to a Δ-4,3-ketosteroid configuration. The latter steroids, which are biologically active and highly significant, include testosterone and corticosteroids.
   c. They inhibit maternal pituitary gonadotropin synthesis and release, thus making *placental* gonadotropins responsible for gonadotropic function.

4. **The ability of the placenta to regulate molecular transport** by permitting or restricting passage and transfer of oxygen and nutrients from the mother to the fetus and metabolic wastes and carbon dioxide from the fetus to the mother

B. Hormones that are significant during pregnancy are understood best in terms of the following five characteristics:

1. **Chemical nature**
   a. Steroids (e.g., progesterone and estriol)
   b. Protein hormones (e.g., HCG and prolactin)

2. **Source**
   a. The placenta is an important source of hormones, including HCG and HPL.
   b. The mother is the exclusive source of certain hormones early in pregnancy; however, as the pregnancy progresses, the fetus (after the first trimester) produces thyroid substances, pituitary tropic hormones, and gonadal steroids; and the placenta (at the end of the first trimester) secretes large quantities of progesterone.
   c. Occasionally there are multiple sources of hormones; for example, estriol is produced by the mother, the placenta, and the fetus.

3. **Mode of determination.** Measurements of certain hormone levels are important in following

the progression of a pregnancy or in determining abnormalities in fetal well-being. The following studies are used:

a. Single urine analysis (e.g., urine pregnancy testing)

b. Twenty-four–hour urine analysis (e.g., urinary estriol). Full-day specimens compensate for diurnal variations in hormone secretions.

c. Maternal blood studies. Blood specimens are valuable if possible diurnal variation in hormone secretion is taken into consideration. HCG and estriol can be measured in blood.

d. Measurement of amniotic fluid hormone levels. Measurement of amniotic fluid androgens determines fetal sex and fetal adrenal hypoplasia.

e. Dynamic tests. Although rarely used, these tests have been employed to determine placental sulfatase deficiency by administering dehydroepiandrosterone sulfate (DHEASO$_4$) to the mother and measuring estrogen production.

4. Normal patterns. Recognizing normal patterns of hormone activity during pregnancy can help to distinguish abnormal pregnancies and fetal compromise.

5. Significance. Understanding the function of a particular hormone may illuminate its role in reproductive physiology, in particular in maintaining pregnancy and fetal well-being; for example, hormone deficiencies that are deleterious to the pregnancy can be corrected by exogenous hormones, and the presence of certain hormones may serve as markers for gestational abnormalities.

a. High levels of HCG suggest a trophoblastic neoplastic disease since HCG originates in trophoblastic tissue.

b. Progesterone deficiency early in pregnancy suggests corpus luteum insufficiency since progesterone is produced by the corpus luteum in early pregnancy.

II. HUMAN CHORIONIC GONADOTROPIN (HCG)

A. Chemical nature. HCG is a glycoprotein composed of two side chains, the α- and β-subunits. This hormone has a molecular weight of approximately 35,000.

1. The α-subunit is biochemically similar to:

a. Luteinizing hormone (LH)

b. Follicle-stimulating hormone (FSH)

c. Thyroid-stimulating hormone (TSH)

2. The β-subunit is relatively unique to HCG.

B. Source. HCG is an almost exclusive product of trophoblastic tissue. It is produced by:

1. Normal placental tissue as early as 6–8 days postconception as demonstrated by immunofluorescent studies

2. Multiple placental development (multiple pregnancies)

3. Hydatidiform moles by virtue of trophoblastic proliferation

4. Choriocarcinoma cells

5. Ectopic pregnancies

C. Mode of determination. Measurements of HCG levels can be made on blood specimens or urine specimens, by biologic and immunologic assays, or by radioreceptor assays. Immunologic assays are more specific and sensitive than the biologic assays and, thus, have replaced them for routine methodology.

1. Biologic assays

a. Friedman rabbit test measures maternal HCG levels by its ability to cause ovulation in rabbits 12 hours after administration.

b. Male frog test measures sperm release into the ejaculatory ducts in male frogs after administration of HCG.

c. Aschheim-Zondek rat test measures ovarian follicular development after exposure to HCG.

2. Immunologic assays

a. Agglutination or latex particle fixation test determines HCG in urine by its competition with standard HCG for a given amount of antibody. It is a rapid assay and is positive in 95% of cases 28 days postconception.

b. Radioimmunoassay is used on blood specimens employing antibodies to the β-subunit of HCG. It is positive 8 days postconception.

    c. Radioreceptor assay measures the amount of HCG in blood that competes with radiolabeled HCG for a given amount of receptor sites on bovine luteal cell membranes. It is a rapid assay, but it is not as specific as the HCG β-subunit radioimmunoassay.

D. Normal patterns

    1. HCG rises rapidly 8 days postconception, doubling every 2–3 days and reaching a peak at approximately 80 days, then dropping to a plateau for the remainder of pregnancy. HCG is detectable throughout a pregnancy.

    2. HCG is increased in the presence of multiple pregnancies.

E. Significance

    1. The major role of HCG is to stimulate progesterone production by the corpus luteum. It, thus, maintains luteal function, which, in the absence of pregnancy, persists for about 14 days.

    2. HCG stimulates Leydig cells of the male fetus to produce testosterone in concert with fetal pituitary gonadotropins. It is, thus, indirectly involved in the development of fetal male external genitalia.

    3. HCG is used as a marker for pregnancy (pregnancy testing).
        a. Low values early in pregnancy suggest poor placental function and may predict abortion or ectopic location of pregnancy.
        b. Significantly high values suggest multiple pregnancy or trophoblastic neoplasia (e.g., hydatidiform mole and choriocarcinoma).

    4. HCG determinations are used to follow the course of patients treated for trophoblastic neoplasia.

    5. HCG is used clinically for induction of ovulation to treat anovulation based upon its biologic similarities to LH.

    6. HCG contains some TSH-like activities.

III. HUMAN PLACENTAL LACTOGEN (HPL)

    A. Chemical nature. HPL is a protein hormone with growth hormone– and prolactin-like effects. Its molecular weight is 22,000.

    B. Source. HPL is formed by the placenta as early as 3 weeks postconception and can be detected in maternal serum as early as 6 weeks. It disappears promptly from the blood following delivery. It has a half-life of about 30 minutes.

    C. Mode of determination. HPL is measured by radioimmunoassay.

    D. Normal patterns

        1. HPL can be detected in the serum of pregnant women as early as the sixth week of pregnancy. It rises steadily during the first and second trimesters with little variation, disappearing rapidly after delivery.

        2. HPL levels vary directly with placental mass and are, thus, affected by multiple pregnancies.

    E. Significance

        1. HPL, the "growth hormone" of the latter half of pregnancy, has the following properties:
            a. It induces lipolysis and elevates plasma free fatty acids, which provide energy for the mother.
            b. It inhibits glucose uptake and gluconeogenesis in the mother.
            c. It has an insulinogenic action, elevating plasma insulin levels, which favors protein synthesis, ensuring a source of amino acids for the fetus.

        2. HPL determinations have been used as a test for placental function.

IV. PROLACTIN

    A. Chemical nature. Prolactin is a protein hormone with a molecular weight of 22,000.

    B. Source. Three potential sources of prolactin during pregnancy are the:

    1. Anterior lobe of the maternal pituitary gland

    2. Anterior lobe of the fetal pituitary gland

    3. Decidual tissue of the uterus

C. Mode of determination. Prolactin is assayed by radioimmunoassay of blood specimens or amniotic fluid.

D. Normal patterns

    1. Prolactin levels in the normal nonpregnant female range between 8 and 25 ng/ml. Levels above this range are related to the following factors:
        a. Ingestion of certain drugs that elevate prolactin (e.g., phenothiazines)
        b. Hypothyroidism
        c. Pituitary adenomas
        d. Hypothalamic disease

    2. During pregnancy, maternal prolactin levels rise to a maximum of 100 ng/ml near term as a result of increased maternal pituitary production.

    3. Amniotic fluid levels of prolactin increase significantly during pregnancy. The source of amniotic fluid prolactin is neither the maternal nor the fetal pituitary gland but the uterine decidua.

E. Significance

    1. Prolactin prepares the mammary glands for lactation.

    2. Prolactin in amniotic fluid is thought to regulate salt and water metabolism in the fetus.

    3. Levels of prolactin in pregnancy, which are considerably higher than in the nonpregnant state, should not be interpreted as indicative of pituitary adenoma growth. However, patients with prolactin-secreting adenomas who conceive should be monitored by visual field determinations for possibility of enlargement.

V. PROGESTERONE

A. Chemical nature. Progesterone is a Δ-4,3-ketosteroid hormone that contains 21 carbon atoms. It has two angular methyl groups at the 10 and 13 positions and a two-carbon side chain at the 17 position.

B. Source

    1. In the nonpregnant state, progesterone is produced by all steroid-forming glands, including the ovaries, testes, and adrenal cortex. It serves as an intermediary and a precursor for other hormones (e.g., testosterone, corticosteroids, and 17-hydroxyl progesterone) and as an end product when it is produced by the corpus luteum.

    2. In the pregnant state, progesterone has a dual source: It is produced by the corpus luteum until the seventh to eighth week of pregnancy after which time the placenta assumes its production until parturition. This shift in production occurs at about the sixth week of pregnancy, and by the ninth week, the corpus luteum becomes an insignificant source of progesterone. This point is clinically significant since progesterone produced by the corpus luteum is essential for pregnancy maintenance until the eighth week.

C. Mode of determination

    1. Progesterone can be measured in blood by radioimmunoassay and competitive protein-binding assay. There does not seem to be diurnal variation in blood levels.

    2. Some laboratories prefer to measure pregnanediol, the major metabolite of progesterone, in 24-hour urine specimens, using chromatographic techniques after extraction.

D. Normal patterns

    1. Since progesterone originates initially from the corpus luteum, it is present at ovulation. In a nonconception cycle, the peak production of progesterone reaches 25 mg/day and measures approximately 20–25 ng/ml in peripheral blood.

    2. In the late luteal phase in a conception cycle, progesterone levels rise slowly as a result of HCG stimulation.

   3. As placental progesterone supplements corpus luteum progesterone, levels rise more rapidly.

   4. A transient decline in peripheral progesterone levels has been described in the seventh to eighth weeks of pregnancy, the time of the luteoplacental shift; however, this subtle change can be appreciated only when daily measurements are made.

   5. Progesterone concentrations in the blood continue to increase up until the time of parturition at which time the placenta produces 250 mg/day.

   6. Progesterone is produced in large quantities in the presence of multiple pregnancies.

E. Significance. Progesterone has all of the following properties:

   1. It prepares the endometrium for nidation.

   2. It maintains the endometrium.

   3. It relaxes the myometrium.

   4. It is thought to be instrumental in preventing the uterus from contracting, and interference with its production or action on the myometrium is thought to result in the onset of parturition.

   5. It has natriuretic actions and, thus, stimulates the increased production of aldosterone during pregnancy.

   6. It serves as a major precursor for critical fetal hormones during pregnancy.
      a. The fetus has a relative deficiency in 3-β-hydroxysteroid dehydrogenase, an enzyme necessary to convert steroids to a Δ-4,3-ketosteroid configuration.
      b. Placental progesterone is, thus, used by the fetal adrenal cortex as a precursor for corticosteroids and by the testes as a precursor for testosterone.

VI. ESTROGENS

A. Chemical nature

   1. Estrogens are phenolic steroids with 18 carbon atoms, characterized by an aromatic A ring. They lack an angular methyl group at the 10 position.

   2. There are three classic estrogens, which differ by the number of hydroxyl groups they contain.
      a. Estrone, a relatively weak estrogen, has one hydroxyl group at the 3 position.
      b. Estradiol, the most potent estrogen, contains two hydroxyl groups at positions 3 and 17.
      c. Estriol, a very weak estrogen, contains three hydroxyl groups at positions 3, 17, and 16. Estriol is produced in very large quantities during pregnancy (1000-fold larger than during the nonpregnant state)—larger than all of the other estrogens.

B. Source

   1. The production of estriol, which depends on the presence of metabolic steps in the mother, the placenta, and the fetus, is complex and takes into consideration two important biochemical principles:
      a. Ample levels of precursor are necessary to produce a specific steroid.
      b. Tissues involved in converting a precursor to a specific steroid must possess the appropriate enzymes to carry out the conversion.
         (1) The fetus has the following enzyme capabilities not possessed by the placenta:
            (a) Cholesterol-synthesizing enzyme
            (b) 16-Hydroxylase
            (c) Sulfokinase
         (2) The placenta has the following enzyme capabilities not possessed by the fetus:
            (a) Sulfatase
            (b) 3-β-Hydroxysteroid dehydrogenase
         (3) The placenta is virtually unable to manufacture cholesterol, as are the fetus and the mother.

   2. Steps in estriol synthesis are as follows:
      a. Cholesterol, mainly of maternal origin, is converted by the placenta to pregnenolone and then to progesterone.
      b. Placental pregnenolone enters the fetal circulation where, together with pregnenolone synthesized by the fetal adrenals, it is converted in part to pregnenolone sulfate.
      c. Pregnenolone sulfate is converted by the fetal adrenals to DHEASO$_4$, the most important

precursor of placental estrone and estradiol. Estrone and estradiol are produced in the placenta from $DHEASO_4$ by reactions involving hydrolysis of the sulfate, conversion of dehydroepiandrosterone to androstenedione, and aromatization.

  d. $DHEASO_4$, formed by the fetal adrenals, is converted to 16-α-hydroxy $DHEASO_4$ mainly in the fetal liver.

  e. 16-α-Hydroxy $DHEASO_4$ is converted by two steps to estriol by the placenta:
  (1) Sulfatase activity, which removes the sulfate radical
  (2) Aromatase activity, which converts the A ring to the phenolic structure characteristic of estrogens

  f. The estriol molecule, which accounts for 90% of the estrogens produced during pregnancy, enters the maternal circulation.

  3. Production of estriol involves integration of maternal, placental, and fetal contributions.

C. Mode of determination. Estriol is measured by assay of peripheral blood specimens and 24-hour urine specimens.

  1. Blood determinations are carried out using radioimmunoassay. While results can be obtained rapidly (i.e., no 24-hour delay from onset of collection to onset of assay), there is a distinct diurnal variation with peak amounts early in the morning.

  2. Determinations on 24-hour urine specimens are carried out using chromatography after extraction. There is no diurnal variation with this method.

D. Normal patterns

  1. Significant amounts of estriol are produced early in the second trimester, and levels continue to rise until parturition.

  2. Values in the urine reach 25–30 mg/day at or near term.

  3. Extremely low levels or no estriol may be associated with:
  a. Fetal demise
  b. Anencephaly
  c. Maternal ingestion of corticosteroids
  d. Congenital adrenal hypoplasia
  e. Placental sulfatase deficiency

  4. The decline in estriol production or the failure of estriol levels to rise may be due to:
  a. Maternal renal disease
  b. Hypertensive disease during pregnancy
  c. Preeclampsia and eclampsia
  d. Intrauterine growth retardation

  5. Large quantities of estriol are produced during multiple pregnancies and Rh isoimmunization.

E. Significance

  1. Estriol is an index of normal function of the fetus. Its production is dependent upon biochemical steps carried out in the adrenal cortex and the liver, which must be functioning normally.

  2. Estriol is an index of normal placental function. Its production is dependent upon pregnenolone and then conversion of 16-α-hydroxy $DHEASO_4$ from the fetus to estriol.

  3. When estriol levels are reduced below normal or fail to rise during pregnancy, fetal and placental well-being should be studied by supplemental tests, including sonography, fetal heart rate testing, and, possibly, amniocentesis.

STUDY QUESTIONS

Directions: Each question below contains five suggested answers. Choose the **one best** response to each question.

1. All of the following hormones are products of placental synthesis or production EXCEPT

(A) human chorionic gonadotropin
(B) human placental lactogen
(C) prolactin
(D) progesterone
(E) estriol

2. A woman states that her last menstrual period was 7 weeks ago and that she has had several days of light bleeding and lower abdominal discomfort. She has previously had a positive home pregnancy test. Measurement of which of the following hormone levels would be appropriate at this time?

(A) Human chorionic gonadotropin
(B) Human placental lactogen
(C) Progesterone
(D) Estriol
(E) Prolactin

3. Human placental lactogen, the growth hormone of pregnancy, is characterized by all of the following statements EXCEPT

(A) it elevates free fatty acids
(B) it elevates plasma insulin levels
(C) it induces lipolysis
(D) it inhibits gluconeogenesis in the mother
(E) it stimulates glucose uptake in the mother

4. Characteristics of progesterone include all of the following EXCEPT

(A) it is an intermediary product in steroid metabolism
(B) it contains 21 carbon atoms
(C) its main source during early pregnancy is the corpus luteum of pregnancy
(D) it is a precursor of testosterone
(E) its ovarian source is important after the first 9 weeks of pregnancy

Directions: Each question below contains four suggested answers of which **one or more** is correct. Choose the answer

A   if **1, 2, and 3** are correct
B   if **1 and 3** are correct
C   if **2 and 4** are correct
D   if **4** is correct
E   if **1, 2, 3, and 4** are correct

5. Hormones produced exclusively by the placenta include which of the following?

(1) Human chorionic gonadotropin
(2) Progesterone
(3) Human placental lactogen
(4) Estriol

6. Functions of human chorionic gonadotropin (HCG) include

(1) stimulation of the granulosa cells
(2) development of male fetal external genitalia
(3) treatment for trophoblastic disease
(4) production of progesterone from the corpus luteum

7. Excessively high levels of human chorionic gonadotropin would be expected in which of the following conditions?

(1) Choriocarcinoma
(2) Hydatidiform mole
(3) Twin gestation
(4) Ectopic pregnancy

8. Elevated prolactin levels can be expected in which of the following circumstances?

(1) Pregnancy
(2) Hypothyroidism
(3) Pituitary adenoma
(4) Phenothiazine use

SUMMARY OF DIRECTIONS

A	B	C	D	E
1, 2, 3 only	1, 3 only	2, 4 only	4 only	All are correct

9. Estriol production during pregnancy depends on the

(1) mother
(2) fetus
(3) placenta
(4) amniotic fluid

ANSWERS AND EXPLANATIONS

1. The answer is C. (*II B; III B; IV B 1–3; V B 2; VI B 1*) Human chorionic gonadotropin (HCG) and human placental lactogen (HPL) are totally manufactured by the placenta during pregnancy. HCG appears early and declines to low levels after the first trimester. HPL rises during the first and second trimesters and declines rapidly after delivery. During pregnancy, progesterone is produced in large quantities by the placenta after the ninth week; prior to that time, progesterone is produced by the corpus luteum of pregnancy. Estriol synthesis is a complex process that involves the mother, the placenta, and the fetus; the placenta does not have all the enzymes necessary to synthesize estrogen and depends on the fetus for some of the intermediate metabolites. Prolactin is not produced by the placenta; for the most part, it is a product of the anterior lobe of both the maternal and fetal pituitary glands.

2. The answer is A. (*II E 3*) Serum human chorionic gonadotropin (HCG) can be very helpful as a marker to evaluate the health or normalcy of a pregnancy, because in a healthy pregnancy HCG rises at a predictable rate; the HCG value should double every 2 days. Therefore, a quantitative HCG value, when lower than normal for the expected gestational age, is often indicative of an abnormal pregnancy, such as a threatened abortion or an ectopic pregnancy.

3. The answer is E. (*III E 1 a–c*) Human placental lactogen induces changes in the maternal physiology, which encourage growth of the fetus. It induces lipolysis, elevating free fatty acids, which provide energy for the mother. It elevates plasma insulin levels, which favors protein synthesis, ensuring a source of amino acids for the fetus, and it inhibits gluconeogenesis and glucose uptake in the mother, which allows for the transfer of materials to the fetus, thus contributing to fetal growth.

4. The answer is E. (*V A, B 1, 2, D 4*) Progesterone, a steroid hormone that contains 21 carbon atoms, is produced in all steroid-forming glands and serves as an intermediary and a precursor for other steroid hormones, such as testosterone and the corticosteroids. The main source of progesterone during the first 6–7 weeks of pregnancy is the corpus luteum of pregnancy; this structure ensures adequate progesterone for implantation and maintenance of the early pregnancy. The placenta is the main source of progesterone during the major part (9–40 weeks) of pregnancy.

5. The answer is B (1, 3). (*I B 2; II B 1; III B; V B 1, 2; VI B 1*) Human chorionic gonadotropin and human placental lactogen are produced only by the placenta. Progesterone is produced by the placenta but is also produced by the corpus luteum with or without pregnancy. Estriol is also a product of the placenta, but in pregnancy, its production depends on metabolic steps in the mother and the fetus as well.

6. The answer is C (2, 4). (*II E 1–5*) As human chorionic gonadotropin (HCG) is secreted from the early trophoblastic tissue, it stimulates the corpus luteum to continue to produce progesterone until such time (about 9 weeks) that the placenta takes over the production of progesterone for the pregnancy. HCG stimulates the Leydig cells in the fetal testis to produce testosterone and, thus, is indirectly involved with the development of the external genitalia of the male fetus. HCG stimulates the luteal cells of the corpus luteum to produce progesterone. Follicle-stimulating hormone stimulates the granulosa cells of the follicle. HCG is not used as a treatment for trophoblastic disease. It is an excellent marker to observe the regression or recurrence of trophoblastic disease as HCG is secreted by a choriocarcinoma and a hydatidiform mole; the disappearance of HCG with treatment of the disease signifies regression or cure.

7. The answer is A (1, 2, 3). (*II E 3 a, b*) Choriocarcinoma, hydatidiform mole, and twin gestations are associated with higher than normal levels of human chorionic gonadotropin (HCG). On the other hand, lower than normal levels of HCG are expected in an ectopic pregnancy, which is abnormally implanted. A slowly rising HCG level may suggest a threatened abortion or an ectopic pregnancy.

8. The answer is E (all). (*IV D 1, 2*) Prolactin levels rise sharply during pregnancy as a result of increased pituitary production. Use of drugs, such as the phenothiazines, and conditions, such as hypothyroidism, are associated with increased levels of prolactin as a result of the interaction between the hypothalamus and the pituitary gland, which causes the pituitary to secrete high levels of prolactin. A pituitary adenoma is also a source of increased prolactin secretion.

9. The answer is A (1, 2, 3). (*VI B 1–3*) Amniotic fluid is not involved in the synthesis of estriol. Steps in the mother, fetus, and placenta affect the production of estriol. Cholesterol from the mother is converted by the placenta to pregnenolone and then to progesterone. Within the fetus, pregnenolone is converted to pregnenolone sulfate and then dehydroepiandrosterone sulfate ($DHEASO_4$) by the fetal adrenal. This then is converted to 16-α-hydroxy $DHEASO_4$ in the fetal liver. The final two steps in the production of estriol occur in the placenta via sulfatase and aromatase activity.

2
Normal Pregnancy, the Puerperium, and Lactation
William W. Beck, Jr.

I. DIAGNOSIS OF PREGNANCY

A. Presumptive symptoms

1. **Cessation of menses**. The abrupt cessation of spontaneous, cyclic, and predictable menstruation is strongly suggestive of pregnancy. Because ovulation can be late on any given cycle, the menses should be at least 10 days late before being considered a reliable indication.

2. **Breast changes**. In very early pregnancy, women complain of tenderness and tingling in the breasts. Breast enlargement and nodularity are evident as early as the second month of pregnancy. The nipples and areolae enlarge and become more deeply pigmented.

3. **Nausea** (with or without vomiting). Morning sickness of pregnancy usually begins early in the day and lasts for several hours. Gastrointestinal disturbances begin at 4–6 weeks gestation and usually last no longer than the first trimester. Excessive nausea and vomiting can result in dehydration, weight loss, and even hospitalization.

4. **Disturbances in urination**. Early in pregnancy the enlarging uterus puts pressure on the bladder, causing frequent urination. This condition improves as the uterus grows and becomes an abdominal organ but returns late in pregnancy when the fetal head settles into the pelvis against the bladder.

5. **Fatigue**. Tiredness is one of the earliest symptoms of pregnancy. This usually persists into the second trimester with the woman getting back to normal by the sixteenth to eighteenth week.

6. **Sensation of fetal movement**. Between the sixteenth and the twentieth week after the last menstrual period, a woman begins to feel movement in the lower abdomen described as a fluttering or gas bubbles. This is known as **quickening**.

B. Clinical evidence

1. **Enlargement of the abdomen**. By the end of the twelfth week of pregnancy, the uterus can be felt above the symphysis pubis. By the twentieth week, the uterus should be at the level of the umbilicus.

2. **Changes in the uterus and cervix**. The uterus enlarges and softens early in pregnancy, and lateral uterine vessel pulsations are palpable. Because of the softening between the cervix and the uterine fundus, there is the sensation that these are two separate structures (**Hegar's sign**). The cervix has a bluish color within the first 6–8 weeks of pregnancy (**Chadwick's sign**).

3. **Endocrine tests** for pregnancy depend on human chorionic gonadotropin (HCG) levels in maternal plasma and excretion of HCG in the urine, which are identified by a number of immunoassays and bioassays.
   a. **Urine pregnancy tests** detect the presence of HCG and luteinizing hormone (LH). Although LH levels are high at midcycle and at menopause, the lowest sensitivity levels to HCG in the urine tests do not pick up LH levels at midcycle or menopause. Significant amounts of urinary protein can give false–positive results.
   b. **Serum pregnancy tests** quantify the β-subunit of HCG, which differs from the β-subunit of LH, thus providing greater sensitivity than the urine tests.

C. Positive signs

1. **Identification of a heart beat**. The diagnosis of pregnancy is assured with the identification of

the fetal heart beat, which ranges from 120–160 beats per minute. The fetal heart can be identified at 12–14 weeks by an ultrasound fetal heart monitor and at 17–19 weeks by auscultation with a stethoscope.

2. **Sonographic recognition of the fetus**. The small white gestational ring can be seen by the new vaginal ultrasound probes after 5 weeks of amenorrhea and by sonography after 6 weeks of amenorrhea. The embryo can be demonstrated within the gestational ring after 8 weeks of amenorrhea, and fetal heart action is seen by real-time ultrasonography at 7–8 weeks of gestation.

D. **Pregnancy dating**. Estimation of the date of confinement (EDC) is based on the assumption that a woman has a 28-day cycle with ovulation on day 14 or 15. Pregnancy lasts for 280 days (40 weeks) from the last menstrual period. The **EDC is therefore 9 months plus 7 days** from the start of the last menstrual period (Näegele's rule). Because ovulation does not always occur at midcycle, the EDC must be adjusted accordingly. The postovulatory phase in any cycle lasts for 14 days; for example, ovulation in a woman with a 35-day cycle occurs on about day 21; therefore, the EDC in such a woman must be pushed back 1 week.

- 3 mon + 7 day

II. PREGNANCY

A. **The first trimester** extends from the last menstrual period through the first 12–13 weeks of pregnancy.

1. **Signs and symptoms**
   a. Nausea, fatigue, and breast tenderness
   b. Frequent urination
   c. Minimal abdominal enlargement because the uterus is still a pelvic organ

2. **Bleeding**. About 25% of all pregnancies have bleeding in the first trimester; half of these pregnancies spontaneously abort, and the other half remain viable without problems. Uterine cramping with bleeding in the first trimester is much more suggestive of impending abortion than is either bleeding or cramping alone.

B. **The second trimester** extends from the end of the first trimester through 27 weeks of pregnancy.

1. **Signs and symptoms**
   a. **General well-being**. This is often the best part of a pregnancy because the symptoms of the first trimester are gone, and the discomfort of the last trimester is not yet present.
   b. **Pain**. As the uterus grows, there is a certain amount of pulling and stretching of pelvic structures. **Round ligament pain**, which results from the stretching of the round ligaments that are attached to the top of the uterus on each side and the corresponding lateral pelvic wall, is very common.
   c. **Contractions**. Palpable uterine contractions **(Braxton-Hicks contractions)** that are painless and irregular can begin during the second trimester.

2. **Bleeding.** A low-lying placenta that causes bleeding at this stage usually moves away from the cervix as the uterus grows.

3. **Fetus**. The fetus attains a size of almost 1000 g (more than 2 lbs) by the twenty-eighth week.
   a. **Motion**. Perceptible fetal activity (quickening) begins between the sixteenth and twentieth week.
   b. **Viability**. There is a 70%–80% survival of infants born at the end of the second trimester. If death occurs, it is usually from respiratory distress due to lung immaturity.

4. **Complications** of second-trimester pregnancies
   a. **Incompetent cervix**, the premature dilation of the cervix in the second trimester, can result in either premature labor or rupture of the membranes.
   b. **Premature rupture of the membranes** without labor or an incompetent cervix can result in serious bacterial infections in both the mother and fetus.
   c. **Premature labor** can present without an incompetent cervix.

C. **The third trimester** extends from the end of the second trimester until term or 40 weeks gestation.

1. **Symptoms**
   a. **Braxton-Hicks contractions** are painless, palpable, irregular contractions that become more apparent in the third trimester.

b. Pain in the lower back and legs is often caused by pressure on muscles and nerves by the third-trimester uterus and fetal head, which fill the pelvis at this time.

c. Lightening is the descent of the fetal head to or even through the pelvic inlet due to the development of a well-formed lower uterine segment and a reduction in the volume of amniotic fluid.

2. Fetus. The fetus gains weight at a rate of about 224 g (½ lb) a week for the last 4 weeks to an average of 3300 g (7–7½ lbs). Decrease in fetal motion is usually due to the size of the fetus and a lack of room within the uterus. However, some decreased fetal activity may be an indication of fetal compromise due to uteroplacental insufficiency.

3. Bleeding
  a. Bloody show, a discharge of a combination of blood and mucus caused by thinning and stretching of the cervix, is a sure sign of the approach of labor.
  b. Heavy bleeding suggests a more serious condition, such as placenta previa or abruptio placentae.

4. Rupture of membranes is either a sudden gush or a slow leak of amniotic fluid that can happen at any time without warning.
  a. Labor usually begins within 24 hours after rupture of membranes.
  b. Induction of labor is indicated if there is no labor within 48 hours or if there is any evidence of infection (chorioamnionitis).

5. Labor. Contractions that occur at decreasing intervals with increasing intensity cause the progressive dilation and effacement of the cervix.

III. STATUS OF THE FETUS

A. Growth and development. A fetus weighs approximately 1000 g (more than 2 lbs) at 26–28 weeks, 2500 g (5½ lbs) at 36 weeks, and 3300 g (7–7½ lbs) at 40 weeks. Fetal lung maturity is indicated by measuring surface-active lipid components of surfactant (i.e., lecithin and phosphatidylglycerol), which are secreted by the type II pneumocytes of fetal lung alveoli and which are essential for normal respiration immediately after birth. Studies have demonstrated that when levels of lecithin in amniotic fluid increase to at least twice that of sphingomyelin (at about 35 weeks), the risk of respiratory distress is very low. In addition, it has been shown recently that the presence of phosphatidylglycerol in the amniotic fluid (in addition to an L/S ratio of 2/1) provides *assurance* of fetal lung maturity as infants born before phosphatidylglycerol appears in surfactant, even with an L/S ratio of 2/1, may be at risk for respiratory distress syndrome.

1. Early fetal lung maturation (from 32–35 weeks) is seen with maternal hypertension, premature rupture of membranes, and intrauterine growth retardation, all of which are stressful to the fetus.

2. This stress prior to 35 weeks increases fetal cortisol secretion, which, in turn, accelerates fetal lung maturation.

B. Lie of the fetus is the relation of the long axis of the fetus to the long axis of the mother and is either longitudinal or transverse.

1. Longitudinal lie. In most labors (more than 99%) at term, the fetal head is either up or down, in a longitudinal lie.

2. Transverse lie. The fetus is crosswise in the uterus in a transverse lie.

3. Oblique lie. This indicates an unstable situation that becomes either a longitudinal or transverse lie during the course of labor.

C. Presentation. The presentation of the fetus is determined by the portion of the fetus that can be felt through the cervix.

1. Cephalic presentations are classified according to the position of the fetal head in relationship to the body of the fetus.
  a. Vertex. The head is flexed so that the chin is in contact with the chest, and the occiput of the fetal head presents. A vertex presentation occurs in 95% of all cephalic presentations.
  a. Face. The neck is sharply extended so that the occiput and the back of the fetus are touching and the face is the presenting part.
  c. Brow. The fetal head is partially extended but converts into a vertex or face presentation during labor.

    2. Breech presentations are classified according to the position of the legs and buttocks, which present first. Breech presentations occur in 3.5% of all pregnancies.

      a. Frank breech. The thighs are flexed, and the legs are extended.

      b. Complete breech. The legs are flexed on the thighs, and the thighs are flexed on the abdomen.

      c. Footling breech. One or both feet or knees present.

IV. THE PUERPERIUM is a period of 4–6 weeks that starts immediately after delivery and is completed when the reproductive tract has returned to its nonpregnant condition.

A. Involution of the uterus. The uterus regains its usual nonpregnant size within 5–6 weeks, going from 1000 g immediately postpartum to 100 g. This rapid atrophy is now recognized as due to the marked decrease in size of the muscle cells rather than the decrease in their total number. Nursing accelerates involution of the uterus because stimulation of the nipples releases oxytocin from the neurohypophysis, which leads to increased contractions of the myometrium.

    1. Afterpains. The uterus contracts throughout the period of involution, which produces afterpains, especially in multiparas and nursing mothers. In primaparas, the uterus tends to remain tonically contracted, while in multiparas the uterus contracts vigorously at intervals.

    2. Lochia is the uterine discharge that follows delivery and lasts for 3 or 4 weeks. Foul-smelling lochia suggests infection.

      a. Lochia rubra is blood-stained fluid that lasts for the first few days.

      b. Lochia serosa is a discharge that is paler than lochia rubra after 3–4 days because it is admixed with serum.

      c. Lochia alba. After the tenth day, because of an admixture with leukocytes, the lochia assumes a white or yellowish-white color.

B. Clinical aspects

    1. Urine. The puerperal bladder has an increased capacity and a relative insensitivity to intravesical fluid pressure.

      a. Overdistension, incomplete emptying, and excessive residual urine are possibilities that facilitate the occurrence of a postpartum urinary tract infection.

      b. A diuresis usually occurs between the second and fifth postpartum days.

    2. Blood. A marked leukocytosis occurs during and after labor. The leukocytosis, primarily a granulocytosis, may be as high as 30,000 per mm³.

      a. By 1 week postpartum, the increased blood volume of pregnancy returns to the usual nonpregnant level.

      b. The pregnancy-induced changes in blood coagulation factors persist for variable periods of time after delivery. The elevated plasma fibrinogen level is maintained at least through the first week of the puerperium. The gradual decline of the increased blood coagulation factors explains the occurrence of phlebitis of the lower extremities early in the puerperium.

    3. Menstruation

      a. Nonlactating women. The first menstrual flow usually returns within 6–8 weeks after delivery with ovulation occurring at 2–4 weeks postpartum.

      b. Lactating women. Ovulation has been detected as early as 10 weeks postpartum, so nursing mothers must understand that *the protection afforded by lactation lasts absolutely for only 6 weeks after which time ovulation and pregnancy are possible.*

D. Postpartum hemorrhage is defined as a blood loss in excess of 500 ml during the first 24 hours after delivery.

    1. Causes

      a. Trauma to the genital tract as a result of:

        (1) Episiotomy

        (2) Lacerations of the cervix, vagina, or perineum

        (3) Rupture of the uterus

      b. Failure of compression of blood vessels at the implantation site as a result of:

        (1) A hypotonic myometrium due to general anesthesia; overdistension of the uterus from a large fetus, hydramnios, or multiple fetuses; prolonged labor; very rapid labor; high parity; or after labor vigorously stimulated with oxytocin

        (2) Retention of placental tissue as seen in placenta accreta or succenturiate lobe

      c. Coagulation defects, either congenital or acquired, as seen in hypofibrinogenemia or thrombocytopenia

   2. Management
      a. Vigorous massage of the uterine fundus
      b. Use of uterine contracting agents, such as intramuscular or intravenous ergonovine (Ergo-trate, 0.2 mg), intravenous oxytocin (Pitocin, 20 units in 1000 ml of lactated Ringer's solution), or intramuscular prostaglandin (75 mg)
      c. Manual exploration of the uterine cavity for retained placental fragments or uterine rupture
      d. Inspection of the cervix and vagina for lacerations
      e. Curettage of the uterine cavity
      f. Hypogastric artery ligation and, rarely, hysterectomy

  E. Puerperal infection is defined as any infection of the genital tract during the puerperium accompanied by a temperature of 100.4°F (38°C) or higher that occurs for at least 2 of the first 10 days postpartum, exclusive of the first 24 hours. Prolonged rupture of the membranes with multiple vaginal examinations during labor is a major predisposing cause of puerperal infection.

   1. Pelvic infections
      a. Endometritis (childbed fever), the most common form of puerperal infection, involves primarily the endometrium and the adjacent myometrium.
      b. Parametritis, infection of the retroperitoneal fibroareolar pelvic connective tissue, may occur by:
        (1) Lymphatic transmission of organisms
        (2) Cervical lacerations that extend into the connective tissue
        (3) Extension of pelvic thrombophlebitis
      c. Thrombophlebitis results from an extension of puerperal infection along veins.

   2. Urinary infections are quite common during the puerperium as a result of:
      a. Trauma to the bladder from a normal vaginal delivery
      b. A hypotonic bladder from conduction anesthesia
      c. Catheterization

   3. Management
      a. Culture and sensitivity of the urine, the endometrial cavity, and the blood
      b. Antibiotics according to sensitivities
      c. Broad-spectrum antibiotics in pelvic infection where accurate identification of the offending organism is impossible
      d. Heparin with suspected thrombophlebitis when a spiking temperature does not respond to intravenous antibiotics

V. LACTATION

  A. Physiology

   1. Breast changes. Progesterone, estrogen, placental lactogen, prolactin, cortisol, and insulin act together in stimulating the growth and development of the breast's milk-secreting apparatus.

   2. Initiation of lactation. With delivery of the placenta, there is a *sharp decrease in the levels of estrogens and progesterone with the release of prolactin,* which stimulates milk production.

   3. Prolactin. A stimulus from the breast curtails the release of prolactin-inhibiting factor from the hypothalamus, which induces a transiently increased secretion of prolactin by the pituitary gland.

   4. Oxytocin. Stimulation of the nipples during nursing causes the release of oxytocin, which is responsible for the let-down reflex and the subsequent release of breast milk.

  B. Nursing. Breast milk is ideal for the newborn because it provides a balanced diet, it contains protective maternal antibodies, and the maternal lymphocytes in breast milk may be important to the infant's immunologic processes. Most drugs given to the mother are secreted in low concentrations in the breast milk. Water-soluble drugs are excreted in high concentration into colostrum, while lipid-soluble drugs are excreted in high concentration into breast milk.

  C. Mastitis is parenchymatous inflammation of the mammary glands that presents at some point after lactation has begun.

   1. Symptoms. Engorgement of the breasts is accompanied by a temperature rise, chills, and a hard, red tender area on the breast.

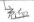

2. Etiology. The most common offending organism is *Staphylococcus aureus* from the infant's nose and throat, which usually enters the breast through the nipple at the site of a fissure or abrasion during the nursing process.

3. Therapy
   a. **Gram-positive antibiotic coverage.** Ampicillin or erythromycin for penicillin-resistant organisms
   b. **Heat to breast**
   c. **Continuation of nursing from the affected breast** to decrease engorgement
   d. **Drainage of the abscess** if the mastitis has progressed to suppuration

STUDY QUESTIONS

Directions: Each question below contains five suggested answers. Choose the **one best** response to each question.

1. All of the following signs or symptoms are present in a 12-week pregnancy EXCEPT

(A) Chadwick's sign
(B) quickening
(C) sonographic fetal heart action
(D) amenorrhea
(E) Hegar's sign

2. All of the following complications are typical of the second trimester of pregnancy EXCEPT

(A) premature labor
(B) cervical incompetence
(C) premature rupture of membranes
(D) placental abruption
(E) round ligament pain

3. Characteristics of a 28-week pregnancy include all of the following EXCEPT

(A) viability
(B) a fetal weight of 1000 g (move than 2 lbs)
(C) lecithin/sphingomyelin ratio of less than 2/1
(D) the absence of type II fetal lung alveoli cells
(E) the presence of phosphatidylglycerol

4. A complete breech presentation is best described by which of the following statements?

(A) The legs and thighs of the fetus are flexed
(B) The legs are extended and the thighs are flexed
(C) The arms, legs, and thighs are completely flexed
(D) The legs and thighs are extended
(E) None of the above

5. Which of the following statements about birth control following delivery is correct?

(A) It is not important until after the first menses
(B) It is not necessary in a woman who is nursing
(C) It should begin immediately in a nonlactating woman
(D) It is not necessary for 1 month following a cesarean section
(E) None of the above statements is correct

6. Postpartum hemorrhage could be a reasonable possibility in all of the following situations EXCEPT

(A) hydramnios
(B) triplets
(C) long labor
(D) erythroblastosis
(E) thrombocytopenia

Directions: Each question below contains four suggested answers of which **one or more** is correct. Choose the answer

    A if **1, 2, and 3** are correct
    B if **1 and 3** are correct
    C if **2 and 4** are correct
    D if **4** is correct
    E if **1, 2, 3, and 4** are correct

7. A woman in her second trimester of pregnancy is likely to experience

(1) round ligament pain
(2) lightening
(3) Braxton-Hicks contractions
(4) bloody show

8. Normal fetal lung maturity would be expected in which of the following clinical presentations?

(1) The presence of phosphatidylglycerol
(2) The presence of type II fetal lung alveoli cells
(3) A lecithin/sphingomyelin ratio of 3/1
(4) A 33-week pregnancy

9. Oxytocin in the puerperium is associated with the

(1) involution of the uterus
(2) initiation of lactation
(3) let-down reflex
(4) resumption of menses

ANSWERS AND EXPLANATIONS

1. The answer is B. *(I A 1, 6, B 2, C 2)* Chadwick's and Hegar's signs occur as early as 6 weeks gestation and are associated with changes in the cervix and the lower uterine segment. Real time ultrasonographic fetal heart action can be seen at about 7–8 weeks. Amenorrhea is an ongoing sign of pregnancy from the last menstrual period. Quickening, the woman's sensation of fetal movement, occurs sometime between 16 and 20 weeks of pregnancy.

2. The answer is D. *(II B 1 b, B 4, C 3 b)* Of the possibilities listed in the question, cervical incompetence is the biggest concern during the second trimester. The incompetence can be accompanied by either premature labor or premature rupture of the membranes, or both. However, any of the three complications can occur as a unique entity. Round ligament pain occurs between 16 and 22 weeks. Placental abruption rarely occurs before 28 weeks at which time the fetus is viable; thus, it is possible to salvage the fetus in this emergency situation.

3. The answer is E. *(II B 2 a, b; III A)* At 28 weeks gestation, the normal fetal weight is about 1000 g, which is a little over 2 lbs. There is a 70%–80% survival of infants born at the beginning of the third trimester. Because of fetal lung immaturity, one would expect a lecithin/sphingomyelin (L/S) ratio of 1/1 or lower and an absence of type II fetal lung alveoli cells, which secrete increasing quantities of lecithin and phosphatidylglycerol at 35–36 weeks. Therefore, the presence of phosphatidylglycerol would not be expected at 28 weeks gestation.

4. The answer is A. *(III C 2)* In a complete breech, the legs are flexed on the thighs and the thighs are flexed on the abdomen. In a frank breech, the legs are extended, and in a footling breech, both the thighs and the legs are extended. The arms have nothing to do with the description of a breech.

5. The answer is C. *(IV B 3)* Ovulation following delivery can occur as early as 2–4 weeks postpartum in a nonlactating woman and 10–12 weeks in a lactating woman. The method of delivery does not influence birth control; therefore, a woman should not delay birth control until after the first menses since ovulation may have occurred. Nursing mothers ovulate and often do so before the fourth postpartum month. Because a nonlactating woman can ovulate so soon after delivery, she must use birth control with her first coitus, which is usually 4 weeks postpartum.

6. The answer is D. *(IV D 1)* Any obstetric situation that overdistends the pregnant uterus can be responsible for postpartum hemorrhage. The bleeding occurs because the myometrium does not contract well after delivery, and the vessels in the placental bed continue to bleed. Thus, triplets and hydramnios can cause such bleeding because of overdistension. A long labor also contributes to uterine atony after delivery because of the inability of the myometrial fibers to contract well due to fatigue. Thrombocytopenia can cause postpartum hemorrhage because of the faulty clotting mechanism inherent in that disease. Erythroblastosis, the presence of erythroblasts in the blood, is not associated with postpartum hemorrhage.

7. The answer is B (1, 3). *(II B 1 b, c, C 1 c, 3)* Round ligament pain is common between 14 and 20 weeks of gestation and subsides thereafter; it is caused by the stretching of the round ligaments as the uterus grows. The irregular, nonlabor Braxton-Hicks contractions can begin before the third trimester. Lightening, the sensation of the fetus dropping into the pelvis, occurs at about 38 weeks if it occurs at all, and bloody show, the appearance of a bloody mucus discharge, occurs just before labor begins at the end of the pregnancy.

8. The answer is A (1, 2, 3). *(III A)* The type II fetal alveoli cells secrete the lecithin and phosphatidylglycerol that mature the fetal lungs. A lecithin/sphingomyelin (L/S) ratio of 3/1 means there is ample lecithin, when compared to sphingomyelin, to insure fetal lung maturity. This ratio must be 2/1 or greater. The presence of phosphatidylglycerol is the most positive available assurance of lung maturity. The fetal lung does not spontaneously mature until 35–36 weeks of gestation; at that time the L/S ratio attains a value of 2/1.

9. The answer is B (1, 3). *(IV A; V A 2–4)* With the stimulation of the nipple during nursing, oxytocin is released from the neurohypophysis. The released oxytocin causes the uterus to contract, which helps with the involution of the uterus, and the breasts to letdown (release) the milk. Oxytocin has nothing to do with the resumption of menses, and prolactin initiates the lactation process.

3
Antepartum Care
William W. Beck, Jr.

I. INTRODUCTION. Pregnancy is a normal physiologic state, not a disease state. It is important for physicians to be familiar with the normal as well as the abnormal changes caused by pregnancy. The objective of prenatal care is the delivery of a healthy infant and maintenance of the health of the mother.

A. Components of antepartum care

1. **Periodic assessment** begins with a comprehensive history and physical examination to identify risk factors or abnormalities and continues at regular intervals.

2. **Patient education** fosters optimal health, good dietary habits, and proper hygiene.

3. **Psychosocial support** is very important during such a profound emotional experience as pregnancy.

B. Definitions of parity

1. A **nulligravida** is a woman who is not and has never been pregnant.

2. A **gravida** is a woman who is or has been pregnant irrespective of the pregnancy outcome. With the first pregnancy she becomes a **primigravida** and with subsequent pregnancies, a **multigravida**.

3. A **nullipara** is a woman who has never completed a pregnancy to the stage of viability; she may or may not have aborted previously.

4. A **primipara** is a woman who has been delivered once of a fetus or fetuses (multiple gestation) who reached the stage of viability.

5. A **multipara** is a woman who has completed two or more pregnancies to the stage of viability. It is the number of pregnancies reaching viability, not the number of fetuses delivered, that determines parity.

II. HISTORY

A. Expected date of confinement (EDC). The EDC is calculated by adding 9 months plus 7 days (Näegele's rule) to the date of the last menstrual period.

1. This calculation assumes a 28-day menstrual cycle with ovulation around the fourteenth day of the cycle.

2. This calculation is unreliable in women with irregular cycles (4–6 weeks apart) because the day of ovulation could range from the fourteenth to the twenty-eighth day of the cycle. In such cases, the calculated EDC would be earlier than the true biologic EDC.

3. This calculation is unreliable in women using birth control pills for contraception who get pregnant in the first postpill cycle. Ovulation may have occurred later than 2 weeks after the onset of the last withdrawal bleeding (i.e., birth control menses).

B. Review of past pregnancies should include:

1. A history of full-term and premature deliveries, including the route of each delivery

2. A history of repeated spontaneous or induced abortions

3. A history of high parity because of the increased risk for puerperal hemorrhage, multiple gestation, and placenta previa

4. The length of each previous pregnancy as well as the sex and weight of the fetus

5. The indication for a previous cesarean section

6. Complications of previous pregnancies or deliveries, such as premature labor, premature rupture of membranes, shoulder dystocia, postpartum hemorrhage, fetal or neonatal deaths, and perinatal morbidity

C. Identification of risk factors, such as maternal health problems, alcohol consumption, cigarette smoking, hypertension, and exposure to environmental hazards (e.g., radiation, heat, anesthesia, or chemicals). Consultation and counseling may be helpful when there has been exposure to possible teratogenic agents.

D. Review of patient and family health histories should include:

1. Information on metabolic disorders, cardiovascular disease, malignancy, congenital abnormalities, mental retardation, and multiple births

2. The family history of congenital anomalies to identify a fetus at risk for an inherited disease

3. The birth of a previous child with congenital anomalies, indicating the need for prenatal genetic counseling and studies

III. PHYSICAL EXAMINATION

A. General examination. A general examination should include an evaluation of height, weight, blood pressure, eye fundus, breasts, heart, lungs, abdomen, rectum, extremities, and current nutritional status.

1. A systolic flow murmur at the left sternal border in pregnancy is within normal limits.

2. Edema of the feet and ankles during the day is normal; generalized edema of the face, hands, abdomen, and ankles is abnormal.

B. Pelvic examination

1. The speculum examination permits visualization of the vagina and the cervix.
  a. Evaluation of cervical and vaginal lesions is done with the Pap smear (Papanicolaou's test), biopsy, or culdoscopic examination.
  b. The bluish-red passive hyperemia of the cervix is characteristic of pregnancy.
  c. A dilated cervix may reveal membranes at the internal os.
  d. A moderate amount of white mucoid discharge in pregnancy is normal.
  e. A foamy yellow liquid in the vagina is suggestive of a *Trichomonas* infection; a white curd-like discharge is consistent with a *Candida* infection.

2. The bimanual examination permits the evaluation of the pelvis and the uterus.
  a. The configuration and capacity of the bony pelvis should be evaluated.
  b. Early pregnancy is the best time to correlate accurately uterine size and duration of gestation; the uterus is usually a pelvic organ until 12 weeks gestation.

C. Abdominal examination. This allows the ongoing evaluation of the growth and status of the fetus.

1. Between 18 and 30 weeks, there is an excellent correlation between the size of the uterus and the gestation by weeks. The measurement in centimeters from the symphysis pubis to the top of the fundus should approximate the weeks of gestation.

2. At midpregnancy (20 weeks gestation), the fundus of the uterus is at the level of the umbilicus.

3. Fetal heart tones can be identified by a Doppler (sonar) device at 12–14 weeks and by a fetoscope at 18–20 weeks.

4. With real-time ultrasonography, fetal heart activity can be seen as early as 2–3 weeks after the first missed menses.

IV. ANTEPARTUM MANAGEMENT

A. Laboratory tests

1. Initial screening should include the following studies:
  a. Hemoglobin or hematocrit level

       b. Urinalysis for protein and glucose
       c. Blood group and Rh type
       d. Irregular antibody screen
       e. Rubella antibody titer, if previous immunity has not been determined
       f. Cervical cytology
       g. Serologic testing for syphilis

  2. The following evaluations should be performed if indicated by ethnic, racial, social, or health histories:
       a. Urine culture
       b. Cervical culture for gonorrhea
       c. Plasma glucose determination, particularly with a positive family history for diabetes or a history of glucosuria or previous large infants (more than 4000 g)
       d. Sickle cell test
       e. Skin test for tuberculosis

  3. α-Fetoprotein levels are measured at 16 weeks, and values are reported as the multiple of the mean (MOM).
       a. Elevated (2.5 MOM and above)
          (1) Open neural tube defects (e.g., anencephaly, spina bifida, and meningomyelocele)
          (2) Omphalocele
          (3) Multiple gestation
          (4) Duodenal atresia
       b. Depressed (0.5 MOM and below). Fifteen to twenty percent of infants with Down's syndrome have these low values.

  4. Third-trimester routine testing should include the following studies:
       a. Repeat hemoglobin or hematocrit level
       b. Repeat antibody testing in unsensitized Rh-negative patients at 28–32 weeks
       c. Prophylactic Rh₀ (anti-D) immune globulin administration (RhoGAM, 300 µg) to reduce the incidence of Rh isoimmunization in an Rh-negative woman with a negative antibody screen and an Rh-positive husband

B. Office visits

  1. Frequency. In an uncomplicated pregnancy, a woman should be seen every 4 weeks for the first 28–30 weeks of pregnancy, every 2 weeks until 36 weeks, and weekly thereafter until delivery. Women with medical or obstetric problems require close surveillance at intervals determined by the nature and severity of the problems.

  2. Monitoring
      a. Mother
          (1) Blood pressure with notation of any change
          (2) Weight with notation of any change
          (3) Presence of headache, altered vision, abdominal pain, nausea, vomiting, bleeding, fluid from the vagina, and dysuria
          (4) Height of the uterine fundus above the symphysis pubis
          (5) Position, consistency, effacement, and dilation of the cervix (late in pregnancy)
      b. Fetus
          (1) Fetal heart rate
          (2) Size of fetus (actual and rate of change)
          (3) Amount of amniotic fluid
          (4) Fetal activity
          (5) Presenting part and station (late in pregnancy)

C. Special instructions. Patients are instructed about the following danger signals, which should be reported immediately whenever they occur.

  1. Any vaginal bleeding

  2. Swelling of the face or fingers

  3. Severe or continuous headache

  4. Dimness or blurring of vision

  5. Abdominal pain

  6. Persistent vomiting

  7. Chills or fever

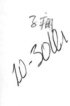 **8.** Dysuria

9. Escape of fluid from the vagina

V. NUTRITION

A. Weight gain. It is unreasonable to advise rigid caloric restriction during pregnancy. Restricted weight gain does little to prevent preeclampsia and eclampsia (excessive weight gain is a prominent feature of preeclampsia and eclampsia). The weight gain of preeclampsia and eclampsia results from edema rather than caloric intake. Twenty to thirty pounds is the recommended weight gain during pregnancy.

   1. Pregnancy-induced changes account for 20 lbs of weight gain in normal conditions: fetus (7½ lbs); placenta plus membranes (1½ lbs); amniotic fluid (2 lbs); increases in the weight of the uterus (2½ lbs), blood (3½ lbs), and breasts (2 lbs); and an increase in lower extremity interstitial fluid (2–3 lbs).

   2. Failure to gain weight may be a dangerous sign; every pregnant woman should gain at least 15–20 lbs.

   3. If there has been less than a 10-lb weight gain by the twentieth week of gestation, dietary habits should be reviewed.

B. Calories. The pregnant woman of average weight requires about 2400 cal/day during pregnancy. This represents an increase of 300 cal/day over her nonpregnant requirements.

   1. Inadequate caloric intake may be associated with an increased risk of fetal difficulties in utero and low-birth-weight neonates who have problems in the intrapartum and postpartum periods.

   2. Whenever caloric intake is inadequate, protein may be metabolized as a source of energy rather than being spared for growth and development.

   3. Inadequate caloric intake seems to have its greatest effect in women who are of low weight prior to pregnancy.

   4. All patients, especially those who are obese, should be reminded that they should not begin a weight reduction program during pregnancy.

C. Protein. Cell growth requires protein. Animal studies suggest that inadequate intake during pregnancy can lead to suboptimal growth of the fetus, decrease in size of various fetal organs, and increase in perinatal morbidity and mortality.

   1. Most mothers store an additional 200–350 g of protein in preparation for losses that occur during labor and parturition.

   2. During pregnancy, an adult woman needs about 1.3 g/day/kg of body weight and an adolescent, 1.5 g/kg.

   3. Most of the protein should come from animal sources, such as meat, milk, eggs, cheese, poultry, and fish since they furnish sufficient amino acids for protein synthesis.

D. Minerals

   1. Iron. Many women have inadequate iron stores because of blood loss during menses. During pregnancy, iron stores may be depleted even further.
      a. Supplemental iron is needed for both the fetus and the expanded maternal blood volume.
      b. The fetus maintains normal hemoglobin levels at the mother's expense, and this may leave her severely anemic.
      c. Elemental iron (30–60 mg) should be given daily to supplement the diet. Iron is found in liver, red meat, dried beans, green leafy vegetables, whole grain cereal, and dried fruits.

   2. Calcium. The recommendation for calcium of 1200 mg/day can be met by drinking a quart of milk every day.
      a. The classic symptom of calcium deficiency in a pregnant woman is leg cramps, especially at night.
      b. Other sources of calcium are tofu (soybean curd) and dairy foods, including cheese and yogurt.

   3. Sodium. A restriction of sodium intake, which was advocated in the past, is no longer advised because of the natriuretic effect of progesterone. There is no justification for the use of diuretics in pregnancy.

E. **Vitamins.** The practice of prescribing supplemental vitamins is common among obstetricians even though there is little evidence that vitamins benefit either the mother or the fetus. Vitamins should not be regarded as a substitute for food.

   1. **Folic acid.** Folic acid is required in the formation of heme, the iron-containing protein of hemoglobin. Deficiencies in folic acid can affect red cell formation and cause megaloblastic anemia.

      a. Approximately 800 μg of folic acid daily are required during pregnancy. Folic acid can be found in many of the foods that provide iron and protein.

      b. An adequate daily supplement of oral folic acid is 1 mg.

      c. Studies have implicated maternal folate deficiencies in a variety of reproductive problems, including abruptio placentae, pregnancy-induced hypertension, and fetal abnormalities, such as neural cord defects.

   2. **Vitamin B$_{12}$.** This vitamin occurs naturally only in foods of animal origin. Since vegetarians may produce infants whose B$_{12}$ stores are low, pregnant vegetarians should be identified so that B$_{12}$ supplements can be provided.

   3. **Vitamin C.** During pregnancy, 80 mg daily of vitamin C is recommended, and a reasonable diet should provide this amount. Large doses (1 g or more) of vitamin C taken for common cold prophylaxis may be harmful to the fetus.

VI. FURTHER CONSIDERATIONS

A. **Exercise.** It is not necessary for the pregnant woman to limit her exercise, providing she does not become excessively tired. Severe restrictions may be necessary in such situations as suspected or actual cervical incompetence, pregnancy-induced hypertension, premature labor, and multiple gestations.

B. **Travel.** No harmful effects have been ascribed to travel; pressurized aircraft present no risk. A pregnant woman should move around every 2 hours to guard against lower extremity venous stasis and thrombophlebitis.

C. **Bowel habits.** Bowel habits during pregnancy tend to become irregular because of the progesterone-induced gastrointestinal smooth muscle relaxation and the pressure of the enlarging uterine mass. A woman may avoid constipation with liberal fluid intake, exercise, mild laxatives, stool softeners, and bulk-producing substances.

D. **Coitus.** Sexual intercourse does no harm at any time during pregnancy unless there is a pregnancy complication, such as ruptured membranes, premature labor, or cervical incompetence. Prostaglandins in the seminal plasma and female orgasm may be responsible for the occasional transient contractions that occur with coitus.

E. **Smoking.** Mothers who smoke often have smaller (by an average of 250 g) infants with an increased perinatal mortality. The adverse effects due to smoking are thought to be a function of:

   1. Carbon monoxide and its functional inactivation of fetal and maternal hemoglobin

   2. The vasoconstrictor action of nicotine, causing reduced perfusion of the placenta

   3. Reduced appetite and reduced caloric intake by women who smoke

F. **Alcohol.** The current recommendation is that no alcohol be consumed during pregnancy. The fetal abnormalities of the fetal alcohol syndrome, which are associated with heavy drinking during pregnancy, are craniofacial defects, limb and cardiovascular defects, and prenatal and postnatal growth and mental retardation.

G. **Medication.** Any drug administered during pregnancy will cross the placenta and reach the fetus; therefore, if a drug must be used, its advantages must outweigh the risks.

   1. The possibility of long-term adverse effects of a medication on a developing fetus (the DES story) must be remembered.

   2. Because of the adverse effects on the hemostatic mechanism of the fetus and its displacement of bilirubin from protein-binding sites, aspirin use, especially late in pregnancy, is contraindicated.

STUDY QUESTIONS

Directions: Each question below contains five suggested answers. Choose the **one best** response to each question.

1.   Näegele's rule for estimating a woman's due date is based on all of the following factors EXCEPT

(A) regular monthly menstrual cycles
(B) a pregnancy of 280 days
(C) ovulation about day 14
(D) cycle regulation with birth control pills prior to conception
(E) conception at midcycle

2.   An abnormal finding during a normal pregnancy is

(A) a weight gain of 11 lbs at 20 weeks
(B) fetal heart tones at 13 weeks detected by Doppler
(C) the fundus of the uterus at the level of the umbilicus at 20 weeks
(D) the uterus as a pelvic organ at 12 weeks
(E) Real-time ultrasonographic evidence of fetal heart motion 4 weeks after the last menstrual period

3.   Appropriate screening tests in an early, uncomplicated pregnancy include all of following EXCEPT

(A) repeat human chorionic gonadotropin levels
(B) hemoglobin
(C) serology
(D) cervical cytology
(E) blood type and Rh factor

4.   All of the following signs or symptoms should be reported immediately as a potential danger signal in a pregnant woman EXCEPT

(A) vaginal bleeding
(B) severe headache
(C) swelling of the ankles and feet
(D) blurring of vision
(E) escape of fluid from the vagina

5.   A pregnant vegetarian is likely to be deficient in which of the following substances?

(A) Calcium
(B) Folic acid
(C) Iron
(D) Protein
(E) Vitamin B_{12}

Directions: Each question below contains four suggested answers of which **one or more** is correct. Choose the answer

A   if **1, 2, and 3** are correct
B   if **1 and 3** are correct
C   if **2 and 4** are correct
D   if **4** is correct
E   if **1, 2, 3, and 4** are correct

6.   Maternal folate deficiency has been implicated in the etiology of

(1) abruptio placentae
(2) anencephaly
(3) preeclampsia and eclampsia
(4) intrauterine growth retardation

7.   Standard protocol in an unsensitized Rh-negative pregnancy at 28 weeks should include

(1) repeat Rh antibody titer
(2) ultrasound examination of the fetus
(3) intramuscular Rh_o immune globulin (300 μg)
(4) analysis of the husband's blood type

8.   Incompatible combinations include which of the following?

(1) 40-week pregnancy and fetal weight of 7½ lbs
(2) 14-week pregnancy and fetal heart tones by fetoscope
(3) 40-week pregnancy and maternal weight gain of 30 lbs
(4) 30-week pregnancy and top of the uterus 27 cm above the symphysis

ANSWERS AND EXPLANATIONS

1. The answer is D. (*II A 1–3*) The expected date of confinement is calculated by adding 9 months and 7 days to the date of the last menstrual period, which is a total of 280 days. This calculation assumes a 28–30-day cycle with ovulation and conception around midcycle or day 14. This calculation would not be accurate in a woman with regular 35-day cycles because her ovulation occurs around day 21, which then affects the true due date. Because of an occasional delay in ovulation in the cycle after stopping the birth control pills, ovulation may occur later than 2 weeks after the last pill period.

2. The answer is E. (*III B 2 b, C 1–4; V A 2, 3*) In a normal gestation, the uterus is still a pelvic organ at 12 weeks. Fetal heart tones can be detected by Doppler at 12–14 weeks, and the fundus of the uterus is at the level of the umbilicus at 20 weeks. A weight gain of 20–30 lbs during a pregnancy is normal, and at least 10 lbs should be gained by 20 weeks. It is not possible to see fetal heart motion by real-time ultrasonography until 6–7 weeks after the last menstrual period or 2–3 weeks after the first missed menses.

3. The answer is A. (*IV A 1 a–g*) With a previous positive pregnancy test, there is no need to repeat it under normal conditions. If the uterus is too small on examination or if there is bleeding, a repeat human chorionic gonadotropin (HCG) would be advisable to diagnose a threatened abortion with inappropriately rising HCG levels. All of the other tests listed in the question (i.e., hemoglobin, serology, cervical cytology, blood type, and Rh factor) are indicated.

4. The answer is C. (*IV C 1–9*) Severe headache and blurred vision may be signs of preeclampsia, which needs immediate attention. Vaginal bleeding could indicate abruptio placentae or placenta previa. Rupture of membranes usually presents as a large or small amount of fluid from the vagina. Swelling of the ankles and feet is common in most pregnancies due to increased venous pressure in the lower extremities; however, generalized swelling, especially of the hands and face, may indicate preeclampsia.

5. The answer is E. (*V E 2*) A vegetarian eats no meat, and vitamin B_{12} occurs naturally only in foods of animal origin. Thus, a physician should assume a lack of B_{12} in the diet of a vegetarian. If a vegetarian drinks milk and eats cheese, beans, fruits, green leafy vegetables, and whole grain cereal, she should not have folic acid, protein, calcium, or iron deficiencies.

6. The answer is A (1, 2, 3). (*V E 1 c*) Folic acid deficiencies are known to cause megaloblastic anemia and have been implicated in reproductive problems, such as abruptio placentae, pregnancy-induced hypertension (preeclampsia and eclampsia), and fetal abnormalities, such as neural tube defects (e.g., spina bifida, meningomyelocele, and anencephaly).

7. The answer is B (1, 3). (*IV A 4*) A small percentage of Rh-negative women become sensitized during a pregnancy that was initially unsensitized. To prevent this from occurring, an injection of Rh_o immune globulin is offered to all unsensitized Rh-negative women during the twenty-eighth week if a repeat Rh antibody titer is still negative. There is no need to perform an ultrasound examination of the fetus or to check the husband's blood type. An injection of Rh_o immune globulin in an Rh-negative fetus does no harm. This would be the case if the husband's Rh-negative status were known; however, that determination is not necessary at 28 weeks.

8. The answer is C (2, 4). (*III C 1, 3; V A 1*) At 40 weeks in a normal pregnancy, one can expect a maternal weight gain of 20–30 lbs and a fetal weight of about 7½ lbs. The sonar device can identify fetal heart tones at 12–14 weeks, while the fetoscope cannot pick up the fetal heart tones until 18–20 weeks. At 30 weeks gestation, the top of the uterus should be about 30 cm from the symphysis pubis as the measurement in centimeters approximates the weeks of gestation between 18 and 30 weeks.

4

Labor and Delivery
William W. Beck, Jr.

I. CAUSES OF LABOR: THEORIES

A. Oxytocin stimulation. Although oxytocin is known to cause uterine contractions when administered late in pregnancy, it is natural to assume that endogenously produced oxytocin may play a role in the onset of spontaneous labor. However, there is a fixed level of oxytocin in maternal blood before and during labor; increased levels are found only during the second stage of labor. Thus, oxytocin does not seem to be responsible for the spontaneous onset of labor.

B. Progesterone withdrawal. Although the withdrawal of progesterone is followed by the prompt evacuation of the contents of the pregnant uterus in rabbits, there is no fall in the human maternal blood levels of progesterone at term. The progesterone level at the placental site, however, may decrease prior to the onset of labor.

C. Fetal cortisol infusion. In pregnant sheep, hypophysectomy, adrenalectomy, or transection of the hypophyseal portal vessels on the fetus results in prolonged gestation. Conversely, infusion of either cortisol or adrenocorticotropic hormone (ACTH) into the fetus with an intact adrenal causes premature labor. In humans, a naturally prolonged gestation results in an anencephalic fetus with faulty fetal brain–pituitary–adrenal function. However, in humans prolonged gestations do not result from the naturally occurring instances of failure of cortisol production as seen in the hydroxylation deficiencies.

D. Prostaglandin release

1. Prostaglandins are known to cause uterine contractions as demonstrated in second trimester abortions.

2. Fetal membranes and decidua vera have prostaglandin synthetase and produce prostaglandins.

3. Nonesterified arachidonic acid is an absolute percursor of prostaglandins.
   a. The esterified form of arachidonic acid is thought to be stored in the fetal membranes.
   b. Phospholipase liberates arachidonic acid from its esterified form in the fetal membranes.
   c. There is a sixfold increase of nonesterified arachidonic acid in the amniotic fluid during labor.

4. Withdrawal of progesterone at the level of the fetal membranes may be important in unmasking phospholipase with the liberation of arachidonic acid and the manufacture of prostaglandins leading to labor.

5. Stimuli known to cause the release of prostaglandins (e.g., cervical manipulation, stripping of the membranes, and rupture of the membranes) augment or induce uterine contractions.

II. LABOR: DEFINITION AND CHARACTERISTICS

A. Definition. Labor is characterized by contractions that occur at decreasing intervals with increasing intensity, causing dilation of the cervix.

B. Myometrial physiology

1. Contraction of uterine smooth muscle is due to the interaction of the proteins actin and myosin.
   a. The interaction of actin and myosin is regulated by the enzymatic phosphorylation of myosin light chains.

b. The phosphorylation of myosin light chains is catalyzed by the enzyme myosin light-chain kinase, which is activated by calcium ion (Ca^{2+}).

2. Gap junctions are important cell-to-cell contacts that facilitate communication between coupled cells via electrical, ionic, or metabolic coupling.

   a. Gap junctions, which are virtually absent during pregnancy, increase in size and number prior to and during labor.

   b. Progesterone appears to prevent and estrogen appears to promote gap-junction formation.

   c. Prostaglandins are believed to be important stimulators of gap-junction formation. If prostaglandins are inhibited, then so is gap-junction formation.

   d. Gap-junction formation is not stimulated by oxytocin.

3. Substances that interfere with the physiology of the myometrium can inhibit contractions.

   a. Antiprostaglandin agents, such as indomethecin and acetylsalicylic acid, inhibit the synthesis of prostaglandin, which, in turn:

   (1) Decreases uterine contractions

   (2) Inhibits gap-junction formation

   (3) Does not cause premature closure of the fetal ductus arteriosus if discontinued by 34 weeks gestation

   b. Magnesium sulfate at sufficient concentrations acts as an antagonist of Ca^{2+} (because of the magnesium) and inhibits the activation of myosin light-chain kinase, thereby preventing premature labor.

C. Stages of labor

1. First stage. The first stage of labor entails **effacement** and **dilation**. It begins when uterine contractions become sufficiently frequent, intense, and long to initiate obvious effacement and dilation of the cervix.

2. Second stage. The second stage of labor involves the **expulsion of the fetus**. It begins with the complete dilation of the cervix and ends when the infant is delivered.

3. Third stage. The third stage of labor involves the **separation** and **expulsion of the placenta**. It begins with the delivery of the infant and ends with the delivery of the placenta.

D. True versus false labor

1. True labor

   a. Contractions occur at regular intervals, and the intervals gradually shorten to 2–4 minutes apart.

   b. The intensity of the contractions gradually increases with contractions lasting 1 minute.

   c. The discomfort is in both the back and the abdomen.

   d. Progressive dilation of the cervix occurs.

   e. Contractions are not affected by sedation.

2. False labor

   a. Contractions occur at irregular intervals.

   b. The contraction intervals are long and do not establish a regular pattern.

   c. The intensity of the contractions remains the same.

   d. The discomfort is chiefly in the lower abdomen.

   e. Contractions are usually relieved and are often stopped by sedation.

   f. Contractions do not cause dilation of the cervix because they are not coordinated and lack fundal dominance.

E. Character of uterine contractions

1. Effective uterine contractions last for 30–90 seconds, create 20–50 mm Hg of pressure, and occur every 2–4 minutes.

2. The pain of contractions is thought to be due to one or more of the following:

   a. Hypoxia of the contracted myometrium (as in angina pectoris)

   b. Compression of nerve ganglia in the cervix and lower uterus by the tightly interlocking muscle bundles

   c. Stretching of the cervix during dilation

   d. Stretching of the peritoneum overlying the uterus

3. During labor, contractions cause the uterus to differentiate into two parts.

   a. The upper segment of the uterus becomes thicker as labor progresses and contracts down with a force that expels the fetus with each contraction.

   b. The lower segment of the uterus passively thins out with contractions of the upper segment and causes effacement of the cervix.

F. Changes of the cervix before or during labor

   1. Effacement of the cervix is the shortening of the cervical canal from a structure of approximately 2 cm in length to one in which the canal is replaced by a more circular orifice with almost paper-thin edges. The process takes place from above downward. It occurs as the muscle fibers in the vicinity of the internal os are pulled upward into the lower uterine segment.

   2. Dilation of the cervix involves the gradual widening of the cervical os. For the head of the average fetus at term to be able to pass through the cervix, the canal must dilate to a diameter of about 10 cm. When a diameter sufficient for the fetal head to pass through is reached, the cervix is said to be completely or fully dilated.

III. NORMAL LABOR IN THE OCCIPUT PRESENTATION

A. Occiput (vertex) presentations occur in about 95% of all labors. The occiput may present in the transverse, anterior, or posterior positions. Position refers to the relation of an arbitrarily chosen portion of the fetus (in this case the occiput of the fetal head) to the right or left side of the maternal birth canal. Positions of the occiput presentation include the following:

   1. Occiput transverse (OT). On vaginal examination, the saggital suture (in the midline front to back) of the fetal head occupies the transverse diameter of the pelvis more or less midway between the sacrum and the symphysis.
   a. In left occiput transverse (LOT) positions, the smaller posterior fontanelle is to the left in the maternal pelvis, and the larger anterior fontanelle is directed to the opposite side.
   b. In right occiput transverse (ROT) positions, the reverse is true.

   2. Occiput anterior (OA). The head either enters the pelvis with the occiput rotated 45 degrees anteriorly from the transverse position, right (ROA) or left (LOA), or subsequently does so.

   3. Occiput posterior (OP). The incidence of posterior positions is approximately 10%. The right occiput posterior (ROP) position is much more common than the left (LOP). The posterior positions are often associated with a narrow forepelvis.
   a. In the ROP position, the sagittal suture occupies the right oblique diameter. The small posterior fontanelle is directed posteriorly to the right of the midline, while the large anterior fontanelle is directed anteriorly to the left of the midline.
   b. In the LOP position, the reverse holds true.

B. Cardinal movements of labor and delivery. A process of adaptation of suitable portions of the fetal head to the various segments of the pelvis is required for the completion of childbirth. These positional changes of the presenting part constitute the mechanism of labor and involve seven cardinal movements, which occur sequentially in the following order:

   1. Engagement. This is the mechanism by which the biparietal diameter of the fetal head, the greatest transverse diameter of the head in occiput presentations, passes through the pelvic inlet. When engagement occurs, the lowest point of the presenting part is, by definition, at the level of the ischial spines, which is designated as **O station.**
   a. This phenomenon may take place during the last few weeks of pregnancy, or it may not do so until after labor begins. It is more likely to happen prior to the onset of labor in a primigravida than in a multigravida.
   b. When the fetal head is not engaged at the onset of labor and the fetal head is freely movable above the pelvic inlet, the head is said to be floating.

   2. Descent. The first requirement for the birth of an infant is descent. In the primigravida who is engaged at the onset of labor, descent may not occur until the start of the second stage. In the multiparous woman, descent usually begins with engagement.

   3. Flexion. When the descending head meets resistance from either the cervix, the walls of the pelvis, or the pelvic floor, flexion of the fetal head normally occurs.
   a. The chin is brought into close contact with the fetal thorax.
   b. This movement causes a smaller diameter of fetal head to be presented to the pelvis than if the head were not flexed.

   4. Internal rotation. This movement is always associated with descent of the presenting part and is not usually accomplished until the head has reached the level of the ischial spines (O station). The movement involves the gradual turning of the occiput from its original position anteriorly towards the symphysis pubis.

5. **Extension.** Extension of the fetal head is essential during the birth process. When the sharply flexed fetal head comes in contact with the vulva, the occiput is brought in direct contact with the inferior margin of the symphysis.
   a. Since the vulvar outlet is directed upward and forward, extension must occur for the head to pass through it.
   b. The expulsive forces of the uterine contractions and the patient's pushing, along with the resistance of the pelvic floor, result in the anterior extension of the vertex in the direction of the vulvar opening.

6. **External rotation.** Following delivery of the head, restitution occurs. In this movement, the occiput returns first to the oblique position from which it started and then to the transverse position, left or right. This movement corresponds to the rotation of the fetal body, bringing the shoulders into an anteroposterior diameter with the pelvic outlet.

7. **Expulsion.** After external rotation, the anterior shoulder appears under the symphysis and is delivered. The perineum soon becomes distended by the posterior shoulder. After delivery of the shoulders, the rest of the body of the child is quickly extruded.

IV. CONDUCT OF LABOR

A. **Detection of ruptured membranes.** Ruptured membranes are signified at any time during pregnancy by either a sudden gush or a steady trickle of clear fluid from the vagina. In a term pregnancy, labor usually follows within 24 hours of membrane rupture. There is a real possibility of intrauterine infection (chorioamnionitis) if the patient has ruptured membranes for longer than 24 hours, with or without labor.

   1. **Nitrazine test.** Nitrazine paper changes color, depending on the pH of the fluid being tested. Amniotic fluid, which is alkaline, turns nitrazine paper deep blue.

   2. **Ferning.** Amniotic fluid, like many body fluids, has a high sodium content, which causes a ferning pattern when the fluid is air dried on a slide. Other vaginal secretions do not have such a ferning pattern.

B. **First stage of labor.** On the average, the first stage lasts for about 12 hours in the primigravida and about 7 hours in the multigravida, although there is great variability from patient to patient.

   1. **Fetal monitoring.** The fetal heart tones should be monitored by any device immediately after a uterine contraction because a sudden drop to less than 120 beats per minute or above 180 beats per minute may be an indication of fetal distress.

   2. **Amniotomy.** Artificial rupture of the membranes permits the observation of the color of the amniotic fluid (whether or not it is meconium-stained) and often shortens the length of labor if a woman is already contracting regularly.

   3. **Latent phase of labor.** During the latent phase, the uterine contractions typically are infrequent, somewhat uncomfortable, and may be irregular, but generate sufficient force to cause slow dilation and some effacement of the cervix. A prolonged latent phase is greater than 20 hours in the primigravida and greater than 14 hours in the multigravida.

   4. **Active phase of labor.** The active phase, or clinically apparent labor, follows the latent phase and is characterized by progressive cervical dilation. A prolonged active phase is seen in the primigravida who dilates at less than 1.2 cm/hr and in the multigravida who dilates at less than 1.5 cm/hr.

   5. **Dysfunctional labor patterns.** Uterine dysfunction in any phase of cervical dilation is characterized by lack of progress as one of the cardinal features of normal labor is its progression.
      a. **Hypotonic uterine dysfunction.** The uterine contractions have a normal gradient pattern but a pressure increase during a contraction of less than 15 mm Hg. This type of dysfunction is usually corrected by stimulating the contractions with an intravenous infusion of oxytocin.
      b. **Hypertonic uterine dysfunction.** The uterine contractions have an abnormal gradient, possibly due to contraction of the midsegment of the uterus with more force than the fundus. The result is painful contractions that result in little or no cervical dilation. Oxytocin is not indicated in a hypertonic uterus. Sedation with morphine relieves the pain, relaxes the patient, and usually results in a normal labor pattern.

C. **Second stage of labor.** On the average, the second stage lasts for about 50 minutes in the primigravida and about 20 minutes in the multigravida. However, second stages lasting 2 hours, espe-

Tima *Math*

Latent 720 714

Active 50" <1.2c/o <1.5 cm/o

70 20"

cially in the primigravida, are not uncommon. This stage is characterized by intense pushing on the part of the patient.

1. Spontaneous vaginal delivery

    a. Delivery of the head. With each contraction, the vulvar opening is dilated by the head. The encirclement of the largest diameter of the fetal head by the vulvar ring is known as *crowning*. The head is then delivered slowly with the base of the occiput rotating around the lower margin of the symphysis pubis.

    b. Delivery of the shoulders. In most cases, the shoulders appear at the vulva just after external rotation and are born spontaneously. If the shoulders are not born spontaneously, *gentle traction* is used to engage and deliver first the anterior and then the posterior shoulder. Excessive traction with extension of the infant's neck can result in temporary or permanent injury to the brachial plexus.

2. Episiotomy. The episiotomy is the most common operation in obstetrics. It is an incision in the perineum that is either in the midline (a median episiotomy) or begun in the midline but directed laterally away from the rectum (a mediolateral episiotomy). The episiotomy substitutes a straight, clean surgical incision for the ragged laceration that may otherwise result. It is easier to repair and heals better than a tear. It shortens the second stage of labor and spares the infant's head from prolonged pounding against the perineum.

    a. Median episiotomy

        (1) Advantages

            (a) Ease of repair

            (b) Rare faulty healing

            (c) Rare dyspareunia

            (d) Good anatomic result

            (e) Small blood loss

        (2) Disadvantage. Extension through the anal sphincter and into the rectum is relatively common.

    b. Mediolateral episiotomy. The main reason for cutting a mediolateral episiotomy is the need for space when delivering a breech or when shoulder dystocia is anticipated.

        (1) Advantage. Extension through the anal sphincter is rare.

        (2) Disadvantages

            (a) Difficult to repair

            (b) Common faulty healing

            (c) Occasional dyspareunia

            (d) Occasional faulty anatomic result

            (e) Greater blood loss than the median episiotomy

D. Third stage of labor. The placenta usually delivers within 5 minutes of the delivery of the infant.

1. Signs of placental separation

    a. The uterus becomes globular and firmer.

    b. There is often a sudden gush of blood.

    c. The uterus rises in the abdomen because the placenta, having separated, passes down into the lower uterine segment and vagina, where its bulk pushes the uterus upward.

    d. The umbilical cord protrudes farther out of the vagina, indicating that the placenta has descended.

2. Uterine hemostasis. The mechanism by which hemostasis is achieved at the placental site is vasoconstriction produced by a well-contracted myometrium. Intravenous or intramuscular oxytocin (10 units intramuscularly or 20 units in a 1000 ml intravenous bottle) or ergonovine (0.2 mg intramuscularly or intravenously) help the uterus to contract down and decrease blood loss. These medications are administered *after* the placenta has delivered.

E. Lacerations of the birth canal. There are four types of vaginal or perineal lacerations, all of which are less likely to occur with an appropriate episiotomy.

1. First-degree lacerations involve the fourchette, the perineal skin, and vaginal mucosa, but not the fascia and muscle.

2. Second-degree lacerations involve the skin, the mucosa, the fascia and muscles of the perineal body, but not the rectal sphincter.

3. Third-degree lacerations extend through the skin, mucosa, perineal body, and involve the anal sphincter.

4. Fourth-degree lacerations are extensions of the third-degree tear through the rectal mucosa to expose the lumen of the rectum.

STUDY QUESTIONS

Directions: Each question below contains five suggested answers. Choose the **one best** response to each question.

1. Characteristics of arachidonic acid include all of the following EXCEPT

(A) the nonesterified form is a precursor of prostaglandin
(B) the esterified form is stored in the decidua vera
(C) it is found in high levels in the amniotic fluid
(D) it is liberated from the esterified form by phospholipase
(E) it combines with prostaglandin synthetase to produce prostaglandin

2. The cardinal movements of labor and delivery involve a certain sequence of events that occurs in an orderly fashion. Which of the following sequences is correct?

(A) Descent/internal rotation/flexion
(B) Engagement/flexion/descent
(C) Engagement/internal rotation/descent
(D) Engagement/descent/flexion
(E) Descent/flexion/engagement

Directions: Each question below contains four suggested answers of which **one or more** is correct. Choose the answer

A if **1, 2, and 3** are correct
B if **1 and 3** are correct
C if **2 and 4** are correct
D if **4** is correct
E if **1, 2, 3, and 4** are correct

3. Synthesis of prostaglandin involves which of the following substances?

(1) Amniotic fluid
(2) Phospholipase
(3) Esterified arachidonic acid
(4) Prostaglandin synthetase

4. Engagement is said to have occurred when the

(1) vertex is at 0 station
(2) biparietal diameter of the infant's head is through the plane of the inlet
(3) presenting part is at the level of the ischial spines
(4) vertex is in the transverse position

5. Ruptured membranes are always associated with

(1) a positive nitrazine test
(2) uterine contractions
(3) ferning of dried amniotic fluid
(4) chorioamnionitis

6. The first stage of labor is characterized by

(1) cervical dilation
(2) pushing
(3) the active phase
(4) crowning

Directions: The group of questions below consists of lettered choices followed by several numbered items. For each numbered item select the **one** lettered choice with which it is **most** closely associated. Each lettered choice may be used once, more than once, or not at all.

Questions 7–9

For each activity listed below, select the substance that is most likely to be responsible for it.

(A) Oxytocin
(B) Prostaglandin
(C) Indomethecin
(D) Magnesium sulfate
(E) Progesterone

7. Stimulates gap-junction formation

8. Influences calcium ion flux in the treatment of premature labor

9. Prevents gap-junction formation directly

ANSWERS AND EXPLANATIONS

1. The answer is B. *(I D 1–3)* The esterified form of arachidonic acid is stored in the fetal membranes. Prostaglandin synthetase is stored in the fetal membranes and the decidua vera. Phospholipase liberates arachidonic acid from its esterified form in the fetal membranes. The nonesterified form is an absolute precursor of prostaglandin. The synthetase combines with the free arachidonic acid to produce prostaglandin.

2. The answer is D. *(III B 1–7)* There are seven cardinal movements in labor and delivery, and they occur sequentially. In order they are: engagement, descent, flexion, internal rotation, extension, external rotation, and expulsion.

3. The answer is C (2, 4). *(I D 3 a–c)* Esterified arachidonic acid is not involved in the synthesis of prostaglandin. It is the nonesterified form that combines with prostaglandin synthetase to form prostaglandin. The phospholipase splits off the nonesterified arachidonic acid from the esterified form. Esterified arachidonic acid is stored in the fetal membranes, not in the amniotic fluid.

4. The answer is A (1, 2, 3). *(III B 1)* Engagement occurs when the presenting part is at the level of the ischial spines, which is designated as 0 station. By definition, this means that the largest diameter of the infant's head, the biparietal diameter, is through the plane of the inlet. The position of the infant's head has nothing to do with engagement as this can occur in any position.

5. The answer is B (1, 3). *(IV A 1, 2)* Because of the alkaline nature of amniotic fluid, it turns nitrazine paper blue, registering a positive test. When amniotic fluid is dried on a slide and observed through a microscope, a ferning pattern appears because of tiny crystals that form due to the salt content of the fluid. Uterine contractions usually begin within 24 hours of rupture of the membranes but may not occur at all. Chorioamnionitis is an unusual accompaniment of ruptured membranes, but its occurrence increases significantly after 24 hours of rupture.

6. The answer is B (1, 3). *(IV B 3, 4)* During the first stage of labor, the cervix gradually dilates up to 10 cm. The active phase is characterized by progressive cervical dilation. Pushing begins with the second stage of labor when the cervix is completely dilated. Crowning occurs late in the second stage just before the infant's head is delivered.

7–9. The answers are: 7-B, 8-D, 9-E. *[II B 1 b, 2 a–d, 3 a (1), (2), b]* Gap junctions are important cell-to-cell contacts that facilitate communication between coupled cells. These junctions, which are absent during pregnancy, increase in size and number prior to and during labor. Prostaglandins appear to be important stimulators of gap-junction formation. Progesterone seems to prevent the formation of gap junctions, and oxytocin appears to have no effect. Indomethecin indirectly prevents the formation of gap junctions by inhibiting the synthesis of prostaglandin, in whose absence gap-junction formation is not possible.

Magnesium sulfate affects calcium ion (Ca^{2+}) metabolism by antagonizing Ca^{2+}, which prevents the activation of myosin light-chain kinase, which, in turn, inhibits the phosphorylation of myosin light chains; uterine contractions are, thus, inhibited, which is the goal of the treatment of premature labor.

5
Intrapartum Fetal Monitoring
William W. Beck, Jr.

I. FETAL MONITORING

A. **Fetal distress** is defined in terms of the manifestations of fetal hypoxia—that is, by changes in the fetal heart rate (FHR) or fetal pH. Adequate fetal oxygenation is essential for a healthy neonate. Assessment of the fetus during labor is essential to characterize the hypoxia that underlies fetal distress. Two methods by which it is possible to predict reliably the extent and etiology of fetal distress include the following:

1. **Continuous FHR monitoring** by which the variability, baseline, and any changes of the FHR are recorded

2. **Fetal scalp capillary blood sampling** by which the pH of the fetal blood is recorded

B. **Significance of hypoxia.** Hypoxic damage to the fetus is difficult to quantitate, but the effects can be devastating.

1. **Neurologic abnormalities.** Cerebral palsy and mental retardation represent the sublethal effects of asphyxia that may not be observed at birth.
   a. There is an association between birth asphyxia, measured by Apgar scores, and the subsequent neurologic outcome.
   b. It has been estimated that between 20% and 40% of all neurologic disorders are influenced by intrapartum events.

2. **Death.** Severe intrapartum asphyxia can cause fetal death.

II. PATHOPHYSIOLOGY OF FETAL HYPOXIA

A. **Nonstressed fetus.** In the absence of stress, the fetus is neither acidotic nor hypoxic. There is an adequate delivery of oxygen to the fetal tissues despite the low fetal arterial PO_2. The transfer of oxygen across the placenta to the fetus is enhanced by the following mechanisms:

1. Fetal cardiac output and systemic blood flow rates that are considerably higher than those of the adult

2. The affinity of fetal blood for oxygen and the fetal oxygen–carrying capacity that are greater than that of an adult

B. **Stressed fetus.** When perfusion is decreased because of impaired uterine or umbilical blood flow, the transfer of oxygen to the fetus is diminished, and the result is an accumulation of carbon dioxide in the fetus.

1. Increased carbon dioxide causes an increase in the PCO_2 and a concomitant fall in pH, analogous to adult respiratory acidosis.

2. Continued hypoxia deprives the fetus of sufficient oxygen to carry out the aerobic reactions of intermediary metabolism, resulting in a buildup of organic acids.

3. With the accumulation of pyruvic and lactic acids, there is a further fall in fetal pH, resulting in metabolic acidosis.

4. Transient falls in fetal or uterine perfusion usually cause a short-lived respiratory acidosis, whereas more prolonged or profound falls result in a combined respiratory and metabolic acidosis.

5. Fetal oxygen deprivation usually results in a decrease in the FHR or **fetal bradycardia**. Bradycardia appears to be an adaptive response to hypoxia, which allows the fetal myocardium to work more efficiently than it does at higher rates.

III. FHR MONITORING. Either an external ultrasound device or an internal electrode attached to the fetal scalp is used to monitor the FHR in conjunction with uterine contractions.

A. Elements of the FHR pattern

1. **Baseline.** The baseline FHR is the steady rate that occurs during and between contractions in the absence of accelerations or decelerations. The normal baseline FHR is between 120 and 160 beats/min.

2. **Beat-to-beat variability.** The beat-to-beat variability represents the continuous interaction of the sympathetic and parasympathetic nervous systems in adjusting the FHR to fetal metabolic or hemodynamic conditions.
   a. **Decreased variability** may signify loss of fine autonomic control of the FHR.
   b. **Good variability** usually predicts a good fetal outcome.

3. **Reactivity.** When a healthy fetus is stimulated, there is a transient increase in variability or baseline acceleration (10–15 beats/min). The stimulation can be external or internal as seen with spontaneous fetal movement.

B. Abnormal FHR changes. There are many reasons for variability and baseline FHR changes.

1. **Decreased variability**
   a. Asphyxia
   b. Drugs, such as atropine, scopolamine, tranquilizers, narcotics, barbiturates, and anesthetics
   c. Prematurity
   d. Tachycardia
   e. Physiologic fetal "sleep states"
   f. Cardiac and central nervous system anomalies
   g. Arrhythmias

2. **Fetal tachycardia** (i.e., rates above 160 beats/min)
   a. Asphyxia (early)
   b. Maternal fever
   c. Fetal infection
   d. Prematurity
   e. Drugs, such as ritodrine and atropine
   f. Idiopathic
   g. Fetal stimulation
   h. Arrhythmias
   i. Maternal anxiety
   j. Maternal thyrotoxicosis

3. **Fetal bradycardia** (i.e., rates below 120 beats/min)
   a. Asphyxia (sudden or profound)
   b. Idiopathic
   c. Drugs
   d. Reflex
   e. Arrhythmias
   f. Hypothermia

C. FHR decelerations. Periodic changes in the FHR assume importance in defining the mechanism and intensity of asphyxial insults. There are **three patterns of periodic decelerations** based on the configuration of the wave form and the timing of the deceleration in relation to the uterine contraction.

1. **Early decelerations:**
   a. Are not caused by systemic hypoxia
   b. Do not appear to be associated with poor fetal outcome
   c. Occur with fetal head compression
   d. Begin with the onset of uterine contractions
   e. Reach their lowest point at the peak of the contraction
   f. Return to baseline as the contraction ends

2. **Late decelerations:**
   a. Are usually found in association with acute or chronic fetoplacental vascular insufficiency

  b. Occur after the peak and extend past the length of the uterine contraction, often with a slow return to the baseline
  c. Are precipitated by hypoxemia, which slows the fetal heart rate as a result of central nervous system asphyxia, direct myocardial depression, or both
  d. May be associated with a mixed respiratory and metabolic acidosis
  e. Are found with increased frequency in patients with preeclampsia, hypertension, diabetes mellitus, intrauterine growth retardation, or other disorders associated with chronic placental insufficiency.
  f. Occur in situations in which there is an acute decrease in the intervillous space flow, such as abruptio placentae, maternal hypotension from conduction anesthesia, or excessive uterine activity, often associated with hyperstimulation during an oxytocin infusion.

3. Variable decelerations:
  a. Are inconsistent in configuration
  b. Have no uniform temporal relationship to the onset of the contraction
  c. Are usually the result of transient compression of the umbilical cord between fetal parts or between the fetus and surrounding maternal tissues
  d. Are often associated with oligohydramnios with or without ruptured membranes
  e. Cause a short-lived respiratory acidosis if they are mild
  f. May be associated with profound combined acidosis if they are prolonged and recurrent

IV. FETAL SCALP BLOOD SAMPLING

A. Rationale. Information about fetal acid–base balance can be obtained by sampling capillary blood from the fetal scalp.

  1. Normal fetal capillary pH is 7.25–7.35 in the first stage of labor.

  2. Fetal scalp pH is lower than maternal pH by approximately 0.1–0.15.

  3. There is generally good agreement between scalp blood pH, cord pH, and Apgar scores.

B. Interpretation of fetal scalp pH

  1. Most authorities consider pH values less than 7.20 indicative of significant asphyxia and values between 7.2 and 7.24 as preacidotic and needing further evaluation. A low-normal or low-scalp pH should be repeated in 20–30 minutes.

  2. Because a pathologic fetal pH may reflect a severe maternal acidosis, fetal acidemia need not necessarily reflect an asphyxial insult if the maternal pH is low.

C. Predictive value of fetal scalp pH

  1. Accuracy. The accuracy of predicting Apgar scores is only about 80%, using fetal capillary pH alone.
    a. False-normal pH values are found in 6%–20% of infants tested.
    b. False-low pH values are found in 8%–10% of infants tested.

  2. False normals. Most false-normal fetal pH values in the presence of low Apgar scores result from:
    a. Sedatives or anesthetics, resulting in poor respiratory effort and flaccidity at birth but normal pH in utero
    b. Prematurity, fetal infection, or any traumatic insult or meconium that happens at delivery
    c. A hypoxic episode that has occurred between the sampling period and the delivery period

  3. False-low pH values may be related to:
    a. Maternal acidosis
    b. Local scalp edema or vasoconstriction
    c. Fetal recovery in utero from an episode of documented acidosis prior to delivery

V. IATROGENIC CAUSES OF FETAL DISTRESS

A. Maternal position. Blood flow through the abdominal aorta and the inferior vena cava may be obstructed by the pregnant uterus when the mother is in the supine position.

  1. There is a 10% incidence of supine hypotension with decreased cardiac output.

  2. Supine hypotension can lead to a decreased placental perfusion and consequent fetal distress.

3. Improvement in fetal oxygenation occurs when the mother is placed in one of the lateral recumbent positions; the uterus then falls away from the great vessels and the hypotension is relieved.

B. Oxytocin stimulation. Use of uterotonic agents has been associated with an increased incidence of late decelerations and decreased placental perfusion secondary to the effects of hyperstimulation and incomplete relaxation of the uterus after a contraction. Hyperstimulation with oxytocin can be minimized with the use of an infusion pump and an internal pressure catheter.

C. Peridural anesthesia. The use of epidural or caudal anesthesia creates a sympathetic blockade, which may result in decreased venous return, consequent diminished cardiac output, maternal hypotension, decreased uteroplacental perfusion, and late decelerations. Laboring patients with peridural anesthesia:

1. Need to be well hydrated so that there is a normal intravascular volume with hypotension being less likely

2. Should be in the lateral position so that the potential effects of the sympathetic blockade are not compounded by pressure of the uterus on the great vessels

VI. INTRAUTERINE RESUSCITATION. Fetal distress may occasionally demand immediate delivery either vaginally or by cesarean section. However, there is usually time to attempt intrauterine resuscitation.

A. Improvement of uterine blood flow. Late decelerations are usually related to impaired intervillous space blood flow. Fetal hypoxia and late decelerations may be improved by maneuvers that maximize uterine blood flow.

1. **Maternal position.** All patients with suspected fetal distress should be placed in one of the lateral recumbent positions.

2. **Maternal hydration.** It is not unusual for women in labor to have been without oral intake for long periods. This can result in a total body water deficit. Even though maternal pulse and blood pressure may be stable, blood flow may be diverted from the uterus to maintain flow in vital organs.
   a. With signs of fetal distress, an infusion of intravenous fluids should begin or should be increased if an intravenous infusion is in place.
   b. In the presence of late decelerations, an infusion of lactated Ringer's or physiologic saline to replace depleted intravascular volume is sometimes curative.

3. **Uterine relaxation.** If oxytocin is being used to stimulate labor, it should be discontinued. Further attempts at tocolysis (relaxation of uterine contractions) with agents, such as intravenous ritodrine or subcutaneous terbutaline, may allow the fetus to recover prior to delivery and be in a more favorable physiologic state than if it had been delivered at the height of its distress.

B. Improvement in umbilical blood flow. Attempts to improve severe variable decelerations should include all of the measures for improving uterine blood flow with additional attention paid to the following:

1. **Maternal position.** Changing the mother's position by moving her from side-to-side, to the Trendelenburg position, or even to the knee-chest position frequently corrects the patterns.

2. **Fetal head position.** When overt cord prolapse has occurred, manual elevation of the fetal head out of the pelvis to take pressure off the cord is an effective method of buying time while preparations are being made for a cesarean section.

C. Improvement of fetal oxygenation. Increasing the concentration of inspired oxygen to the mother results in a small increment in fetal P_{O_2} and may be a useful measure in treating fetal distress. Though fetal P_{O_2} may increase by a small degree, fetal oxygen content may increase considerably because of the affinity of fetal blood for oxygen.

D. Amnioinfusion involves the infusion of fluid into the amniotic cavity through the dilated cervix to expand the cavity and relieve the pressure on a compressed umbilical cord.

STUDY QUESTIONS

Directions: Each question below contains five suggested answers. Choose the **one best** response to each question.

1. All of the following fetal mechanisms compensate for the normal-low fetal arterial PO_2 EXCEPT increased

(A) fetal cardiac output
(B) fetal systemic blood flow rates
(C) fetal pulmonary blood flow
(D) affinity of fetal blood for oxygen
(E) fetal oxygen–carrying capacity

2. Explanations for a decreased variability in the fetal heart rate tracing include all of the following EXCEPT

(A) fetal "sleep state"
(B) prematurity
(C) barbiturate ingestion
(D) fetal stimulation
(E) asphyxia

3. Characteristics or associated findings with late decelerations include all of the following EXCEPT

(A) they are seen in patients with preeclampsia
(B) they may be associated with respiratory alkalosis
(C) they are associated with a decreased uteroplacental blood flow
(D) they usually are accompanied by a decreased PO_2
(E) they usually are accompanied by an increased PCO_2

Directions: Each question below contains four suggested answers of which **one or more** is correct. Choose the answer

A if **1, 2, and 3** are correct
B if **1 and 3** are correct
C if **2 and 4** are correct
D if **4** is correct
E if **1, 2, 3, and 4** are correct

4. With uteroplacental insufficiency during labor, the fetus would be expected to show a decrease in

(1) PO_2
(2) PCO_2
(3) pH
(4) lactic acid

5. Variable decelerations are characterized by which of the following statements?

(1) They occur late in the contraction cycle
(2) They occur with a nuchal cord
(3) They are associated with head compression
(4) They may improve with the Trendelenburg position

6. A patient in the active phase of labor is 5 cm dilated and has decreased variability on the fetal heart rate monitor. Correct statements concerning a fetal scalp pH of 7.22 include which of the following?

(1) It is indicative of severe asphyxia
(2) It should be repeated in 20 minutes
(3) It suggests significant fetal metabolic acidosis
(4) It could be due to maternal acidosis

7. Epidural anesthesia can produce fetal distress by decreasing

(1) maternal venous return
(2) maternal cardiac output
(3) uterine blood flow
(4) maternal heart rate

Directions: The group of questions below consists of lettered choices followed by several numbered items. For each numbered item select the **one** lettered choice with which it is **most** closely associated. Each lettered choice may be used once, more than once, or not at all.

Questions 8–10

For each clinical situation listed below, select the most appropriate form of management.

(A) Intravenous hydration
(B) Nasal oxygen
(C) Fetal heart rate (FHR) monitoring
(D) Fetal scalp pH
(E) Cesarean section

8. A patient with chronic hypertension presents to the labor floor at term in active labor. Her blood pressure is 140/100, and she has 1+ urinary protein. She is 4 cm dilated.

9. FHR monitoring reveals persistent late decelerations in a patient whose cervix now is 8 cm dilated.

10. Fetal scalp pH in a patient having late decelerations with slow recovery over a 30-minute period is returned as 7.19.

ANSWERS AND EXPLANATIONS

1. The answer is C. (*II A 1, 2*) Despite the normal-low fetal arterial PO_2, the nonstressed fetus is neither hypoxic nor acidotic. It compensates with a physiology that exhibits all of the possibilities listed in the question (i.e., increased cardiac output, fetal systemic blood flow rates, affinity of fetal blood for oxygen, and fetal oxygen–carrying capacity) except an increased pulmonary blood flow. In fact, there is very little pulmonary blood flow because there is no oxygenation of blood in the lungs of the fetus; the blood bypasses the lungs and is shunted into the general circulation through the patent ductus arteriosus.

2. The answer is D. (*III B 1 a–c, e*) Decreased fetal heart rate (FHR) variability can be seen in a number of benign and ominous situations during labor, such as fetal "sleep states," prematurity, drug ingestion, asphyxia, tachycardia, arrhythmias, and fetal anomalies. With fetal stimulation in a healthy fetus, there is a transient tachycardia and no change in the FHR variability.

3. The answer is B. (*III C 2 d, e*) Late decelerations are indications of a decreased uteroplacental blood flow and often reflect hypoxemia or acidosis in the fetus. Preeclampsia is one of the several clinical entities that may have a decreased uteroplacental blood flow. The pathophysiology involves a fetal respiratory acidosis (not alkalosis) and metabolic acidosis, which means there is a decreased PO_2 and an increased PCO_2.

4. The answer is B (1, 3). (*II B 1–4*) With uteroplacental insufficiency, fetal hypoxia can develop, resulting in a decrease in PO_2. At first, a respiratory acidosis develops in the fetus, which means that the PCO_2 rises; there is a concomitant decrease in the fetal pH. As the hypoxia continues, a metabolic acidosis develops with which there is a rise in the lactic and pyruvic acids.

5. The answer is C (2, 4). (*III C 3 c; VI B 1*) Variable decelerations have no uniform temporal relationship to the onset of a contraction and are associated with cord compression, such as a cord around the infant's neck (a nuchal cord). Early decelerations are associated with head compression. Variable decelerations may improve with changes in maternal position (moving from side-to-side and the knee-chest or Trendelenburg positions), which takes pressure off the compressed cord.

6. The answer is C (2, 4). (*IV B 1, 2, C 3*) A fetal scalp pH of 7.2–7.24 is worrisome, but it is not indicative of severe distress, asphyxia, or acidosis in the fetus. A scalp pH at this level must be repeated in 20–30 minutes. One of the reasons for a false-low pH in the fetus is maternal acidosis, a situation in which the fetus is acidemic but not necessarily asphyxic. A fetal scalp pH of less than 7.2 indicates significant asphyxia, which demands immediate delivery.

7. The answer is A (1, 2, 3). (*V C*) Epidural anesthesia creates a sympathetic blockade that allows the pooling of blood in the lower extremities. As a result of this, maternal hypotension can develop as a result of a decreased venous return and a reduced cardiac output. These two factors lead to a decreased uterine blood flow, which may translate into fetal distress. With hypotension secondary to epidural anesthesia, there is actually an increased maternal heart rate as a compensatory mechanism for decreased venous return.

8–10. The answers are: 8-C, 9-D, 10-E. (*II A, B; III C 2; IV B 1*) In a patient with chronic hypertension, the index of suspicion about fetal distress must be high. However, no therapy is justified without first making the diagnosis of fetal distress. Thus, the first step would be fetal heart rate (FHR) monitoring to see if there is any distress.

In a woman who is 8 cm dilated, delivery is still some time off. There must be an accurate assessment of fetal well-being to see if labor can continue. A fetal scalp pH would be indicated with further management dependent on its value.

Immediate delivery is indicated in the patient with FHR monitoring and fetal scalp pH indications of significant fetal distress and acidosis. No further intrauterine resuscitation is indicated at this point.

6

Postdates Pregnancy

PonJola Coney

I. INTRODUCTION. Postdatism is the term that most commonly describes a syndrome of dysmaturity in a pregnancy that continues for more than 42 weeks. Synonyms for postdatism include: post-term pregnancy and postmaturity. Approximately 10% of all pregnancies continue beyond 42 weeks, and 4% continue beyond 43 weeks. This chapter examines the **significance of postdatism**, the **risk to the fetus**, and the **management of a postdates pregnancy**.

A. The average duration of a pregnancy is 280 days (or 40 weeks) from the first day of the last menstrual period or 266 days from ovulation, based on a 28-day cycle (Näegele's rule)*. The length of gestation increases approximately 1 day for each day the menstrual cycle is more than 28 days.

B. Determination of the exact duration of pregnancy is of foremost importance and is possible in a number of ways at various stages of pregnancy. When the last menstrual period is certain and occurs normally in a cyclic fashion, it is still very useful in pregnancy.

    1. A first visit early in pregnancy is helpful for correlation of uterine size, first detectable fetal heart rate (FHR), quickening, and serial measurements of the uterine fundus. Ultrasound examination is very accurate in the second trimester.

    2. A first visit late in pregnancy; erroneous last menstrual date; oligo-ovulation; ultrasound late in pregnancy; recent pregnancy, abortion, or oral contraceptive use without resumption of menses; acute illness; intrauterine growth retardation; metabolic disturbances; severe emotional disturbances; and heavy drug use complicate accurate pregnancy dating.

C. Etiology of postdatism. From animal experiments, the etiology of postmaturity appears to be a combination of maternal, fetal, and genetic factors, all of which are predetermined.

    1. A deficiency of adrenocorticotropic hormone in the fetus, placental sulfatase deficiency, and extrauterine pregnancy have been hypothesized as potential causative factors.

    2. The exact mechanism of spontaneous onset of labor is unclear, but the fetus, placenta, and mother are all involved. The longest pregnancy on record is 1 year and 24 days ending in a liveborn anencephalic infant. Central nervous system abnormalitites, such as anencephaly, are associated with prolonged pregnancy.

II. CLINICAL SIGNIFICANCE OF POSTDATISM

A. Incidence. Postdatism occurs more frequently in the young and elderly primigravidas and in the grandmultiparas. Although postdates pregnancy occurs infrequently, it carries a higher perinatal mortality than a term gestation. The fetal mortality for all groups is:

    1. 40–41 weeks: 1.1%

    2. 43 weeks: 2.2%

    3. 44 weeks: 6.6%

B. Dysmaturity syndrome. Normally, there is little growth of the fetus post-term (after 40 weeks); however; there is some growth, but it plateaus at 42 weeks. Dysmaturity syndrome is observed

---

*To estimate the expected date of delivery, count back 3 months from the first day of the last menstrual period and add 7 days.

in 30% of postdates infants and in 3% of term infants. The clinical features of the syndrome include:

1. Loss of subcutaneous fat
2. Dry, wrinkled, and cracked skin
3. Meconium staining of the skin, membranes, and umbilical cord
4. Long nails
5. An unusual degree of alertness

C. **Fetal compromise secondary to placental insufficiency**, resulting from placental aging or senescence, which critically reduces the metabolic and respiratory support to the fetus, is the major concern in postdates pregnancy. Asphyxia is frequently responsible for the perinatal morbidity and mortality in postdatism. Findings at autopsy of postdates infants suggestive of hypoxia include:

1. Petechiae of the pleura and pericardium
2. Amniotic debris in the lung

D. **Histology.** There is no pathognomonic histologic picture for postdatism. However, since placental insufficiency is the major concern, placental changes have been noted histologically and may correlate with insufficiency. These changes, which may be simply physiologic but can reduce the placental surface area available for nutritional and endocrine support to the fetus, include the following:

1. Calcification
2. Edema of villi
3. Syncytial pseudohyperplasia
4. Syncytial knots
5. Fibroid degeneration of villi
6. Placental microinfarction

III. ANTEPARTUM RISK ASSESSMENT FOR THE POSTDATES FETUS. A number of studies are available that group the fetus according to risk for increased morbidity and mortality and that facilitate the decision to intervene or wait for the onset of spontaneous labor.

A. **Biochemical evaluation**

1. **Maternal urinary estriol.** The production of estrogens in pregnancy is interdependent on placental, maternal, and fetal factors (Fig. 6-1). Approximately 90% of the precursors of estriol are formed in the fetal adrenal glands, and over 90% of maternal urinary estrogens are estriol. Thus, maternal urinary levels of estriol have long been recognized as reliable indices of fetoplacental function.
   a. **Estriol excretion.** Absolute values of estriol are not as important as the serial values of estriol excretion over days or weeks. Generally less than 12 mg/24 hr or a drop below the

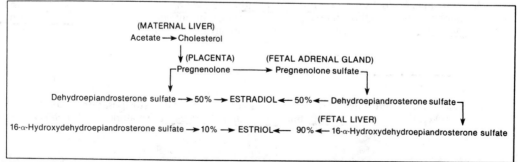

Figure 6-1. Estrogen synthesis in pregnancy in fetoplacental units. Estradiol secreted into the maternal circulation is conjugated in the maternal liver and excreted in several forms in maternal urine.

tenth percentile indicates fetal jeopardy. Maternal plasma estriols also can be used to indicate fetal compromise.

    (1) Thirty percent of fetuses with normal levels of estriol may still experience intrapartum fetal distress, including:

        (a) Tachycardia

        (b) Bradycardia

        (c) Late decelerations

        (d) Severe variables

        (e) A scalp pH of less than 7.25

    (2) Decreased levels of estriol may also represent other disease states, such as:

        (a) Diabetes

        (b) Intrauterine growth retardation

  b. Accurate measurement of urinary estriol may be complicated by:

    (1) Difficulty obtaining a complete collection over a 24-hour period

    (2) Individual differences in excretion

    (3) Day-to-day variation in excretion

  2. Human placental lactogen (HPL) is a protein hormone secreted by the placenta. It is currently a major subject of interest but is still under investigation in the study of placental function. The HPL level is proportional to the weight of the fetus and the placenta. One study reported that HPL levels were significantly lower in 75% of postdates pregnancies in which the infant had signs of dysmaturity. Determinations should be done serially just as with estriols.

B. Amniotic fluid evaluation

  1. Ultrasonography is used to estimate amniotic fluid volume, which is an indirect index of placental function. Oligohydramnios is correlated with placental insufficiency.

  2. Amniocentesis is helpful when gestational age is in question for maturity studies. Amniotic fluid levels of estriol and HPL have no predictive value. The finding of meconium-stained amniotic fluid raises concern, but its true significance when the patient is not in labor is controversial.

C. Fetal heart rate (FHR) testing

  1. Nonstress test (NST), or fetal activity test (FAT), is a noninvasive test of fetal activity, which correlates with fetal well-being. Fetal heart acceleration is observed during fetal movement. An external monitor is used to record the FHR, and the mother participates by indicating fetal movements.

    a. A reactive test reveals three or more fetal movements over 30 minutes with fetal heart acceleration of at least 15 beats amplitude of 15 seconds duration.

    b. In one study, 99% of oxytocin challenge tests were negative for signs of fetal distress when performed after a reactive NST.

  2. Contraction stress test (CST), or nipple stimulation test*, is a test of the FHR in response to oxytocin administered intravenously prior to labor, which indirectly measures placental function. A CST is performed when the NST is nonreactive.

    a. Criteria for a negative CST is three uterine contractions per 10 minutes with no evidence of late decelerations, severe variables, or loss of beat-to-beat variability.

    b. More often a favorable outcome follows a negative CST, but as many as 25% of fetuses may experience intrapartum fetal distress following a negative CST.

    c. CSTs have a 25% false–positive rate.

D. Biophysical profile. This is a composite of tests designed to identify a compromised fetus during the antepartum period.

  1. Components of the profile (performed ultrasonographically)

    a. Nonstress test

    b. Fetal breathing

    c. Fetal tone

    d. Fetal motion

    e. Quantity of amniotic fluid

  2. Scoring of the profile. Each test is given either 2 or 0 points for a maximum of 10 points. An important feature in the postdates profile is the amniotic fluid component. An acceptable score is 6 unless one of the two negative assessments is a deficient amount of amniotic fluid.

---

*The nipple stimulation test is an endogenous means of releasing oxytocin in response to manual stimulation of the patient's breast nipples. It is a noninvasive contraction stress test.

IV. MANAGEMENT OF THE POSTDATES PREGNANCY

A. Expectant. Because the induction of labor is accompanied by a high incidence of uterine inertia, long labor, cervical trauma, forceps delivery, and cesarean delivery, expectant management is warranted in some cases. Since 60% of patients will go into labor spontaneously between 40 and 41 weeks and 80% by 43 weeks, the pregnancy should simply be monitored as long as the fetus is deemed "doing well" by prenatal testing. However, the ability of antepartum testing to identify accurately the fetus at risk is far from ideal. As no single test is adequate, a combination of tests is desirable. Electronic intrapartum fetal heart monitoring is still the mainstay for intrapartum management of labor. Antenatal testing is temporal and has no predictive interval of safety for a fetus from the time performed; therefore testing must be repetitive, frequent, and expertly interpreted.

B. Active. Regardless of the status of the cervix, delivery is indicated for the fetus identified as at risk. In spite of sophisticated testing, the postdates group has more induced labors, prolonged labors, uterine inertia, high incidences of intrapartum fetal distress, and high cesarean birth rates. Nonetheless, with careful antepartum, intrapartum, and neonatal monitoring, the perinatal mortality for the postdates infant can almost approach that of the term population.

C. Methods of induction. In the postdates pregnancy, delivery is indicated if there is evidence of deteriorating fetal well-being or if the pregnancy is passed 42 weeks.

   1. Oxytocin infusion. This method may or may not be successful due to the condition of the cervix. An uneffaced, unripe cervix may not respond to oxytocin stimulation because of the absence of gap junctions in the cervix (see Chapter 4, section II B).

   2. Prostaglandin gel. Application of prostaglandin gel on the cervix the day before attempting the oxytocin infusion often induces changes in the cervix, such as gap-junction formation, that result in a successful stimulation of labor the following day.

BIBLIOGRAPHY

Aladjem S, et al: *Clinical Perinatology*, 2nd ed. St Louis, CV Mosby, 1980, p 257

Anderson G: Postmaturity: a review. *Obstet Gynecol Survey* 27:65, 1972

Clifford SH: Postmaturity with placental function: clinical syndrome and pathologic findings. *J Pediatr* 44:1, 1954

Devoe L, Sholl J: Postdates pregnancy: assessment of fetal risk and obstetric management. *J Reprod Med* 28:576, 1983

Josimovitch J, et al: Evaluation of post-term pregnancies with maternal serum placental lactogen and alpha fetoprotein concentrations in normal and prolonged pregnancies. *Obstet Gynecol* 50:445, 1977

Koller WS Jr, Curet LB: Fetal activity determinations and OCT for the assessment of fetal well-being. *Obstet Gynecol* 52:176, 1978

Vintzileos AM, et al: The fetal biophysical profile and its predictive value. *Obstet Gynecol* 62:271, 1983

STUDY QUESTIONS

Directions: Each question below contains five suggested answers. Choose the **one best** response to each question.

1. The first step in the assessment of postdatism is

(A) ultrasound examination
(B) determination of the true length of gestation
(C) measurement of fetal heart rate
(D) determination of amniotic fluid volume
(E) contraction stress test

2. All of the following factors have been associated with postdates pregnancy EXCEPT

(A) deficiency of adrenocorticotropic hormone
(B) central nervous system abnormalities
(C) placental sulfatase deficiency
(D) insufficient oxytocin level
(E) extrauterine pregnancy

3. The perinatal mortality rate at 44 weeks gestation is

(A) less than 1%
(B) 1%–2%
(C) 2%–3%
(D) 4%–5%
(E) 6%–7%

4. Estriol levels are an indicator of fetal well-being because the majority of its precursors are formed in the

(A) placenta
(B) fetal adrenal gland
(C) maternal adrenal gland
(D) amniotic fluid
(E) maternal liver

5. Amniocentesis in the management of postdatism is used for measurement of

(A) human placental lactogen
(B) estriol
(C) maturity
(D) meconium staining
(E) fetal cells

Directions: Each question below contains four suggested answers of which **one or more** is correct. Choose the answer

A   if **1, 2, and 3** are correct
B   if **1 and 3** are correct
C   if **2 and 4** are correct
D   if **4** is correct
E   if **1, 2, 3, and 4** are correct

6. Maternal estriol levels that represent fetal compromise are accurately described by which of the following statements?

(1) The serial values of estriol excretion are more important than the absolute values
(2) Absolute values are less than 12 mg/24 hr
(3) Excretion values are below the tenth percentile
(4) Excretion is variable from day to day

7. Which of the following tests would be indicated following a nonreactive nonstress test?

(1) Contraction stress test
(2) Biophysical profile
(3) Nipple stimulation test
(4) Amniocentesis for fetal lung maturity

ANSWERS AND EXPLANATIONS

1. The answer is B. *(I A, B)* Before embarking on postdates testing, it is essential to determine the true length of the pregnancy. A "postdates" pregnancy may, in fact, not be postdates due to uncertain dates of the last menstrual period or an irregular menstrual cycle in which the pregnant woman ovulated later than the usual day 14 of the cycle. Review of such features as quickening, uterine size at first visit and serial measurements thereafter, and the date of the first detectable fetal heart tones can be helpful in establishing the due date.

2. The answer is D. *(I C)* There is no evidence to support the theory that oxytocin may be insufficient in prolonged pregnancy. Animal studies testing adrenocorticotropin or cortisol do support an association with the failure of the onset of spontaneous labor. The absence of placental sulfatase and the high incidence of central nervous system abnormalities, particularly anencephaly, with prolonged pregnancy are well documented. With an extrauterine pregnancy, there is no mechanism for the onset of labor because the fetus is not in the uterus.

3. The answer is E. *(II A 1–3)* As pregnancy progresses beyond 40 weeks, perinatal morbidity and mortality increase. The perinatal mortality at term is 1.1%, and by 44 weeks gestation, there is a six-fold increase (6%–7%).

4. The answer is B. *(III A 1; Figure 6-1)* Under normal circumstances, estriol levels increase with advancing gestation. It is derived from 16-α-hydroxydehydroepiandrosterone sulfate (16-α-OHDHEAS), whose primary source is the fetal adrenal gland. There is a maternal source (liver) of estriol, but this comprises less than 10% of the total. Thus, maternal urinary levels of estriol have long been recognized as a reliable index of fetoplacental function.

5. The answer is C. *(III B 2)* Amniocentesis is helpful when gestational age is in question for maturity studies. Amniotic fluid levels of human placental lactogen and estriol have not proven predictive of fetal jeopardy or well-being in prolonged pregnancy. Certainly maturity studies (lecithin/sphingomyelin ratio and phosphatidylglycerol levels) are helpful when the exact duration of the pregnancy is unknown. The finding of meconium-stained amniotic fluid raises concern, but its true significance is controversial.

6. The answer is A (1, 2, 3). *(III A 1)* The multiple factors involved in measuring urinary estriols in regard to collection suggest that a single value to assess the fetus at risk should not be used. Absolute values of estriol are not as important as serial values of estriol excretion over days or weeks. In addition, values below 12 mg/24 hr or below the tenth percentile are suggestive of a fetus at risk. It is important to note, however, that 30% of fetuses with normal estriol levels may still exhibit intrapartum fetal distress. Maternal plasma levels may also indicate fetal compromise but also require serial measurement.

7. The answer is A (1, 2, 3). *(III C 1, 2, D)* A nonreactive nonstress test (NST) is an indication of potential fetal distress. Therefore, additional testing for fetal well-being must be accomplished. The contraction stress test (CST) may be performed with either intravenous oxytocin or nipple stimulation. The presence of contractions provides more stress on the uteroplacental unit and, thus, is a good test of its reserve. The biophysical profile is an alternative to the CST in further testing fetal well-being in the presence of a nonreactive NST. There is no need for testing of fetal lung maturity at this point because there is no immediate indication that delivery should be considered.

diabetes
hypertension
anemias
urinary infection
thyroid disease

7
Medical Complications of Pregnancy
William W. Beck, Jr.

I. DIABETES is a medical disease that is made worse by pregnancy and that increases the risks of pregnancy complications.

A. Diagnosis of diabetes during pregnancy

1. There should be a **high index of suspicion** in women who have:
   a. A strong family history of diabetes
   b. Previously given birth to large infants
   c. Persistent glucosuria
   d. A history of unexplained fetal losses

2. **Glucosuria** during pregnancy should be investigated, keeping in mind that it does not always reflect hyperglycemia from impaired glucose tolerance but may reflect a lower renal threshold for glucose, which may be induced by a normal pregnancy.

3. **Glucose testing**
   a. **One-hour glucose tolerance test.** This is a good screening test for high-risk patients and is performed before and after a 50 g glucose load. An abnormal test necessitates a standard glucose tolerance test. Abnormalities are reflected by the following plasma glucose levels:
      (1) Fasting: 105 mg/dl or above   *Fast 105+*
      (2) One hour: 140 mg/dl or above   *1º   140+*
   b. **Standard glucose tolerance test.** This is a 3-hour test with periodic blood determinations after a 100 g glucose load is ingested. Class A diabetes (chemical diabetes) is the diagnosis when two or more plasma glucose levels equal or exceed:
      (1) 105 mg/dl (fasting)
      (2) 190 mg/dl (1 hour)
      (3) 165 mg/dl (2 hour)
      (4) 145 mg/dl (3 hour)

4. **Classification of diabetes in pregnant women**
   a. A: chemical diabetes
   b. B: maturity-onset diabetes; age over 20 years and duration under 10 years
   c. C_1: age 10–19 years at onset
   d. C_2: 10–19 years duration
   e. D_1: under age 10 years at onset
   f. D_2: over 20 years duration
   g. D_3: benign retinopathy
   h. D_4: calcified vessels of legs
   i. D_5: hypertension
   j. F: nephropathy
   k. R: proliferating retinopathy

B. Effect of pregnancy on diabetes

1. **The diabetogenic properties of pregnancy** are reversible but still may induce abnormalities in glucose tolerance in women who have no evidence of diabetes.
   a. Insulin antagonism is due to the action of placental lactogen and the sex steroids, estrogen and progesterone.
   b. Placental insulinase accelerates insulin degradation.

2. **Control of diabetes** may be more difficult in pregnancy.
   a. Nausea and vomiting can lead to insulin shock.
   b. Infection can lead to insulin resistance and ketoacidosis.

    3. Insulin requirements in chemical and overt diabetics decrease rapidly after delivery with the disappearance of placental lactogen and insulinase and estrogen and progesterone.

C. Effect of diabetes on pregnancy

  1. Mother. There is an increased likelihood of:
    a. Preeclampsia and eclampsia
    b. Infection, which can be severe
    c. A large infant, which can present problems with delivery, such as shoulder dystocia
    d. Cesarean section delivery because of the macrosomia of the infant
    e. Hydramnios
    f. Postpartum hemorrhage

  2. Fetus. There is an increased likelihood of:
    a. Perinatal mortality, especially when the pregnant diabetic is not managed appropriately
    b. Perinatal morbidity from birth injury (often due to macrosomia with accompanying shoulder dystocia and brachial plexus injury)
    c. Perinatal hypoglycemia and hypocalcemia
    d. Congenital abnormalities, such as neural tube defects
    e. Diabetes in the offspring

D. Preconception and prenatal care

  1. Hemoglobin A$_{1c}$ determination at the patient's first visit provides an assessment of her prior diabetic regulation.

  2. Strict glucose control prior to and during early pregnancy is thought to reduce the risk of severe malformations, such as neural tube defects, which are seen in fetuses of poorly controlled diabetics. The maternal glucose level should be kept as close to normal as possible.
    a. This may involve one or more antepartum hospitalizations for glucose control.
    b. The pregnancy should continue until the fetus is mature unless the intrauterine environment has deteriorated to the point at which fetal well-being is threatened.

  3. Determination of the precise fetal age is important in a diabetic woman.
    a. Sonographic evaluation is used in conjunction with the last menstrual period to date the pregnancy.
    b. A well-established expected date of confinement (EDC) is necessary to assess accurately:
      (1) Macrosomia
      (2) Hydramnios
      (3) Intrauterine growth retardation, which is seen in diabetics with vascular disease

  4. Insulin requirements cannot be gauged by the degree of glucosuria.
    a. Glucosuria may be present because of an increase in the glomerular filtration of glucose without increased tubular reabsorption.
    b. Significant hypoglycemia could develop if the insulin dosage is manipulated because of the glucosuria rather than blood glucose levels.

E. Third-trimester and delivery management

  1. Class A diabetes. These patients are treated with diet alone with frequent monitoring of blood glucose levels. In gestational diabetes that does not require insulin, the pregnancies are delivered at term; there is no need for early termination.

  2. Overt insulin-dependent diabetes
    a. Admission to the hospital at 34–36 weeks is indicated so that the fetus can be monitored closely to prevent the sudden fetal demise that can occur. Important monitors are:
      (1) The nonstress test (NST) and the contraction stress test (CST), which can be done several times a week. The NST should be reactive, and the CST should be negative if the fetus is healthy.
      (2) Biophysical profile, which includes the following:
        (a) NST
        (b) Fetal breathing
        (c) Fetal tone
        (d) Fetal motion
        (e) Quantity of amniotic fluid
    b. Signs of fetal distress include the following:
      (1) A nonreactive NST
      (2) A positive CST
      (3) A poor biophysical profile

[handwritten: Lung L/S ratio > 37-38 wk]

(4) Decreased insulin requirements

c. The timing of delivery depends on the health and maturity of the fetus. In a diabetic, the lecithin/sphingomyelin (L/S) ratio may take longer to show fetal lung maturity than in a nondiabetic; lung maturity at 37–38 weeks cannot, therefore, be assumed without measuring amniotic fluid levels of L/S and phosphatidylglycerol.

d. Method of delivery

(1) Induction of labor may be attempted if the fetus is not excessively large and if the cervix is capable of being induced, that is, if it is soft, appreciably effaced, and somewhat dilated.

(2) Cesarean section is commonly used to avoid the trauma of a delivery of a large infant and to avoid the stress of labor for the fetus that has shown signs of distress.

(3) The possibility of shoulder dystocia in the macrosomic infant of a diabetic mother should not be forgotten.

II. HYPERTENSIVE DISEASE

A. Definitions

1. Hypertension is a blood pressure reading on two occasions of at least 140/90 or a rise of 30 mm systolic or 15 mm diastolic. *[handwritten: 30|15]*

2. Preeclampsia is hypertension with proteinuria, edema, or both, induced by pregnancy after the twentieth week unless it is a molar pregnancy.

3. Eclampsia is the occurrence of convulsions in a woman who meets the criteria for preeclampsia.

4. Gestational hypertension is hypertension that develops during the latter half of pregnancy or during the first 24 hours after delivery. This is not accompanied by any other evidence of preeclampsia, and it disappears within 10 days following delivery.

5. Chronic hypertensive disease is characterized by the presence of persistent hypertension before the twentieth week of pregnancy in the absence of a hydatidiform mole.

B. Pregnancy-induced hypertension involves hypertension alone, preeclampsia, and eclampsia. It is rare prior to the twentieth week of pregnancy in the absence of a hydatidiform mole.

1. Nulliparity. Preeclampsia is predominantly a disease of nulliparous women, particularly those in the extremes of reproductive life, that is, teenagers and women over 35 years of age.

2. Multiparity. In multiparas, preeclampsia may be associated with:
a. A multiple gestation
b. Fetal hydrops
c. Chronic hypertension
d. Diabetes
e. Coexisting renal disease

3. Classification of pregnancy-induced hypertension
a. Mild
(1) Diastolic blood pressure of less than 110 mm Hg   *[handwritten: /110]*
(2) 1+ proteinuria
(3) Normal serum creatinine
(4) Absence of:
(a) Thrombocytopenia
(b) Fetal growth retardation
b. Severe
(1) Diastolic blood pressure of 110 mm Hg or more   *[handwritten: /110↑]*
(2) 2+ proteinuria or more
(3) Presence of:
(a) Headaches
(b) Visual disturbances
(c) Upper abdominal pain (hepatic edema and stretching of Glisson's capsule)
(d) Oliguria
(e) Thrombocytopenia
(f) Elevated creatinine
(g) Fetal growth retardation
c. Life-threatening. Eclamptic seizures may occur before, during, or after labor. If a seizure appears more than 48 hours after delivery, it is more likely than not to be the result of some other central nervous system disorder.

4. Etiology of preeclampsia (theory)
  a. There is a release of local vasoconstrictors, which are destroyed by placental enzymes in a normal pregnancy but which are deficient in preeclampsia.
  b. Vasoconstrictors lead to vasospasm and poor placental perfusion, which in turn lead to:
    (1) Poor blood supply to the fetus and potential intrauterine growth retardation
    (2) Release of general vasoconstrictors, which results in:
      (a) Hypertension
      (b) Decreased renal blood flow, which results in hypoxia of the glomerulus with resultant:
        (i) Proteinuria
        (ii) Retention of water
        (iii) Edema

C. Consequences of pregnancy-induced hypertension, which are largely due to the vasospasm inherent in the disease process, include:

  1. Rising blood pressure as a result of a steady cardiac output with an increase in arteriolar constriction and peripheral resistance

  2. Hemoconcentration as a result of an increased vascular permeability with too little fluid intravascularly and a marked excess extravascularly

  3. Reduced renal perfusion and glomerular filtration, resulting in:
    a. Elevated plasma uric acid concentration
    b. Elevated plasma creatinine and urea (in severe cases)

  4. Decreased maternal placental perfusion—a major reason for the increased perinatal morbidity and mortality

D. Clinical aspects of preeclampsia

  1. Blood pressure. A rise in blood pressure is the most significant sign of preeclampsia. A persistent diastolic pressure of 90 mm Hg or more is abnormal.

  2. Weight gain. Excessive weight gain, that is, more than 2 lbs per week or 6 lbs per month, may be the first sign of preeclampsia. Weight gain is usually sudden and attributable to an abnormal retention of fluid.

  3. Proteinuria. This may be minimal in preeclampsia. Proteinuria usually develops later than the hypertension.

  4. Headache. This sign is significant in severe preeclampsia because it may be the forerunner of a convulsion. It is often frontal and resistant to mild analgesia.

  5. Epigastric pain. This is a sign of severe preeclampsia and may be rapidly followed by a convulsion.

  6. Visual disturbances. These range from slight blurring of vision to blindness and are due to arteriolar spasm, ischemia, and edema of the retina with occasional retinal detachment.

E. Treatment of pregnancy-induced hypertension. The goals of treatment are termination of the pregnancy with the least possible trauma to the mother and fetus and the birth of an infant who ultimately thrives.

  1. Inappropriate treatment
    a. Diuretics can reduce renal perfusion and uteroplacental perfusion in a situation where there is already a constricted intravascular volume.
    b. Ambulatory care. There is no place for ambulatory treatment of pregnancy-induced hypertension unless the blood pressure elevation is mild (less than 135/85) and there is no proteinuria. If these conditions are met, the patient should be told to:
      (1) Rest in bed in the left lateral position
      (2) Have outpatient examinations twice a week
      (3) Report any symptoms, such as headache, blurred vision, or abdominal pain

  2. Hospitalization is necessary when the patient has a blood pressure of 140/90 or above with or without proteinuria.
    a. The patient is confined to bed with bathroom privileges only.
    b. Weight, urinary protein, blood pressure, serum creatinine, and platelets are monitored daily.

    c. Regular assessment of fetal well-being with frequent NSTs, CSTs, and serial sonography for fetal growth is essential to assure an uncompromised fetus.

    d. In women with severe preeclampsia, anticonvulsants (magnesium sulfate) and antihypertensives (hydralazine) should be used to stabilize the patient prior to delivery.

  3. Delivery

    a. Termination of the pregnancy with removal of the trophoblast cures pregnancy-induced hypertension.

    b. Temporization in the hope of increasing the time in which the fetus is in utero is only appropriate in mild disease. Procrastination can be dangerous as the preeclampsia itself can kill the fetus.

    c. Indications for delivery include:

      Induce   **(1)** Increasing proteinuria

      (2) Worsening hypertension

      (3) Compromise in fetal well-being, as manifested by:

        (a) A nonreactive NST

        (b) A positive CST

        (c) A poor biophysical profile

    d. The L/S ratio may be an important test in the premature fetus. The goal is an L/S ratio greater than 2.0, but it may not be possible to wait for this to happen with hypertension that is getting worse. However, the conversion of the L/S to mature levels may occur earlier than would be normally expected because of the stress of the disease.

    e. Induction of labor with intravenous oxytocin is often successful when there is no fetal distress.

    f. Cesarean section is the usual method of delivery with severe preeclampsia, especially with a cervix that cannot be induced as in a premature gestation.

  4. Postpartum. There is usually rapid improvement in hypertension following delivery, although it may transiently worsen.

    a. Eclampsia may develop any time during the first 24 hours postpartum.

    b. Magnesium sulfate instituted before or during delivery should be continued for 24 hours postpartum.

    c. Antihypertensives, such as hydralazine (Apresoline), should be given intermittently for diastolic blood pressure of 110 mm Hg or higher. *PRN*

    d. Hypertension induced by pregnancy usually disappears by 2 weeks postpartum.

III. ANEMIAS

A. Acquired anemias

  1. Iron deficiency. The iron requirements of pregnancy are considerable, and in most women iron stores are low.

    a. A pregnant woman needs 800 mg of elemental iron of which 300 mg goes to the fetus and 500 mg is used to expand the maternal red cell mass.

    b. Anemia exists with a hemoglobin of less than 10 during pregnancy. ≤ 10

    c. There is a natural decrease in the hematocrit during the second half of pregnancy because the newly formed hemoglobin and red cell mass do not keep pace with the expansion of the maternal blood volume.   *2° Δ ↓Hct.*

    d. Daily elemental iron (200 mg) is necessary to correct the anemia and maintain adequate stores.

    e. Because of the normal transfer of iron from the mother to the fetus, the fetus does not suffer from iron deficiency anemia even in a severely anemic mother.

  2. Megaloblastic anemia is caused by a folic acid deficiency; women with this anemia are also usually iron deficient.

    a. This anemia is found in pregnant women who consume neither fresh vegetables nor foods with a high content of animal protein.

    b. Women with megaloblastic anemia during pregnancy may develop:

      (1) Nausea

      (2) Vomiting

      (3) Anorexia

    c. Treatment includes:

      (1) A well-balanced diet

      (2) Oral iron

      (3) Folic acid (1 mg/day)

B. Congenital anemias, which are characterized by the hemoglobinopathies (i.e., sickle cell anemia, hemoglobin SC disease, β-thalassemia, and sickle cell trait), result in increased maternal morbidity and mortality, spontaneous abortion, and perinatal mortality. Prophylactic red cell transfusions have been used effectively with SS, SC, and β-thalassemia diseases when administered prior to the development of pain. They are given to keep the hematocrit above 25%, decrease the painful crises, and decrease pregnancy wastage and perinatal loss.

1. **Sickle cell anemia–hemoglobin SS disease** (SS disease) occurs when an individual receives the gene for the production of hemoglobin S, an abnormal variant of hemoglobin, from each parent. Since the sickle cell trait commonly appears in 1 out of 12 black individuals, there is a theoretical incidence of SS disease of 1 in 576. The actual rate among pregnant women is somewhat less, because of the high mortality rate among individuals with SS disease, especially during early childhood. Prophylactic transfusions have become common practice in an attempt to maintain nonsickling red cells at 50% or higher.
   a. Pregnancy is a serious burden in women with SS disease.
      (1) The anemia becomes more intense.
      (2) The pain crises become more frequent.
      (3) Infection and pulmonary dysfunction are common.
      (4) Death of the woman and child may result.
   b. There is intense erythropoiesis because of the shortened life span of the red blood cells with the abnormal hemoglobin. Because of this, the folic acid needs of a pregnancy complicated by SS disease are considerable, requiring 1 mg/day.
   c. The hemoglobin concentration does not fall much below 7 g/dl.
   d. Labor is managed with:
      (1) Adequate hydration and oxygen to prevent sickling
      (2) Analgesia
      (3) Packed cell transfusion if a cesarean section is contemplated

2. **Sickle cell–hemoglobin C disease** (SC disease) occurs in 1 in 2000 pregnant black women.
   a. During pregnancy, maternal morbidity and mortality is considerably higher in SC disease than in SS disease; however, there is a lower perinatal mortality with SC disease as compared with SS disease.
   b. One in eight pregnancies ends in maternal death, abortion, stillbirth, or neonatal death.
   c. There is a high incidence of severe pain and pulmonary dysfunction, the latter resulting from embolization of necrotic bone marrow, both fat and cellular components.

3. **Sickle cell–β-thalassemia disease** has a perinatal mortality and morbidity similar to those of SC disease with somewhat less maternal morbidity and mortality.

4. **Sickle cell trait** is characterized by the inheritance of the gene for the production of hemoglobin S from one parent and hemoglobin A from the other. The trait occurs in 8.5% of black individuals.
   a. Sickle trait does not influence the frequency of abortion, perinatal mortality, low birth weight, or pregnancy-induced hypertension.
   b. Urinary tract infection and asymptomatic bacteriuria are twice as common in patients with sickle trait as in those without the trait.

IV. URINARY TRACT INFECTION. Pregnancy, with its functional and anatomic changes of the urinary tract, predisposes women to the development of urinary tract infection. Five percent of pregnant women have bacteriuria at the first prenatal visit.

A. Cystitis is characterized by dysuria, particularly at the end of urination, as well as urgency and frequency. If cystitis is not treated, the upper urinary tract may become involved in an ascending infection.

B. Acute pyelonephritis is one of the most common medical complications of pregnancy. It complicates late pregnancy and the puerperium in 2% of women and usually results from an ascending infection of the bladder.

1. When unilateral, the disease usually is right-sided.

2. It is characterized by:
   a. The abrupt onset of fever
   b. Shaking chills
   c. Aching pain in one or both lumbar regions
   d. Anorexia

  e. Nausea
  f. Vomiting

  3. *Escherichia coli* is the organism most commonly cultured from the urine.

  4. Factors that predispose the pregnant woman to pyelonephritis include the following:
  a. Compression of the ureter at the pelvic brim by the enlarging uterus and by the enlarged ovarian vein leads to a progressive dilation of the renal calyces, pelves, and ureters.
  b. There is a decrease in tone and peristaltic action of the ureters secondary to the levels of progesterone and its relaxation effect on smooth muscle.
  c. A decreased bladder sensitivity to volume in the puerperium may be secondary to spinal or epidural anesthesia and may lead to overdistension of the bladder and the need for catheterization, which can result in the seeding of bacteria.

C. Asymptomatic bacteriuria denotes the presence of actively multiplying bacteria within the urinary tract without the symptoms of a urinary tract infection.

  1. The highest incidence is in black multiparas with sickle cell trait.

  2. Twenty to forty percent of women with asymptomatic bacteriuria during pregnancy subsequently develop an acute urinary tract infection.

  3. Bacteriuria is not a prominent factor in the genesis of low birth weight or prematurity.

  4. Treatment involves one of the following:
  a. Nitrofurantoin (Macrodantin), 100 mg daily for 10 days
  b. Sulfisoxazole (Gantrisin), 1 g four times a day for 10 days
  c. Single dose therapy with:
     (1) Sulfisoxazole, 2 g
     (2) Nitrofurantoin, 200 mg
     (3) Ampicillin, 2 g plus probenecid, 1 g

V. THYROID DISEASE

A. Hyperthyroidism

  1. Diagnosis. Hyperthyroidism during pregnancy can be identified by:
  a. Tachycardia that exceeds the increase caused by normal pregnancy
  b. A high pulse rate while sleeping
  c. An enlarged thyroid gland
  d. Exophthalmos
  e. Failure to gain weight normally
  f. Markedly elevated plasma thyroxine levels as compared with normal values in the nonpregnant state

  2. Treatment. Hyperthyroidism can almost always be controlled with antithyroid medication without any threat to the mother. Treatment may be medical or surgical.
  a. Medical therapy includes the use of propylthiouracil; however, this drug readily crosses the placenta and may induce fetal hypothyroidism and goiter. The common practice of administering supplemental thyroid hormone to protect the fetus does not always protect against the development of goiter in the fetus.
  b. Surgical therapy. Thyroidectomy can be performed after the hyperthyroid condition has been brought under control. Surgery is most properly timed during the period between the beginning of the second trimester and early in the third trimester.

B. Hypothyroidism

  1. Unique features
  a. Hypothyroidism is often associated with infertility.
  b. If pregnancy occurs, there is an apparent increased abortion rate.
  c. Infants of hypothyroid mothers are healthy without evidence of thyroid dysfunction.
  d. Simple colloid goiter in the mother, if unassociated with hypothyroidism, has no influence on the pregnancy.

  2. Diagnosis. Hypothyroidism is diagnosed in pregnancy when the level of circulating thyroxine does not rise as expected and when the level of thyroid-stimulating hormone is elevated.

  3. Treatment is with supplemental thyroid hormone. For the woman already on thyroid replacement, the dosage does not have to be increased.

VI. HEART DISEASE

A. Incidence of heart disease in pregnancy

1. Heart disease occurs in 1% of all pregnancies. Because of the decreased incidence of rheumatic fever, fewer women are seen with rheumatic heart disease. Corrective surgery however, has enabled more women with congenital heart disease to reach childbearing age.

2. There is a 38% incidence of fetal wastage in the pregnancies of women with hypoxic congenital heart disease. Severe maternal hypoxia results in:
   a. Abortion
   b. Premature delivery
   c. Intrauterine demise

B. Diagnosis of heart disease during pregnancy

1. Symptoms that occur in normal pregnancies that can be confused with symptoms of heart disease include:
   a. Systolic murmurs, which are functional
   b. Accentuated respiratory effort, which sometimes represents dyspnea
   c. Edema, especially in the lower extremities during the last half of pregnancy

2. Criteria for the diagnosis of heart disease in pregnancy include:
   a. A diastolic, presystolic, or continuous heart murmur
   b. Unequivocal cardiac enlargement
   c. A loud, harsh systolic murmur, especially if associated with a thrill
   d. Severe arrhythmias

C. Classification of heart disease

1. **Class I**: uncompromised with no limitation of physical activity

2. **Class II**: slightly compromised with slight limitation of physical activity

3. **Class III**: markedly compromised with marked limitation of physical activity

4. **Class IV**: inability to perform any physical activity without discomfort

D. Management of pregnant cardiac patients

1. **Class I and II cardiac patients.** Patients are allowed to go through pregnancy; however, they must be constantly aware of the signs of developing cardiac failure.
   a. **Recommended prenatal care** includes:
      (1) Rest for 10 hours per night and rest after each meal
      (2) No heavy work; light work on one level of the house
      (3) Avoidance of foods rich in sodium
      (4) Weight gain of under 25 lbs
   b. **Congestive heart failure.** The onset may be very subtle, so observation must be constant. Signs and symptoms include:
      (1) Cough with rales on physical examination
      (2) Inability to carry out normal household chores
      (3) Increasing dyspnea on exertion
   c. **Hospitalization before delivery** is common.
      (1) **Labor**
         (a) The semirecumbent position must be assumed.
         (b) The maternal pulse and respiratory rate must be monitored. A pulse of greater than 100 or a respiratory rate of greater than 24/min are signs of cardiac embarrassment.
      (2) **Adequate analgesia.** Continuous epidural anesthesia is good for relief of pain and apprehension. It is important to guard against hypotension because of the possible reversal of blood flow in women with cardiac shunts whereby blood bypasses the lungs.
      (3) **Delivery** should be accomplished vaginally unless there is an obstetrical reason for a cesarean section. There is less morbidity and mortality with the vaginal delivery than with a cesarean section.
   d. **Cardiac failure**
      (1) **Before labor or full dilation of the cervix**
         (a) The failure must be treated before there can be any thought of delivery. Although the fetus can be severely distressed by cardiac failure, the mother will be compromised if delivery is effected prior to therapy.
         (b) Treatment includes:

     (i) Morphine
     (ii) Oxygen
     (iii) Rapid digitalization
     (iv) A potent diuretic
     (v) The Fowler position in bed
   (2) After complete dilation of the cervix and engagement, there should be prompt forceps or vacuum extraction delivery to eliminate the stress of the second stage of labor.
  e. Postpartum
   (1) The autotransfusion that occurs after delivery of the placenta can throw a marginally compensated woman into failure.
   (2) Postpartum infection and hemorrhage are potential problems in women with heart disease.

 2. Class III cardiac patients
  a. One-third of class III patients will decompensate during pregnancy. Therefore, there is the question about performing a therapeutic abortion on these patients who cannot or do not want to be hospitalized or stay in bed for most of the pregnancy.
  b. The method of delivery is vaginal.
   (1) The sick cardiac patient withstands major surgical procedures poorly.
   (2) Severe heart disease is a contraindication for cesarean section.

 3. Class IV cardiac patients must be treated for cardiac failure in pregnancy, labor, and the puerperium. Delivery by any method carries a high maternal mortality rate.

STUDY QUESTIONS

Directions: Each question below contains five suggested answers. Choose the **one best** response to each question.

1. The infant of a diabetic mother is at risk for all of the following EXCEPT

(A) increased perinatal death rate
(B) hypocalcemia
(C) hyperglycemia
(D) neural tube defects
(E) macrosomia

2. A pregnant woman with the sickle cell trait is at risk for an increased incidence of

(A) perinatal mortality
(B) a low-birth-weight infant
(C) pregnancy-induced hypertension
(D) urinary tract infection
(E) spontaneous abortion

3. Factors that can contribute to an acute urinary tract infection during pregnancy, delivery, or the puerperium include all of the following EXCEPT

(A) compression of the ureter by the large uterus at the pelvic brim
(B) increased ureteral tone and peristalsis
(C) asymptomatic bacteriuria
(D) decreased bladder sensitivity after epidural anesthesia
(E) bladder catheterization following delivery

Directions: Each question below contains four suggested answers of which **one or more** is correct. Choose the answer

A   if **1, 2, and 3** are correct
B   if **1 and 3** are correct
C   if **2 and 4** are correct
D   if **4** is correct
E   if **1, 2, 3, and 4** are correct

4. Glucosuria in urine samples during routine prenatal visits indicates

(1) gestational diabetes
(2) an increased glomerular filtration of glucose
(3) a need for dietary control
(4) a need for glucose tolerance screening

5. Indications for delivery at 36 weeks in the pregnancy of an insulin-dependent diabetic include which of the following?

(1) A poor biophysical profile
(2) Increased insulin requirements
(3) A positive contraction stress test
(4) A lecithin/sphingomyelin ratio of 1.8/1

6. Preeclampsia in the multiparous pregnant patient is associated with which of the following conditions?

(1) Multiple gestation
(2) Diabetes
(3) Glomerulonephritis
(4) Chronic hypertension

7. Pathophysiologic consequences of preeclampsia include

(1) decreased glomerular filtration rate
(2) increased plasma uric acid
(3) decreased placental perfusion
(4) increased intravascular volume

8. Signs of heart disease in pregnancy include

(1) lower extremity edema
(2) systolic murmurs
(3) increased respiratory effort
(4) arrhythmias

Directions: The group of questions below consists of lettered choices followed by several numbered items. For each numbered item select the **one** lettered choice with which it is **most** closely associated. Each lettered choice may be used once, more than once, or not at all.

Questions 9–11

For each clinical presentation listed below, select the hematologic condition that is most likely to be associated with it.

(A) Iron deficiency anemia
(B) Megaloblastic anemia
(C) Sickle cell anemia
(D) Hemoglobin SC disease
(E) Sickle cell trait

9. A woman presents at 33 weeks gestation, complaining of severe chest pain and difficulty breathing. When her abdomen is auscultated, there are no fetal heart tones. Ultrasound examination confirms a fetal demise.

10. A woman with a hemoglobin of 9.0 before becoming pregnant has a hemoglobin of 8.0 during her pregnancy despite supplemental oral iron and folic acid. Her infant is born with a normal hemoglobin.

11. A woman at 32 weeks gestation presents for the second time in 6 weeks with premature uterine contractions. A bacteriuria was found in the urine and treated each time, and the contractions stopped on both occasions after the treatment.

ANSWERS AND EXPLANATIONS

1. The answer is C. (*I C 2 a–d*) The effects of diabetes on the fetus and infant can be considerable, especially uncontrolled diabetes. There is an increase in fetal abnormalities, such as neural tube defects. Macrosomia is common, and the perinatal death rate is higher than normal. The newborn may demonstrate hypocalcemia and *hypo*glycemia. The insulin secretion that has been stimulated in the fetus by the high levels of glucose from the mother continues after birth and can drop the newborn blood glucose to dangerously low levels.

2. The answer is D. (*III B 4 a, b*) Sickle cell trait occurs in 1 in 12 blacks or 8.5% of the black population. It is important to know that a woman has sickle cell trait because of the increased incidence of asymptomatic bacteriuria and urinary tract infection in these women. However, sickle cell trait does not influence the frequency of abortion, perinatal mortality, low-birth-weight infants, or pregnancy-induced hypertension.

3. The answer is B. (*IV B 4 a–c, C 1, 2*) There are a number of factors that contribute to the increased incidence of urinary tract infection during pregnancy, delivery, and the puerperium. Asymptomatic bacteriuria leads to acute urinary tract infection in 20%–40% of women. Conduction anesthesia can temporarily denervate the bladder, leading to overdistension and stasis. Catheterization effectively seeds the bladder with bacteria. The large uterus can compress the ureter, leading to dilation of the renal calyces, pelves, and ureters. Progesterone is a smooth muscle relaxant, which leads to a *decrease* in ureteral tone and peristalsis.

4. The answer is C (2, 4). (*I A 1–3*) The finding of glucose in the urine (glucosuria) of a pregnant woman does not mean that she has gestational diabetes. However, it is an indication to perform glucose tolerance testing because gestational diabetes is a distinct possibility. Glucosuria is most often secondary to the pregnancy-related increased glomerular filtration of glucose without an increased tubular reabsorption. It is unnecessary to control dietary glucose intake strictly without a diagnosis of gestational diabetes.

5. The answer is B (1, 3). (*I E 2 a–c*) Because of the significant incidence of fetal demise in diabetic pregnancies, it is essential to terminate the pregnancy when there is evidence of fetal compromise. A poor biophysical profile and a positive contraction stress test are indications of fetal distress. A *decreased* need for insulin is also a dangerous sign, indicating that the pregnancy is no longer a healthy one. A lecithin/sphingomyelin ratio of less than 2/1 (or 2.0) means that the fetal lung is immature, which is a contraindication for delivery.

6. The answer is E (all). (*II B 1, 2 a–e*) Preeclampsia is predominantly a disease of the nulliparous woman, especially at the extremes of reproductive life—the teenager and the woman over the age of 35 years. However, preeclampsia does appear in the multiparous pregnant woman in association with such conditions as diabetes, chronic hypertension, multiple gestation, fetal hydrops, and chronic renal disease.

7. The answer is A (1, 2, 3). (*II C 1–4*) Preeclampsia is thought to be caused by the release of local vasoconstrictors, which leads to vasospasm. This, in turn, results in decreased placental perfusion and the release of general vasoconstrictors, which lead to hypertension and a decreased renal blood flow and glomerular filtration. The rise in uric acid results from the decreased glomerular filtration. Preeclampsia is characterized by a contracted or decreased intravascular volume, which results in hemoconcentration.

8. The answer is D (4). (*VI B 1 a–c, 2 a–d*) Of the answers listed in the question, only arrhythmias are diagnostic of heart disease in pregnancy. Lower extremity edema occurs in most pregnancies due to the pressure of the large uterus on the inferior vena cava. Functional systolic or flow murmurs are common in pregnancy as is an increased respiratory effort due to the elevation of the diaphragm secondary to the pressure upwards from the intra-abdominal contents.

9–11. The answers are: 9-D, 10-A, 11-E. (*III A 1, 2, B 2 a–c, 4 a, b*) One of the congenital hemoglobinopathies should be suspected as the etiology of the death of the infant in utero described in the question. Sickle cell anemia does not have as high a fetal loss rate as does hemoglobin SC disease. In addition, the chest pain and difficulty breathing in the woman could be caused by a pulmonary embolus of necrotic bone marrow, which is characteristic of hemoglobin SC disease.

The woman with a hemoglobin of 9.0 entered pregnancy with a severe iron deficiency that became worse with the demands of pregnancy, that is, with the production of fetal hemoglobin and the expansion of maternal red cell mass. Because the anemia became worse despite oral iron and folic acid, it is not likely to be a megaloblastic anemia. The fetus does not suffer from anemia in iron deficiency no matter how severe the anemia is in the mother.

A clue to the etiology of the problem of the women with premature contractions is the bacteriuria. Urinary tract infection and asymptomatic bacteriuria are very common in patients with sickle cell trait. Also, urinary tract infections are a common reason for premature uterine contractions, which usually disappear with treatment of the infection.

8
Fetal Physiology
PonJola Coney

I. INTRODUCTION

A. Placenta. The placenta consists of blood vessels, vascular spaces, and a small amount of supporting connective tissue. Placental implantation is predominantly on the posterior aspect of the fundus, the area with the most satisfactory blood supply.

1. **The major functions of the placenta** are:
   a. Metabolism of glycogen, cholesterol, and fatty acids
   b. Transfer of substances via simple and facilitated diffusion
   c. Active transport and pinocytosis
   d. Secretion of protein and steroid hormones

2. **The maternal surface of the placenta** is divided into 12–20 cotyledons and appears dark, resembling venous blood. The circulation originates in the endometrial arterioles, and blood is propelled into the cotyledons by the maternal systole.

3. **The fetal surface of the placenta** is shiny and smooth with large blood vessels coursing through the membranous surface. The membrane covering this surface is the **chorion**, which is next to the **amnion** (innermost fetal membrane); the chorion and amnion are separated only by a small amount of connective tissue.

B. Fetal and maternal circulations are separated by the placental membrane interposed between the intervillous space and the fetal capillary. This unit is the site of exchange of water, carbon dioxide, oxygen, electrolytes, amino acids, sugars, vitamins, hormones, and antibodies for the maintenance of fetal biochemical homeostasis, nutrition, and growth. Harmful substances (e.g., drugs, poisons, and infectious agents) also pass through the placental membrane. The intervillous space contains 150 ml of blood that is replenished three to four times per minute.

C. Umbilical structures

1. **Umbilical arteries** on the fetal side have the following characteristics:
   a. They originate from the aorta.
   b. They divide and attach to the membranes.
   c. They subdivide continuously.
   d. They supply arterial blood to all portions of the placenta.

2. **The umbilical cord** is semirigid and through it blood circulates from the placenta to the fetus. Blood is propelled by the fetal heart. The total umbilical cord blood flow is 125 ml/kg/min or 500 ml/min.

II. HEMODYNAMICS OF THE FETUS (Fig. 8-1)

A. Oxygenated, nutriment-bearing blood is carried from the placenta to the fetus through the abdominal wall via the umbilical vein. Shunts, which divert oxygenated blood to the arterial circulation, particularly the brain, are characteristic of blood flow in the fetus.

1. **The ductus venosus** connects the portal sinus to the inferior vena cava and allows a portion of the umbilical and portal blood (via sphincteric mechanism) to bypass the liver (60%). This blood going into the right ventricle is less well oxygenated than blood coming directly from the placenta.

2. **The foramen ovale** is a right to left intracardiac (atrial) shunt. The inferior vena cava communicates with both atria via the foramen ovale.

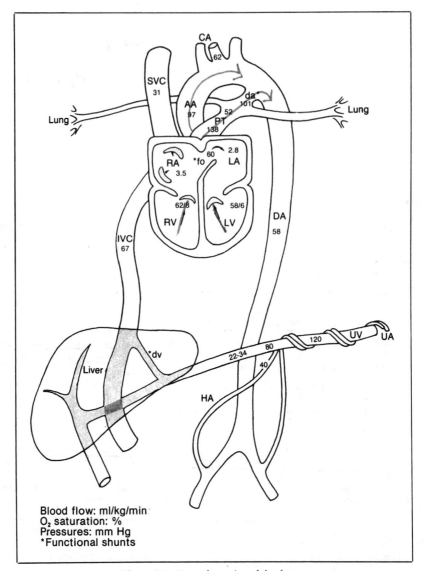

Figure 8-1. Hemodynamics of the fetus.

3. **The ductus arteriosus** is an anastomosis between the left pulmonary artery and the arch of the aorta. The high vascular resistance, which is secondary to increased vasomotor tone and collapsed lungs, in the pulmonary tree is five times total systemic resistance. The pulmonary artery pressure is greater than the aortic pressure directing blood into the ductus and the aorta.

4. **Blood in the right atrium** is received from the coronary sinus (5%), superior vena cava (20%), and inferior vena cava (75%). A portion (45%) is shunted into the left atrium, and the remainder enters the right ventricle. From the right ventricle, blood flows into the lungs (10%), the ductus arteriosus (90%), descending aorta, hypogastric arteries, and the umbilical arteries.

5. **Blood in the left atrium** enters the left ventricle, ascending aorta, and the carotid arteries (see Fig. 8-1).

B. **Cardiac output** of the fetal heart is 200 ml/kg/min, which is higher than the cardiac output of the adult. The cardiac output of the right ventricle is greater than that of the left ventricle, resulting in a right ventricular preponderance as recorded on the fetal electrocardiogram. The distribution of cardiac output is as follows:

　　　1. Placenta: 40%

　　　2. Body: 37%

　　　3. Lungs: 5%

　　　4. Adrenals: 2%

　　　5. Brain: 3%

　　　6. Heart: 4%

　　　7. Miscellaneous (e.g., gut and spleen): 9%

C. Arterial blood pressure increases progressively throughout gestation to 75/55 mm Hg at term. The umbilical venous pressure is 22–34 mm Hg, and a significant decrease results in death of the fetus. The fetal heart rate is 120–160 beats/min.

III. REGULATION OF BLOOD FLOW AND PRESSURES.
The placenta lacks autonomic innervation but acts as a damper to the effects of nervous stimulation from the maternal circulation. Ultimate regulation of fetal blood flow and pressures is by vascular smooth muscle tone, autonomic nervous stimulation, sympathetic amines, and vasodilator metabolites. Muscular contractions, gravity, and respiratory movement have no effect.

A. Stimuli that affect umbilical circulation are:

　　1. **Mild fetal hypoxia.** The arterial blood pressure and umbilical blood flow are increased without a change in umbilical venous resistance.

　　2. **Severe fetal hypoxia.** The umbilical blood flow is decreased and the umbilical venous resistance is increased.

B. The dynamics of the ductus arteriosus are affected by various drugs and stimuli.

　　1. Prostaglandins, especially the E family, and intrauterine, neonatal asphyxia sustain patency. The increased sensitivity of the ductus arteriosus to prostaglandin E_2 suggests a role by this prostanoid in regulating or maintaining patency. Infusions of prostaglandin E_1 and E_2 have been shown to dilate the ductus arteriosus.

　　2. Prostaglandin inhibitors, acetylcholine, histamine, and catecholamines promote closure. Indomethacin is a potent prostaglandin synthetase inhibitor. The efficacy of nonsurgical closure of the patent ductus arteriosus with indomethacin in preterm infants is well established with morbidity and mortality at least as satisfactory as in surgically treated cases.

IV. OXYGEN DELIVERY TO FETAL TISSUES.
Aerobic metabolism is the usual pathway in the fetus but anaerobic glycolysis is operational. The fetal heart can withstand a lack of oxygen for a longer period than the adult heart because of the greater glycogen stores in fetal myocardium. The **oxygen content of fetal blood, hemoglobin concentration,** and **blood flow** determine the adequacy of oxygen delivery to the tissues.

A. Increased oxygen–carrying capacity of fetal blood is possible because of a number of factors.

　　1. The pH of fetal blood is less than that of whole blood. The Bohr effect is applicable (decreased affinity of hemoglobin for oxygen when there is a high concentration of H^+ ions).

　　2. Diphosphoglycerate (2,3-diphospho-D-glycerate) is a by-product of anaerobic glycolysis. It does not bind to the γ chains of fetal hemoglobin; thus, it does not impair the binding and unloading of oxygen.

　　3. Hemoglobin content of fetal blood is high so that oxygen–carrying capacity is increased. Thus, despite the fact that oxygen saturation of fetal blood (see Fig. 8-1) is rarely over 70%, the tissues are not hypoxic. Fetal needs are met because oxygen consumption is high (4 ml/kg/min), which is as much as an adult at rest.

　　4. The PO_2 of intervillous blood is lower than maternal blood, which favorably influences the transfer of oxygen from maternal to fetal blood.

　　5. The tissue PO_2 is low (less than 15 mm Hg), allowing the transfer of oxygen along a decreasing gradient.

　　6. **The oxygen dissociation curve of fetal hemoglobin** is to the left of the adult curve. At a given

temperature and pH, the PO$_2$ saturation of fetal blood is lower than maternal blood, enhancing oxygen transfer across the placenta.

B. Hematopoiesis occurs in the yolk sac in the second week of gestation, in the liver and spleen in the fifth week, and in the bone marrow in the eleventh week. The first hemoglobin types are Portland, Gower I, and Gower II. Fetal hemoglobin (Hb F) appears at 3 months and differs from adult (Hb AA) because of the presence of two γ chains instead of two β chains. Adult hemoglobin appears early in the second trimester, but at term, 70% of the hemoglobin present is fetal. The hemoglobin concentration is high in the fetus, 16–18 g/dl. Erythropoietin is of hepatic origin in the fetus and is highest in utero.

V. FETAL AND NEONATAL METABOLISM

A. Fetus

1. As growth proceeds, **extracellular water** decreases. Early in gestation, 90%–95% of body weight is water. At term, 70%–75% of body weight is water. Fat deposition begins at a fetal weight of 800 g, increases toward term, and extracellular fluid decreases.

2. The fetus synthesizes its own protein from amino acids from maternal blood. **The principal sugar in fetal blood is glucose.** It crosses the placenta via facilitated diffusion. Fetal level is determined by maternal level.

3. Enzymes in early embryonic and fetal development are related primarily to energy production, protein, and lipoprotein synthesis and later to organ differentiation and function. Activity of specific enzyme systems varies with gestational age. There are changes in enzyme form or nature of isoenzyme activity as gestational age progresses. The enzyme studied most is lactate dehydrogenase. The M form, which is predominant in fetal tissue, is active in low oxygen tensions and, thus, is important in anaerobic glycolysis.

B. Neonate. At birth, the following events occur:

1. The lungs become aerated and pulmonary vascular resistance decreases.

2. Pulmonary blood flow increases.

3. The left atrial pressure exceeds right atrial pressure, and the foramen ovale closes.

4. Bradykinin from the aerated lungs constricts the ductus arteriosus, ductus venosus, and umbilical vein. These are no longer functional and are known as the ligamentum arteriosus, ligamentum venosum, and the ligamentum teres, respectively.

5. The intra-abdominal portion of the umbilical arteries becomes the lateral umbilical ligaments.

BIBLIOGRAPHY

Abdul-Karim R: Fetal physiology—review. *Obstet Gynecol Surv* 23:713, 1968

Aladjem S, Brown A, Sureau C: *Clinical Perinatology,* 2nd ed. St. Louis, CV Mosby, 1980, pp 52–63

Danforth DN: *Obstetrics and Gynecology,* 3rd ed. New York, Harper and Row, 1977, pp 247–256

Friedman W, et al: Pharmacologic closure of patent ductus arteriosus in the premature infant. *N Engl J Med* 295:526–529, 1976

Moore KL: *The Developing Human: Clinically Oriented Embryology.* Philadelphia, WB Saunders, 1973, pp 257–264

Obeyesekere HI, et al: Pharmacological closure of ductus arteriosus in preterm infants using indomethacin. *Arch Dis Child* 55:271–276, 1980

STUDY QUESTIONS

Directions: Each question below contains five suggested answers. Choose the **one best** response to each question.

1. The approximate percentage saturation of fetal blood going to the heart, head, and upper limbs is

(A) 40%
(B) 50%
(C) 60%
(D) 70%
(E) 80%

2. Contraction of the sphincter of the ductus venosus results in increased blood flow in which of the following ways?

(A) Through the portal sinus to the portal veins into the hepatic sinusoids
(B) Through the ductus venosus into the right atrium
(C) Reversed through the umbilical vein
(D) By a sphincter mechanism, which is more theoretical than functional
(E) None of the above

3. Which of the following statements best describes the foramen ovale?

(A) It shunts blood from right to left
(B) It connects the pulmonary artery with the aorta
(C) It shunts deoxygenated blood into the left atrium
(D) It is an extracardiac shunt
(E) It is functional after birth

Directions: Each question below contains four suggested answers of which **one or more** is correct. Choose the answer

A   if **1, 2, and 3** are correct
B   if **1 and 3** are correct
C   if **2 and 4** are correct
D   if **4** is correct
E   if **1, 2, 3, and 4** are correct

4. Oxygen delivery to fetal tissues is determined by which of the following factors?

(1) Blood flow
(2) Oxygen content of fetal blood
(3) Hemoglobin concentration
(4) Diphosphoglycerate levels

5. The hemoglobin normally found in the fetus at term includes which of the following chains?

(1) $\alpha_4\alpha_4$
(2) $\alpha_2\gamma_2$
(3) $\alpha_2\gamma_4$
(4) $\alpha_2\beta_2$

Directions: The group of questions below consists of lettered choices followed by several numbered items. For each numbered item select the **one** lettered choice with which it is **most** closely associated. Each lettered choice may be used once, more than once, or not at all.

Questions 6–8

For each statement below, select the stimuli with which it is most likely to be associated.

(A) Severe fetal hypoxia
(B) Neonatal asphyxia
(C) Autonomic nervous stimulation
(D) Mild fetal hypoxia
(E) None of the above

6. Umbilical blood flow is elevated

7. The ductus arteriosus is closed

8. Umbilical venous resistance is increased

ANSWERS AND EXPLANATIONS

1. The answer is C. *(II A 1)* The blood returning from the placenta is very well oxygenated, which is somewhat reduced by the time it reaches the head and neck, secondary to mixing of oxygenated (umbilical vein, inferior vena cava) and deoxygenated (superior vena cava) blood. Consequently, it is approximately 60% saturated, which is still very adequate.

2. The answer is A. *(II A 1)* The sphincter of the ductus venosus is muscular. Contraction diverts blood to the liver, and relaxation allows more blood to pass through the ductus into the inferior vena cava and into the heart. During hypoxia and fetal distress, ductal flow decreases. The ductus venous may also help to maintain umbilical venous pressure.

3. The answer is A. *(II A 2)* The foramen ovale is an intracardiac shunt that shunts oxygenated blood to the left atrium from the right atrium in order to increase delivery of oxygenated blood to the head, neck, and upper limbs. It is not normally functional after birth as with all shunts in the fetal circulation.

4. The answer is A (1, 2, 3). *(IV A, B)* The primary determinant of oxygen supply to the tissues is blood flow to the various organs. Oxygen saturation of the blood as well as the hemoglobin concentration are secondary but very important. Since diphosphoglycerate does not bind to the fetal hemoglobin, it does not effect saturation and delivery of oxygen. At a given PO_2 under identical temperature and pH, fetal blood has a lower oxygen saturation than maternal blood.

5. The answer is C (2, 4). *(IV B)* The first hemoglobin types are Portland, Gower I, and Gower II. Fetal hemoglobin (Hb F) appears first at 3 months gestation and differs from adult hemoglobin (Hb AA) by the presence of two γ chains instead of two β chains. Hb AA is present by the second trimester and increases toward term, but Hb F is still predominant at term (70%).

6–8. The answers are: 6-D, 7-C, 8-A. *(III A, B)* Hypoxia is a major regulator of blood in the fetus. In the early stages of hypoxia or mild cases, the blood pressure and the umbilical blood flow increase with no effect on umbilical venous resistance. As the hypoxia worsens, umbilical venous resistance increases, followed by a decrease in blood flow, which could eventually lead to the death of the fetus.

Closure of the ductus arteriosus is promoted by drugs that act on the autonomic nervous system—that is, acetylcholine and catecholamines. Prostaglandin inhibitors, however, are more potent and, therefore, have greater therapeutic usefulness in the neonatal period when the ductus remains patent.

9

Identification of the High-Risk Patient
Nancy S. Roberts

I. INTRODUCTION. The goals of perinatal care are a healthy mother and a normal infant. Thus, the necessity of identifying the patient at risk cannot be overemphasized. Early identification and management of risk factors are essential to ameliorate long-term sequelae. Pregnancy is a dynamic state that needs continuous surveillance and adjustment of management plans.

II. MATERNAL MORTALITY

A. Definitions

1. **Maternal mortality** is the number of maternal deaths that occur during pregnancy or within 42 days of the termination of pregnancy.

2. **Maternal mortality rate** is the number of maternal deaths per 100,000 live-births. Presently in the United States, the maternal mortality rate is 9/100,000 live-births—a dramatic improvement over the rate of 21.5 in 1972.

B. The major causes of maternal death are in order:

1. Hypertensive disorders of pregnancy

2. Pulmonary embolism

3. Uterine hemorrhage

4. Sepsis

C. Risk factors for maternal mortality include:

1. **Advanced maternal age.** Women in their forties are seven times more likely to die in pregnancy as compared to women in their twenties.

2. **General anesthesia.** Increased mortality is associated with:
   a. An inability to intubate, particularly in women with short necks or women with anatomic airway distortion.
   b. Aspiration of gastric contents due to the relative incompetence of the lower esophageal sphincter and delayed gastric emptying characteristic of pregnant women. Both labor and narcotics further delay gastric emptying.

3. **Race.** The maternal mortality rate for blacks is threefold greater than for whites.

4. **Hypertensive disease**
   a. When preeclampsia progresses to frank convulsions (eclampsia), the patient sometimes lapses into a coma from the convulsion or experiences a cerebrovascular accident and dies. Maternal deaths from eclampsia range from 7%–17% in the 1970s to 0.4% in 1984.
   b. Maternal deaths from severe chronic hypertension range from 0.5%–2%.

5. **Cesarean delivery.** Maternal mortality from a cesarean section should be less than 1%. There is a higher risk of maternal death from cesarean section as compared to vaginal delivery associated with anesthesia complications, severe sepsis, and thromboembolic events. Some centers in the Northeast report a zero maternal mortality rate in 10,000–17,000 deliveries.

6. Cyanotic heart disease. The prognosis for a pregnancy in women with Eisenmenger's syndrome or pulmonary hypertension is poor; there is also a 30% incidence of maternal mortality associated with this syndrome.

III. HISTORY. The first task in risk identification and management is a thorough historical assessment. Continuous assessment for acute problems is imperative since many disease states can be unmasked by pregnancy.

A. General history

1. Socioeconomic status. Socioeconomic status is defined by an interrelated complex group of factors—educational level, marital status, income, and occupation—all of which play an important role in maternal and fetal morbidity and mortality. Low socioeconomic status is related to an increased risk of perinatal morbidity and mortality.

2. Age. Age is an identifiable risk factor for both low and high maternal age.

   a. Maternal age less than 20 years increases the risk for:

      (1) Premature births

      (2) Fetal deaths

      (3) Neonatal deaths

      (4) Preeclampsia and eclampsia

      (5) Uterine dysfunction

      (6) Late prenatal care

   b. Maternal age over 35 years of age increases the risk for:

      (1) First-trimester miscarriage. The miscarriage rate for women over 40 years of age has been found to be 3 times higher than for women under 30.

      (2) Genetically abnormal conceptuses. The risk of fetal chromosomal anomalies increases in direct proportion to maternal age. (This increase may also explain in part the increase in first-trimester miscarriages.) Trisomy 21 represents 90% of the chromosomal abnormalities, but other autosomal trisomies (i.e., 13 and 18) and sex chromosomal anomalies also increase with advancing age.

      (3) Maternal and fetal death

      (4) Medical complications, such as hypertensive disease of pregnancy and diabetes. Women with medical complications also have a higher fetal loss rate.

      (5) Multiple gestation. For example, the rate of dizygotic twins is:

         (a) 3/1000 live-births in women under 21 years of age

         (b) 14/1000 live-births in women 35–40 years of age

      (6) Labor problems, including:

         (a) Increased breech presentations

         (b) Abnormal progress in labor, especially slow cervical dilation

         (c) A high cesarean section rate. In a 1986 study, the rate rose from 16% for women 20–30 years of age to over 35% for women over 40. Part of the increase may be attributed to a greater incidence of:

            (i) Placenta previa

            (ii) Abnormal presentations

            (iii) Multiple gestations

            (iv) Medical complications

3. Addiction

   a. Tobacco. There is a dose-response relationship between heavy cigarette smoking and increased fetal morbidity and mortality. Although the physiologic mechanism is unclear, there is an increased risk for:

      (1) Abruptio placentae

      (2) Placenta previa

      (3) Bleeding during pregnancy

      (4) Premature rupture of membranes

      (5) Prematurity

      (6) Spontaneous abortion

      (7) Sudden infant death syndrome

      (8) Fetal death

      (9) Low birth weight

     (10) A reduction in the supply of breast milk

     (11) Respiratory illness

   b. Drugs. The maternal and fetal consequences of drug addiction in pregnancy are dependent upon the drug ingested. Deleterious effects of drug addiction include:

      (1) Tolerance (i.e., the need to take increasing amounts of the drug to get the same effect)

(2) Withdrawal

(3) Intrauterine growth retardation

(4) Congenital anomalies

(5) Infections associated with unsterile injections, especially hepatitis and human immunodeficiency virus (HIV) infection

(6) Malnutrition

(7) Premature delivery

   c. **Alcohol.** Not only does alcohol abuse undermine maternal health, but a pattern of abnormalities known as the fetal alcohol syndrome manifests in varying degrees of severity in the fetus.

      (1) The severity of fetal involvement is usually related to the quantity of alcohol ingested and the time of gestation during which the fetus is exposed. However, this does not follow a dose-response relationship.

      (2) Because the effects of the occasional use of alcohol on the fetus are not known, most authorities recommend abstinence from alcohol during pregnancy.

4. Employment may be associated with an increased incidence of preterm labor, especially for women in physically demanding or stressful jobs; however, this is a controversial issue. For example, recent studies have delineated the harmful effects of prolonged exposure to computer terminals.

B. Obstetric history. Maternal reproductive history has a strong predictive correlation to the development of future sequelae. Therefore, the following information should be obtained so that appropriate management plans can be made to ameliorate any risk factors.

  1. Parity

   a. **Nullipara.** Nulliparous women are at high risk for developing specific problems, including:

      (1) Preeclampsia and eclampsia

      (2) New physiologic changes and stresses heretofore never experienced and disease states that could be unmasked

      (3) Relative lack of knowledge of the pregnancy state and possible complications

   b. **Multipara.** Grand multiparous women (5 children or more) seem to be at increased risk for:

      (1) Placenta previa

      (2) Postpartum hemorrhage secondary to uterine atony

      (3) Increased incidence of dizygotic twins. This may occur because grand multiparas are usually of advanced age.

  2. Abortion. Cervical trauma from elective dilatation of the cervix may place a woman at an increased risk for:

   a. Spontaneous abortion

   b. Incompetent cervix

   c. Preterm delivery

   d. Low-birth-weight infant

  3. Preterm delivery. The incidence of preterm delivery, which correlates well with past reproductive performance (see Table 9-3):

   a. Increases with each subsequent preterm delivery. The recurrence rate for premature labor is 25%–40%.

   b. Decreases with each birth that is not preterm

  4. A large infant (4000 g or more) may indicate a previously undetected or uncontrolled glucose intolerance and may be associated with subsequent intrapartum complications, such as:

   a. Difficult vaginal delivery due to a shoulder dystocia

   b. Cesarean section for relative cephalopelvic disproportion

   c. Postpartum complications for the neonate, such as hypoglycemia

  5. Perinatal death (stillborn or neonatal). A pregnancy that follows a perinatal death should be followed closely so that a similar outcome can be avoided. Perinatal death may be an indication of an underlying problem that may or may not have been detected previously, such as:

   a. Glucose intolerance

   b. Collagen vascular disease

   c. Congenital anomalies

   d. Preterm delivery

   e. Obstetric injury

   f. Hemolytic disease

g. Abnormal labor

h. Lupus anticoagulant—an immunoglobulin associated with placental infarction, stillbirth, or preeclampsia

6. Congenital anomalies. If a previous child is born with congenital anomalies, there is an increased risk of having another child with congenital anomalies. Evaluation is necessary for future management decisions (e.g., amniocentesis or early termination).

7. Ectopic pregnancy. A woman with a history of ectopic pregnancy has an increased risk of developing another ectopic pregnancy; thus, it is imperative that she be evaluated at 5 or 6 weeks gestation by pelvic examination or vaginal ultrasound so that the site of pregnancy can be confirmed immediately.

8. Cesarean section

a. A woman who has had a previous cesarean section must make a decision as to whether she would like to attempt a vaginal delivery with a subsequent pregnancy, provided there are no medical or surgical contraindications, such as:

(1) An active herpes infection at term

(2) Absolute cephalopelvic disproportion

(3) Vertical uterine incision

(4) Myomectomy with penetration into the endometrium

b. Most experts at this time feel that a woman who has had two prior cesarean sections should have repeat cesarean sections with subsequent pregnancies. However, this is still being evaluated and should not be absolute since various factors (e.g., the intrinsic healing capacity of the woman) play a role in determining the strength of the uterine scar.

9. Hemorrhage. Women with a history of hemorrhage have an increased risk of hemorrhage with subsequent pregnancies regardless of the cause (i.e., placental abruption, placenta previa, or postpartum hemorrhage).

10. Pregnancy-induced hypertension (preeclampsia and eclampsia)

a. There appears to be a familial tendency.

b. Women with a history of preeclampsia or eclampsia have an increased risk of developing it in subsequent pregnancies.

c. Some studies indicate that women with pregnancy-induced hypertension are likely to develop essential hypertension in the future, which may complicate a subsequent pregnancy.

C. Medical history

1. Chronic hypertension (140/90 or higher). Essential hypertension may be present at the first prenatal visit or it may develop during the course of the pregnancy. The prognosis for a successful obstetric outcome in the well-controlled hypertensive patient is very good. However, there does appear to be an association with development of:

a. Preeclampsia

b. Abruptio placentae

c. Perinatal loss

d. Maternal mortality

e. Myocardial infarction

f. Uteroplacental insufficiency

g. Cerebrovascular accident

2. Cardiac disease has both maternal and fetal implications.

a. In the mother, heart disease may develop or worsen. Because of the hemodynamic changes associated with pregnancy some cardiac lesions are particularly dangerous, such as Eisenmenger's syndrome, primary pulmonary hypertension, Marfan's syndrome, and hemodynamically significant mitral stenosis.

b. Fetal growth and development are dependent on an adequate supply of well-oxygenated blood. If this supply is limited, as it appears to be with certain cardiac lesions, then the fetus is at risk for abnormal development and even death.

c. Offspring of parents with cardiac disease have an increased risk of developing cardiac disease in their lifetime. This is sometimes identified in utero with ultrasound.

d. The various medications used to control cardiac disease have potential fetal complications.

3. Pulmonary disease. Maternal respiratory function and gas exchange are affected by the associated biochemical and mechanical alterations that occur with a normal pregnancy. The effect of pregnancy on pulmonary disease is often unpredictable. Thus, when pulmonary disease affects maternal well-being or compromises the supply of well-oxygenated blood to the fetus, there is need for concern.

4. Renal disease
  a. In a normal pregnancy, the renal system undergoes certain physiologic, anatomic, and functional changes that may stress the renal system; therefore, continuous assessment is necessary in patients with preexisting or developing renal disease.
  b. Under proper medical supervision and control of blood pressure, most women with underlying renal disease can have an uneventful pregnancy without adverse effects on either the primary disease or the ultimate prognosis, if the creatinine level is below 2 mg/100 ml.
  c. Fetal mortality is increased, and it is imperative that the patient understand the need for frequent prenatal visits and antepartum testing. Patients should also be aware of the potential complications of antihypertensive medication during pregnancy on the fetus.

5. Diabetes.
The cornerstone of management for the pregnant diabetic is rigid metabolic control to make the patient as consistently euglycemic as possible. Ideally, these efforts should begin before conception and continue throughout the pregnancy. Many maternal and fetal problems may complicate the pregnancy of a diabetic, including:
  a. Maternal mortality (rare)
  b. Fetal mortality
  c. Hydramnios
  d. Congenital anomalies
  e. Chronic hypertension
  f. Preeclampsia
  g. Maternal edema
  h. Maternal pyelonephritis
  i. Intrauterine fetal death
  j. Neonatal mortality (congenital anomalies being the major cause)
  k. Neonatal morbidity, including:
   (1) Respiratory distress syndrome
   (2) Macrosomia
   (3) Hypoglycemia
   (4) Hyperbilirubinemia
   (5) Hypocalcemia

6. Thyroid disease.
Pregnancy with its associated hormonal and metabolic changes makes the evaluation of thyroid function very complex. Untreated hypothyroidism or hyperthyroidism may profoundly alter pregnancy outcome. The fetal thyroid is autonomous and is unaffected by maternal thyroid hormone. Treatment during pregnancy poses a very complicated situation since the fetal thyroid responds to the same pharmacologic agents as does the maternal thyroid.

7. Collagen vascular disease (rheumatic disease).
Many rheumatic diseases are common in women, often during the reproductive years. The effect of pregnancy is unpredictable as precipitation, aggravation, or amelioration of the disease may occur. Rheumatic disease may affect the outcome of the pregnancy (e.g., with systemic lupus erythematosus, there is an increased risk of abortion, premature labor, and intrauterine fetal death), and the particular pharmacologic agents used in the treatment of the disease may affect the fetus adversely.

8. Hematologic disorders
  a. Physiologic alterations and metabolic demands associated with pregnancy may result in anemias secondary to iron or folic acid deficiency.
  b. Hemoglobinopathies (e.g., sickle cell disease) may be severely affected by pregnancy with the development of serious complications in both the mother and the child.
  c. Disorders of blood coagulation and platelets may not only affect the antepartum management and its maternal and fetal effects, but it also may play a role in intrapartum, delivery, and postpartum management because of the possibility of hemorrhage.
  d. Some hematologic disorders have a genetic component; therefore, genetic counseling and management decisions should be discussed prior to conception or in the early stages of pregnancy.

9. Genetic disorders
  a. A genetic disorder of the mother must be evaluated prior to pregnancy or in early pregnancy since the associated changes of pregnancy may so stress the genetic problem as to threaten her health, or the disease itself may compromise the intrauterine growth of the fetus.
  b. Historical factors that may help to identify the high-risk couple include:
   (1) Consanguinity. Marriage between close relations results in a large pool of identical genes, thereby increasing the possibility of sharing similar mutant genes, resulting in:
    (a) An increased risk of miscarriage
    (b) An increased risk of rare recessive genetic disease in offspring

    (2) Ethnicity. Specific ethnic groups are more likely to develop specific diseases (e.g., Tay-Sachs disease in Ashkenazi Jews and sickle cell anemia in blacks).   *CF whites*

    (3) Parental age (maternal and paternal)
        (a) There is an increased risk for Down's syndrome with advanced maternal age (over 35).
        (b) There is an increased risk of de novo single gene mutation with advanced paternal age (over 55).

  c. Once a high-risk couple is identified, genetic counseling should be undertaken to ascertain risks, carrier testing, and early prenatal diagnosis if possible by chorionic villi sampling or amniocentesis. Such testing can lead to wise reproduction planning or the relief of anxiety in high-risk couples.

  d. Women who will be 35 or over at the time of delivery should be offered α-fetoprotein testing and chorionic villus sampling or amniocentesis.

10. Pituitary disorders. Pregnancy is uncommon in women with pituitary abnormalities since pituitary integrity is necessary for conception. However, some pituitary disorders carry an increased health risk during pregnancy (e.g., prolactinoma).

11. Adrenal disorders. Gestational changes in adrenal function do occur, and it is important that adrenal homeostasis be preserved because some complications of inadequate adrenal function may be life-threatening (e.g., acute adrenocortical insufficiency).

12. Parathyroid disorders. Parathyroid homeostasis is essential for maternal and fetal well-being, and serum calcium concentration is the key value in evaluating parathyroid function. Calcium requirements increase during pregnancy and are usually maintained by a normal diet, although supplements are added to ensure adequate intake.

13. Liver disease. As with most organ systems, the liver undergoes anatomic, physiologic, and functional changes during pregnancy, and as with most disease entities, pregnancy may aggravate or make more difficult the ability to follow a particular disease. If a woman has liver disease, it is essential that it be identified, a baseline established, and the patient followed closely. Liver disease may have deleterious effects on the fetus (e.g., viral hepatitis).

14. Neurologic disorders. The effects of pregnancy on preexisting or concurrent neurologic disorders can be quite diverse. As with many other disorders, therapeutic dilemmas often arise between pharmacologic treatment with its associated fetal effects and the risk of uncontrolled disease to the mother and the fetus.

15. Venous thromboembolic disorders. Pregnancy and the immediate postpartum period can predispose women to venous thrombosis. It is important to identify the women at high risk because many thromboembolic events can be prevented.

16. Infectious diseases. In addition to rubella, syphilis, and gonorrhea for which pregnant women are routinely screened, certain viral and parasitic infectious agents are capable of crossing the placenta and producing serious problems for the fetus and the newborn. The following infections during pregnancy place the mother and her child at high risk for potential morbidity and mortality:

  a. Cytomegalovirus
    (1) The pregnant woman who acquires cytomegalovirus as a primary infection has an increased risk of congenital anomalies chiefly in the central nervous system.
    (2) Neonatal death from disseminated disease may occur.
    (3) Postnatal infection may also occur, but it is generally without sequelae.

  b. Herpes simplex virus (HSV)
    (1) This is a sexually transmitted virus.
    (2) Infection during pregnancy increases the risk of fetal loss and prematurity.
    (3) Most neonatal infections are acquired either during passage through an infected birth canal or as an ascending spread of the virus from the cervix after the membranes have ruptured.
    (4) A neonatal infection may go undetected without sequelae, or it may cause fatal disseminated disease. Survivors may manifest ophthalmologic or neurologic sequelae.
    (5) It is important to identify women with a history of HSV or newly acquired HSV so that appropriate management decisions, particularly regarding delivery, can be made.

  c. Hepatitis B
    (1) Infection occurring in the first or second trimester is generally not associated with adverse consequences. However, acute third-trimester infections have been associated with an increased risk of prematurity with resultant fetal morbidity and mortality and transmission of the hepatitis infection to the infant. Affected neonates may:
        (a) Be asymptomatic

      (b) Develop fulminant disease, cirrhosis, or hepatocellular carcinoma, resulting in death

      (c) Become chronic carriers

    (2) Vertical transmission of the disease may occur from mothers who are chronic carriers of HB_s Ag. Transmission rate is 80%–90% for the mother carrying the E antigen.

    (3) Efforts aimed at prevention of the disease in the newborn of mothers who are chronic carriers or who have acute third-trimester disease must be initiated at birth, including:

      (a) Nasogastric aspiration to remove secretions

      (b) Administration of hyperimmune serum globulin

      (c) Hepatitis vaccine prophylaxis

    (4) Treatment of the mothers includes rest, adequate fluids, and a nutritious diet.

  d. Toxoplasmosis

    (1) Toxoplasmosis is a parasitic infection that produces clinically vague maternal symptoms but that can infect the fetus in utero.

    (2) Fetal risk is related to the gestational age at which maternal infection occurs, which may be a reflection of the immune status of the fetus; for example, there is a greater risk of transmission to the fetus in the third trimester, but it is generally without significant sequelae. There is less frequent transmission in the first trimester but the sequelae are usually more severe.

    (3) The mother is at increased risk for:

      (a) Abortion

      (b) Stillbirth

      (c) Severe congenital infection

    (4) Because cats serve as reservoirs for toxoplasmosis, the physician should:

      (a) Inquire about their presence and alert the patient to the potential risks

      (b) Obtain serologic tests for toxoplasmosis if the patient does have a cat

      (c) Encourage the patient to limit her contacts with cats, especially cleaning the litter box

e. Parvovirus infection

    (1) This is a single-stranded DNA virus that causes a wide spectrum of maternal illness including:

      (a) Asymptomatic infection

      (b) Erythema infectiosum (fifth disease), a mascular rash that often occurs in schoolage children. It is preceded by fever, myalgias, and respiratory or gastrointestinal symptoms.

      (c) Arthritis or arthralgias

      (d) Aplastic crises, especially in women with a variety of chronic hemolytic anemias

    (2) The fetal effects include:

      (a) Nothing. Infants born to infected women have had serologic evidence of infection without adverse effects.

      (b) Congenital anomalies. While one aborted fetus was reported to have eye abnormalities, the incidence of abnormalities after maternal parvovirus infection is very rare.

      (c) Miscarriage

      (d) Fetal death (15%) in documented maternal infection. The highest incidence of fetal death occurs when the mother is infected during the first 18 weeks of pregnancy. Fetal deaths have been reported to occur from 1–10 weeks after clinical illness in the mother.

      (e) Hydrops fetalis due to a severe nonimmune hemolytic anemia

f. Human immunodeficiency virus (HIV)

    (1) Women at risk for HIV infection may be infected through:

      (a) Blood products

      (b) Sexual intercourse

      (c) Contaminated needles

    (2) Although certain "high-risk" groups have been identified, such as intravenous drug users, Haitians, prostitutes, people receiving blood products (i.e., hemophiliacs), and women whose partners have had a homosexual experience, over half of all pregnant women infected with HIV are not from a high-risk group.

    (3) Women who are infected with the virus may show no symptoms of the disease and may feel well. In one study, asymptomatic women, identified because their children developed HIV-related disease, were followed for 2 years postpartum. Between 50% and 75% of women developed symptoms.

    (4) Women shown to be infected with HIV should be evaluated for:

      (a) Gonorrhea and syphilis

      (b) *Chlamydia*

      (c) Hepatitis B infection
      (d) Tuberculosis
      (e) Cytomegalovirus
      (f) Toxoplasmosis

(5) Important guidelines to follow during labor and delivery of all potentially infected parturients are listed below.

      (a) Consider all patients infected until testing for HIV is proven negative.

      (b) Use the following protective clothing or techniques:
         (i) Protective eyewear
         (ii) Water-repellent gowns
         (iii) Gloves
         (iv) Frequent handwashing
         (v) Wall suction or bulb suction

      (c) Avoid direct exposure to maternal or neonatal secretions.

      (d) Never resheath needles to avoid a contaminated needle puncture.

      (e) Avoid scalp sampling for fetal pH or scalp electrodes for monitoring the fetal heart rate.

(6) Pregnancies in mothers with HIV infection are also at increased risk for:

      (a) Premature rupture of membranes

      (b) Low-birth-weight infants

(7) The rate of mother-to-infant transmission perinatally has been estimated to be as high as 65%–95%, regardless of maternal symptoms. Infants born to mothers with HIV may become infected:

      (a) In utero

      (b) During delivery

      (c) After birth from:
         (i) Contaminated breast milk
         (ii) Close contact

(8) The perinatal effects of drugs used in pregnant women with HIV are listed in Table 9-1.

D. Family history. There seems to be a familial tendency for the development of the following risk factors:

1. Maternal
    a. Hypertension
    b. Multiple births
    c. Diabetes
    d. Hemoglobinopathy

Table 9-1. Perinatal Effects of Drugs Used in Women with Human Immunodeficiency Virus

Illness	Treatment and Dose	Reported Risks in Pregnancy*
Pneumocystis carinii pneumonia	Sulfamethoxazole, 100 mg/kg/d, and trimethoprim, 20 mg/kg/d (folate antagonist)	Kernicterus and congenital malformations (rare) [Category C]
	Pentamidine, 4 mg/kg/d intravenously	Unknown (Category C)
Herpes simplex	Acyclovir (purine nucleoside analogue), 200 mg 5 times daily	Unknown (Category C)
Toxoplasmosis	Sulfadiazine, 1 g orally four times a day, and pyrimethamine, 25–50 mg each day	One case of gastroschisis, kernicterus; most reports show no effect (Category C)
Candidiasis	Ketoconazole, 400 mg each day for 14 days, then each day for 5 days per month for 6 months	No known risks (Category C)
Symptomatic human immunodeficiency virus (low T-cell count)	Zidovudine, 200 mg every 4 hours (thydmidine analogue, inhibits reverse transcriptase)	Unknown

*Category C indicates either that studies in animals have revealed adverse effects on the fetus (teratogenic, embryocidal, or other) and there are no controlled studies in women or that studies in women and animals are not available. Drugs should be given only if the potential benefit justifies the potential risk to the fetus.

Note.—Reprinted with permission from Minkoff H: Care of pregnant women infected with human immunodeficiency virus. *JAMA* 258:2716, 1987.

      e. Uterine fibroids
      f. Eclampsia

  2. Maternal or paternal
    a. Mental retardation
    b. Congenital anomalies
    c. Congenital hearing loss
    d. Allergies

E. Medications. Various medications have adverse effects on the fetus, and it is imperative that the risks and benefits to the mother and fetus be evaluated and discussed with the patient prior to starting, continuing, or stopping medications (see Chapter 15, Teratology).

IV. PHYSICAL EXAMINATION. The obstetric patient should undergo a thorough physical examination so that her general health can be assessed.

  A. General examination. Maternal size, which may reflect socioeconomic and nutritional status, has become an important predictive index.

    1. Mothers who are short in stature or underweight are at increased risk for:
      a. Perinatal morbidity and mortality
      b. Low-birth-weight infants
      c. Preterm delivery

    2. Obesity presents a medical hazard to the pregnant woman and her fetus. Complications that are more likely to develop in obese woman include:
      a. Hypertension
      b. Diabetes
      c. Aspiration of gastric contents during the administration of anesthesia
      d. Wound complications
      e. Thromboembolism

  B. Pelvic examination

    1. The perineum, vulva, vagina, cervix, and adnexa are the areas that should be examined and any abnormalities noted that may affect future management (e.g., adnexal masses or cervical lesions).

    2. Clinical pelvimetry should also be done to assess adequacy of the maternal pelvis to facilitate vaginal delivery.

    3. Presentation may also affect management and therefore must be assessed continually especially in the later stages of the pregnancy.

  C. Evaluation of the uterus. The size of the uterus is evaluated continuously throughout the course of the pregnancy. The estimated date of confinement (EDC) should be established at the first prenatal visit so that subsequent discrepancies can be properly evaluated. There is good correlation between fundal height in centimeters measured from the symphysis pubis and gestational age in weeks beyond 20 weeks.

    1. If the uterus is smaller than the estimated gestational age, then the physician must determine if:
      a. There has been a miscalculation due to menstrual irregularity.
      b. The infant is small for gestational age. Causative factors include:
        (1) Intrauterine growth retardation
        (2) Intrauterine infection
        (3) Chromosomal abnormalities
        (4) Congenital anomalies

    2. If the uterus is larger than the estimated gestational age, the following factors must be considered:
      a. Improper dates
      b. Uterine anomalies
      c. Polyhydramnios
      d. Multiple gestation
      e. Hydatidiform mole

  D. Reproductive tract abnormalities

    1. Structural uterine anomalies
      a. Generally the prognosis with minor defects is excellent.

   b. In women with major defects, the prognosis is usually fairly good; however, there is an increased risk of:
   - **(1)** Cesarean section (for abnormal presentation)
   - **(2)** Perinatal loss
   - **(3)** Low-birth-weight infant
   - **(4)** Abortion
   - **(5)** Abruptio placentae

   2. Adenomyosis, which is characterized by the presence of ectopic foci of endometrial glands and stroma in the myometrium, increases the risk of:
   - **a.** Uterine rupture
   - **b.** Postpartum hemorrhage
   - **c.** Dystocia

   3. Premalignant and neoplastic lesions. Depending on the extent of the premalignant or neoplastic lesion, management and treatment of the pregnancy and the lesion may be quite complicated. The extent of treatment ranges from close observation to interruption of the pregnancy for more definite treatment.

   4. Fibroids. The location of the myomas is important in determining possible future sequelae. For example, large submucosal myomas are more likely to have deleterious effects on the pregnancy, whereas annoying pain may be more likely the result of fibroids that undergo torsion (pedunculated) or necrosis (parasitic subserosal). Generally the pregnancy has an increased risk of being complicated by:
   - **a.** Abortion
   - **b.** Faulty placental implantation (causing fetal growth delay)
   - **c.** Faulty correlation of uterine size and dates
   - **d.** Entrapment of the placenta
   - **e.** Dysfunctional labor
   - **f.** Postpartum hemorrhage
   - **g.** Obstruction of labor by cervical or lower uterine segment myomas
   - **h.** Unstable lie or compound presentation

   5. Incompetent cervix. This is usually appreciated by a history of a suspicious second-trimester loss with minimal labor contractions and with or without rupture of membranes or cervical trauma.

   6. Diethylstilbestrol-exposed patients. These patients need close observation throughout pregnancy because of the probability of both cervical and uterine anomalies, causing:
   - **a.** Abortion or ectopic pregnancy (first trimester)
   - **b.** Incompetent cervix (second trimester)
   - **c.** Premature labor and rupture of membranes (third trimester)

V. LABORATORY DATA BASE. Routine laboratory studies that may indicate maternal and fetal problems and thus may affect management of the pregnancy include the following:

A. Blood type and antibody screen are essential in all prenatal patients.

   1. Sensitization, although it has very little effect on maternal health, may have profound consequences for the fetus and the management of the pregnancy. If there has been maternal sensitization to red blood cell antigens (e.g., prior tranfusions), the resultant antibodies can be transferred to the fetus, which results in hemolytic disease and its intrauterine and extrauterine consequences (see Chapter 11, Rh Isoimmunization).

   2. The antibody screen is still essential in Rh-positive individuals because other blood group antigens (i.e., Kell, Kidd, and Duffy) can produce severe hemolytic disease in the fetus.

B. VDRL. Syphilis involves a number of different stages, and the evaluation of each stage is important in assessing fetal risk. Pregnancy complicated by preexisting or newly acquired syphilis may result in:

   1. An uninfected live infant

   2. A late abortion (after the fourth month of pregnancy)

   3. A stillbirth

   4. A congenitally infected infant

C. Gonorrhea culture. Whether or not the gonococcal infection is symptomatic or asymptomatic, it can have adverse effects on the course of pregnancy, contributing to both maternal and infant morbidity. Generally, there is an increased incidence of:

1. Intrauterine growth retardation

2. Prematurity

3. Premature rupture of membranes

4. Associated maternal arthritis, rash, or peripartum fever

5. Histologic evidence of chorioamnionitis

6. Clinical diagnosis of sepsis in the neonate

D. Rubella titer

1. The clinical course of rubella is no more severe or complicated in the pregnant woman as compared to the nonpregnant woman of comparable age. However, active maternal infection does carry a risk for the fetus, including:
   a. First-trimester abortion
   b. Fetal infection, resulting in severe congenital anomalies

2. Maternal infection in the first trimester carries with it the greatest risk to the fetus.

3. If a patient is diagnosed as having a rubella titer of less than 1:8, she should be immunized postpartum.

E. Complete blood count

1. Anemia. If present, anemia should be evaluated further and treated. Maternal anemia may be associated with pyelonephritis, prematurity, and fetal growth retardation.

2. Leukocytosis. A mild leukocytosis is normal in pregnancy; however, a grossly abnormal value needs to be investigated.

F. Urinalysis. Although the mechanism is unclear, there are specific physiologic and anatomic changes that occur during pregnancy that predispose the pregnant woman with symptomatic or asymptomatic urinary tract infections to develop pyelonephritis.

1. Asymptomatic bacteriuria is prevalent in 3%–5% of pregnant women, particularly those in lower socioeconomic groups and those at risk because of parity and age.

2. It is important that early detection, treatment, and close follow-up be instituted.

3. Asymptomatic bacteriuria predisposes the pregnant woman to the development of acute systemic pyelonephritis, which has serious complications for the mother and fetus and has been associated with premature labor and delivery. Approximately 20%–40% of pregnant woman with asymptomatic bacteriuria develop systemic pyelonephritis.

4. Few woman acquire asymptomatic bacteriuria who are not bacteriuric at their first prenatal visit. Therefore, it is believed that pregnancy does not increase the incidence of asymptomatic bacteriuria but rather sets the stage for the development of systemic pyelonephritis in those women with preexisting bacteriuria.

G. Pap smear. Baseline cervical cytology should be established and if abnormalities are noted, proper evaluation must be instituted.

H. Blood sugars. Various centers differ on how and when to evaluate women for gestational diabetes. However, since pregnancy is a diabetogenic state and aggressive, early management can help to prevent some of the complications of diabetes, *all* pregnant woman with a family history of diabetes should have at least a 1-hour glucose screen at 26–28 weeks gestation.

I. α**-Fetoprotein screening** should be offered to all pregnant women and drawn at 16–20 weeks gestation.

1. Maternal serum levels are elevated in 80% of pregnancies in which there is a fetal neural tube defect (i.e., anencephaly and spina bifida). Other disorders that elevate maternal serum α-fetoprotein are:
   a. Wrong dates (i.e., the pregnancy is further along than anticipated)
   b. Multiple gestation
   c. Fetal demise

d. Placental abruption
e. Fetal congenital defects (e.g., omphalocele, gastroschisis, and congenital nephrosis)

2. Maternal serum levels may be low in cases where the fetus has Down's syndrome.

VI. RISK ASSESSMENT

A. Antepartum. Pregnancy is a dynamic state; therefore, continued assessment during the prenatal period is necessary to identify problems early and allow prompt intervention. Dr. Calvin J. Hobel has done extensive research with high-risk patients and has identified the major perinatal problems responsible for most neonatal morbidity (Table 9-2).

1. Prematurity. Preterm labor and delivery account for much perinatal morbidity and mortality. Thus, early identification of women at risk for preterm labor and delivery allows appropriate preventive measures to be instituted. Table 9-3 is adapted from R.K. Creasy's work on a system for determining risk of preterm delivery and a grading system to assess relative risks.

2. Intrauterine growth retardation. It is important that the progress of each pregnancy be assessed carefully, including serial weight and fundal height measurements at regular intervals. Intrauterine growth retardation is most often associated with historical factors (see Chapter 16, The High-Risk Neonate, section IV C); however, it is occasionally associated with disease states that affect uterine and placental blood flow. If needed, further antenatal testing should be instituted.

3. Preeclampsia and eclampsia. There are a number of associated historical risk factors (see Table 9-2). In addition, many clinicians use the roll-over test or supine pressor test (rotation of the patient from the left lateral recumbent to the supine position). A rise in the diastolic pressure of more than 20 mm Hg is considered a positive test. It is necessary that close observation and evaluation be done for the early detection of proteinuria, edema, and hypertension.

Table 9-2. Prenatal Assessment Objectives

Major Perinatal Problems to Be Identified Early	Associated Prenatal Problems	
	Historical Factors	**Developing Factors**
Prematurity (less than 37 weeks)	Mother's education Previous stillbirth Previous premature birth Previous neonatal death Multiparity (5 children or more) Uterine malformation Weight less than 100 lbs History of genitourinary infections	Moderate to severe pregnancy-induced hypertension Incompetent cervix Rh sensitization Smoking Pyelonephritis Narcotic use
Intrauterine growth retardation	Previous stillbirth Previous neonatal death Multiparity (5 children or more)	Moderate to severe pregnancy-induced hypertension
Preeclampsia/eclampsia	Chronic hypertension History of renal disease Diabetes Age less than 17 years	Weight gain of more than 2 lbs/week Intrauterine growth retardation Positive roll-over test Multiple pregnancy
Diabetes	Age over 35 years Infant over 9 lbs Family history Fetal anomaly	Polyhydramnios Pregnancy-induced hypertension Genitourinary infections
Congenital anomalies	Age over 35 years Diabetes Habitual abortion Previous fetal anomaly	

Note.—Five major perinatal problems and the significantly related prenatal problems are listed. The prenatal assessment objective is the early identification of the patient at risk for any one of these problems. Data were collected from 1417 pregnancies. (Reprinted with permission from Bolognese RJ, et al: *Perinatal Medicine: Management of the High Risk Fetus and Neonate*, 2nd ed. Baltimore, Williams & Wilkins, 1982, p 10.)

Table 9-3. System for Determining Risk of Spontaneous Preterm Delivery

Points Assigned	Socioeconomic Factors	Previous Medical History	Daily Habits	Aspects of Current Pregnancy
1	Two children at home Low socioeconomic status	Abortion × 1 Less than 1 year since last birth	Works outside home	Unusual fatigue
2	Maternal age less than 20 years or more than 40 years Single parent	Abortion × 2	Smokes more than 10 cigarettes per day	Gain of less than 10 lbs by 32 weeks
3	Very low socioeconomic status Height less than 150 cm Weight less than 100 lbs	Abortion × 3	Heavy or stressful work Long, tiring trip	Breech at 32 weeks Weight loss of 5 lbs Head engaged at 32 weeks Febrile illness
4	Maternal age less than 18 years	Pyelonephritis		Bleeding after 12 weeks Effacement Dilation Uterine irritability
5		Uterine anomaly Second-trimester abortion Exposure to diethystilbestrol Cone biopsy		Placenta previa Hydramnios
10		Preterm delivery Repeated second-trimester abortion		Twins Abdominal surgery

Note.—The score is computed by adding the number of points given any item. The score is computed at the first visit and again at 22–26 weeks gestation. A total score of 10 or more places the patient at high risk for spontaneous preterm delivery. (Reprinted with permission from Creasy RK, et al: A system for predicting spontaneous preterm birth. *Obstet Gynecol* 55:692, 1980.)

4. **Diabetes.** It is essential that the diagnosis of diabetes be made as early as possible. The cornerstone of management is establishing an early, rigid, euglycemic metabolic control to reduce fetal and neonatal morbidity and mortality.

5. **Congenital anomalies.** It is difficult to identify the woman at risk for congenital anomalies. Some laboratory tests can be used to identify the fetus with a particular anomaly (e.g., maternal α-fetoprotein determinations for neural tube defects).

B. **Intrapartum.** Assessment of the pregnant woman must continue into the intrapartum period. Certain prenatal factors are associated with subsequent intrapartum risk and outcome. It is important to identify events associated with poor outcome so that appropriate interventions may reduce fetal and neonatal morbidity and mortality. Table 9-4 represents Dr. Calvin J. Hobel's prospective analysis, which identified three major perinatal problems and their related prenatal, neonatal, or intrapartum complications.

1. **Abnormal labor.** Only three types of abnormal labor (a–c below) have been found to be associated with subsequent neonatal morbidity. However, prenatal factors may be related to the development of the other types of abnormal labor (a, c–e below).
   a. Primary dysfunctional labor
   b. Prolonged second stage (more than 2.5 hours)
   c. Prolonged labor (more than 20 hours total)
   d. Prolonged latent phase of labor
   e. Precipitous labor
   f. Secondary arrest of cervical dilation

2. **Low Apgar scores in the prenatal or intrapartum period.** Many of the factors associated with low Apgar scores at birth can be identified early in the intrapartum period, and appropriate intervention instituted. Umbilical cord gases rather than Apgar scores are a more accurate index of the newborn condition.

3. **Respiratory distress** (see Table 9-3)
   a. **Respiratory distress syndrome** is often related to preterm labor and delivery.
   b. **Transient tachypnea.** Certain prenatal or intrapartum events should be evaluated and where possible ameliorated or controlled so that this type of respiratory distress is avoided.
   c. **Meconium aspiration.** Aggressive management intrapartum and immediately after delivery is necessary if meconium aspiration is to be avoided. Not all meconium aspiration is preventable, no matter what measures are taken.

Table 9-4. Intrapartum Assessment Objectives

Major Problems to Be Prevented	Associated Problems	
	Prenatal	**Neonatal or Intrapartum**
Abnormal labor		
Prolonged latent phase of labor	Age over 35 years	None
Primary dysfunctional labor	Habitual abortion	Fetal anomalies, low 1 minute Apgar score, meconium aspiration
Prolonged second stage (more than 2.5 hours)	None	Hyperbilirubinemia
Precipitous labor	Previous stillbirth Previous premature birth	None
Prolonged labor (more than 20 hours total)	Smoking	Resuscitation at birth Fetal anomalies
Low Apgar scores	Prenatal	Intrapartum
1 minute: less than 5	Moderate to severe preeclampsia* Maternal cardiac disease Diabetes Previous stillbirth Previous neonatal death Abnormal fetal position Multiple pregnancy	Premature infant Premature rupture of membranes Abnormal presentation Multiple pregnancy • Heavy meconium Primary dysfunctional labor Abruptio placetae Fetal acidosis Breech vaginal delivery* Operative forceps Shoulder dystocia
5 minute: less than 5	Moderate to severe preeclampsia* Diabetes Previous stillbirth Rh sensitization Abnormal fetal position	Abruptio placentae • Heavy meconium Abnormal presentation Premature infant Breech delivery* Fetal acidosis Operative forceps
Respiratory distress		
Respiratory distress syndrome	Moderate to severe renal disease Diabetes Previous stillbirth Previous premature birth Previous neonatal death Multiparity Uterine malformation Rh sensitization Moderate to severe preeclampsia Pyelonephritis	Premature labor Moderate to severe toxemia Breech presentation* Abruptio placentae Fetal acidosis Breech vaginal delivery
Other respiratory distress (transient tachypnea)	Diabetes Previous neonatal death Previous cesarean section Infant over 9 lbs Maternal age over 35 years	Prematurity Premature rupture of membranes Cesarean section Heavy meconium*

Table 9-4. Continued

Major Problems to be Prevented	Associated Problems	
	Prenatal	Neonatal or Intrapartum
Meconium aspiration	Diabetes	Moderate to severe preeclampsia*
	Previous stillbirth	Heavy meconium*
	Multiparity (5 children or more)	Multiple pregnancy
	Multiple pregnancy	Primary dysfunctional labor
	Moderate to severe preeclampsia	Abruptio placentae
		Fetal acidosis
		Breech delivery
		Shoulder dystocia

Note.—Three major perinatal problems and the significantly related prenatal and intrapartum risk factors determined by a prospective analysis of perinatal data collected from 1417 pregnancies (1968–1972). The intrapartum objectives are to identify pregnancies and neonates at risk for developing any of these perinatal problems by the recognition of the listed prenatal or intrapartum risk factors. (Reprinted with permission from Bolognese RJ, et al: *Perinatal Medicine: Management of the High Risk Fetus and Neonate*, 2nd ed. Baltimore, Williams & Wilkins, 1982, p 18.)

*An analysis of 1977 data identified factors that are no longer associated with poor outcome.

STUDY QUESTIONS

Directions: Each question below contains five suggested answers. Choose the **one best** response to each question.

1. Maternal mortality rate is defined as the number of maternal deaths per

(A) 1000 live-births
(B) 10,000 live-births
(C) 100,000 live-births
(D) 1000 pregnancies
(E) 100,000 pregnancies

2. All of the following factors are associated with an increased risk of perinatal morbidity EXCEPT

(A) low socioeconomic status
(B) low maternal age (less than 20 years old)
(C) heavy cigarette smoking
(D) alcohol abuse
(E) exercise

3. Maternal age less than 20 years increases the risk for all of the following conditions EXCEPT

(A) preeclampsia
(B) fetal death
(C) uterine dysfunction
(D) genetically abnomal conceptus
(E) premature births

4. All of the following statements about urinary tract infections during pregnancy are true EXCEPT

(A) asymptomatic bacteriuria in pregnancy needs to be treated
(B) pregnancy increases the risk of developing asymptomatic bacteriuria
(C) acute systemic pyelonephritis is associated with premature labor and delivery
(D) few women develop asymptomatic bacteriuria who are not bacteriuric at their first prenatal visit
(E) The incidence of asymptomatic bacteriuria is higher in pregnant women with a low socioeconomic status and increased parity and age

Directions: Each question below contains four suggested answers of which **one or more** is correct. Choose the answer

A   if **1, 2, and 3** are correct
B   if **1 and 3** are correct
C   if **2 and 4** are correct
D   if **4** is correct
E   if **1, 2, 3, and 4** are correct

5. Correct statements about risk factors during pregnancy include which of the following?

(1) A woman with a prior ectopic pregnancy is at risk for another ectopic
(2) A grand multiparous woman is at risk for postpartum hemorrhage
(3) The incidence of preterm delivery increases with each subsequent preterm delivery
(4) Once a cesarean section, always a cesarean section

6. Historical factors that are helpful in identifying the couple at risk for a genetic disorder include

(1) consanguinity
(2) parental age
(3) ethnicity
(4) previous spontaneous abortion

7. Disease entities for which pregnant women are routinely screened include

(1) hepatitis B
(2) toxoplasmosis
(3) cytomegalovirus
(4) syphilis

8. Factors associated with an increased risk for uterine rupture include

(1) fibroids
(2) exposure to diethylstilbestrol
(3) cervical carcinoma
(4) adenomyosis

ANSWERS AND EXPLANATIONS

1. The answer is C. (*II A 2*) The definition of the maternal mortality rate is the number of maternal deaths per 100,000 live-births. Over the past 50 years, there has been a significant decline in maternal mortality in the United States. As recently as 1975, the maternal mortality rate was 12.8/100,000 live-births, that is, 6.7 for whites and 19.8/100,000 for others. The dramatic difference between rates is attributed to economic and social factors, including lack of skilled personnel and appropriate delivery facilities, lack of good early antepartum care, poor nutrition, and faulty health education.

2. The answer is E. (*III A 1–3*) Alcohol abuse undermines maternal health as well as produces a pattern of abnormalities in the fetus known as the fetal alcohol syndrome; the severity of the fetal involvement is related to quantity and the time during gestation of fetal exposure. The effects of the occasional social use of alcohol on the fetus are not known, so most physicians advise their patients to avoid alcohol during pregnancy. Low socioeconomic status, low maternal age, and heavy cigarette smoking have all been shown to be closely associated with an increased risk of perinatal morbidity. Exercise during pregnancy has not been associated with an increased risk of perinatal morbidity and mortality as long as it is done in moderation.

3. The answer is D. (*III A 2 a*) Young mothers have an increased risk of many complications for unknown reasons. Speculative reasons include poor nutrition, low socioeconomic status, and late or substandard prenatal care. It is older women (i.e., older than 35 years of age), not younger, who are at risk for genetically abnormal conceptuses.

4. The answer is B. (*V F 1–4*) Few women develop asymptomatic bacteriuria who are not bacteriuric at their first prenatal visit. It is believed that pregnancy does not increase the incidence of asymptomatic bacteriuria but rather sets the stage for the development of systemic pyelonephritis in those women with bacteriuria. Asymptomatic bacteriuria does predispose the pregnant woman to the development of acute systemic pyelonephritis, which has been associated with premature labor and delivery. In addition, asymptomatic bacteriuria is more prevalent in pregnant patients with low socioeconomic status and increased parity and age.

5. The answer is A (1, 2, 3). (*III B 1 b, 3 a, b, 7, 8 a, b, 9*) A woman with a prior ectopic pregnancy is at increased risk for a subsequent ectopic pregnancy and must be evaluated early in the pregnancy. A woman with greater that five previous vaginal deliveries is at increased risk for postpartum hemorrhage secondary to uterine atony. Also, the incidence of preterm delivery increases with each previous preterm delivery; however, it does seem to decrease with each birth that is not preterm. A patient with one prior cesarean section may opt to attempt a vaginal delivery as long as there are no medical or surgical contraindications. Current studies reveal that greater than 50% of patients who have undergone cesarean section because of cephalopelvic disproportion may have a subsequent vaginal delivery.

6. The answer is A (1, 2, 3). [*III C 9 b (1)–(3)*] Consanguinity and ethnicity are helpful in identifying the high-risk patient because in each case a large pool of identical genes are shared, increasing the possibility of sharing similar mutant genes. Paternal age over 55 may increase the risk of a de nova single gene mutation. Advanced maternal age (over 35) increases the risk of chromosomal anomalies. One spontaneous abortion is not necessarily a rare event and is not likely to help in identifying the high-risk patient.

7. The answer is D (4). (*III C 16 a, c, d*) The infectious disease entities listed in the question— hepatitis B, toxoplasmosis, cytomegalovirus, and syphilis—play a role in increasing perinatal morbidity; however, only gonorrhea, syphilis, and rubella are common enough to make routine screening necessary. If sufficient clinical suspicion exists, the patient may need to be evaluated for hepatitis, cytomegalovirus, toxoplasmosis, and herpesvirus.

8. The answer is D (4). (*IV D 2 a, c, 3, 4, 6*) Adenomyosis is not only associated with increased risk of uterine rupture but also with postpartum hemorrhage and dystocia. Fibroids, cervical neoplasia, and exposure to diethylstilbestrol have not been associated with uterine rupture, but each places the patient at high risk for other complications.

10
Premature Labor
Luciano Lizzi

I. PREMATURITY

A. Definition. Prematurity denotes a lack of development and is manifested by low birth weight (500–2499 g), physical signs of immaturity, and gestational age less than 37 weeks (259 days). Infants who are of low birth weight but physically mature (e.g., growth-retarded infants) and infants who are large for gestational age but physically immature (e.g., infants of diabetic mothers) are not considered premature.

B. Epidemiology. Over the last 10 years, the incidence of prematurity has remained stable, but the neonatal outcome has improved. Between 1968 and 1978, the neonatal death rate declined to a rate of 10 per 1000 live births.

1. In the United States, 7.5% of all live-born children are premature.

2. Approximately 2%–3% of these children are born prior to 33 weeks gestation.

3. Approximately 50% of all perinatal deaths are among the children born before 33 weeks gestation.

4. Additionally, 50%–70% of all perinatal deaths are secondary to complications arising from a preterm birth.

II. RISK FACTORS FOR PREMATURE DELIVERY. A patient who has had a previous premature birth faces a recurrence risk of 20%–30% in the next pregnancy. Fifty percent of the patients who deliver prematurely have no risk factor.

A. Predisposing factors for prematurity include the following:

1. Low socioeconomic status, which may involve low income, low level of education, and poor nutrition. Black Americans, for example, tend to have infants with gestational ages 1 week less than white Americans.

2. Maternal age less than 16 years or primigravid women greater than 30 years of age.

3. Previous obstetric history of premature birth. One premature birth increases the risk fourfold, and two premature births increase the risk sixfold.

4. Work that is physically demanding or that is stressful and anxiety-provoking
    a. High-risk jobs include clerical, sales, service, and manufacturing positions.
    b. Intermediate-risk jobs are in the technical and professional sectors.
    c. Low-risk jobs include housekeeping and positions in agricultural and fishing industries.

5. Smoking more than 10 cigarettes per day

6. A complicated past medical history, including:
    a. Previous elective termination of pregnancy, especially after 12 weeks gestation
    b. Exposure in utero to diethylstilbesterol (DES), resulting in a cervical or uterine structural abnormality
    c. Congenital uterine anomalies or uterine fibroids
    d. Maternal renal disease

7. Multiple gestations. Thirty to fifty percent of twins are delivered prior to 36 weeks gestation.

8. Psychosocial stress

B. Complications of pregnancy resulting in prematurity

1. Upper urinary tract infection
   a. Asymptomatic bacteriuria
   b. Pyelonephritis

2. Maternal diseases
   a. Hypertension
   b. Preeclampsia and eclampsia
   c. Asthma
   d. Hyperthyroidism
   e. Heart disease
   f. Drug addiction
   g. Cholestasis
   h. Anemia with hemoglobin levels less than 9 g/dl

3. Conditions that overdistend the uterus
   a. Multiple gestations
   b. Gross fetal anomalies, leading to hydramnios
   c. Diabetes
   d. Rh isoimmunization

4. Antepartum hemorrhage

5. Placental abruption or fetal death

6. Maternal abdominal surgery or generalized sepsis

7. Intrauterine infection

III. MECHANISMS OF THE INITIATION OF LABOR. The exact mechanism by which labor begins is unknown, but it appears to be the result of the interplay of a number of physiologic changes in the mother and the fetus.

A. Placental steroids. It has been proposed that the onset of labor occurs in response to changes in target tissue sensitivity to placental steroids.

B. Estrogen–progesterone ratio. It appears that an increase in the estrogen–progesterone ratio may initiate labor.

1. In sheep, a fall in the production of progesterone by the placenta seems to remove a local hormonal block to myometrial activity beneath the placental implantation site.

2. In humans, progesterone does not fall significantly although estrogen rises.

C. Prostaglandins play a significant role in the initiation of labor. Their contribution to precipitating labor is suggested by the increase in uterine activity noted after rupture of the membranes, amniocentesis, amnionitis, and uterine manipulation during abdominal surgery. Also, drugs that inhibit prostaglandin synthesis, such as indomethacin, are effective agents for stopping preterm labor.

D. Fetal oxytocin release has been documented by higher oxytocin levels in the umbilical artery (from the fetus) than in the umbilical vein (to the fetus). Fetal adrenal function and cortisol production may also play a role in the initiation of labor, but it is of uncertain significance at this time.

E. Decreased uterine blood flow may be responsible for increased uterine contractility noted in many conditions, such as preeclampsia, eclampsia, multiple gestation, poor nutrition, dehydration, heavy smoking, and maternal vascular insufficiency.

F. Changes in steroid hormones that precede labor initiate and propagate the formation of myometrial gap junctions, which allow for the propagation of contractions throughout the cellular elements of the uterus.

G. Current model of labor

1. The amnion and the chorion are the site of storage of arachidonic acid.

2. Phospholipase A_2 is present within the lysosomes of the fetal membranes.

3. Changes in steroid hormone concentration or concentration ratios induce lysosomal perturbation with resultant accelerated expression of phospholipase A$_2$ activity.

4. Phospholipase A$_2$ catalyzes the hydrolysis of glycerophospholipids, resulting in the release of arachidonic acid.

5. Arachidonic acid diffuses to the uterine decidua where it is converted to prostaglandin by a prostaglandin synthetase enzyme complex.

6. Prostaglandin then diffuses into the amniotic fluid and myometrium, decreasing the level of cyclic adenosine monophosphate, which increases the concentration of free calcium ion at the level of the myometrial sarcoplasmic reticulum. The increasing intracellular calcium concentration becomes available to myosin light-chain kinase, which then allows for myometrial contraction.

IV. MANAGEMENT OF PREGNANCIES AT RISK FOR PRETERM LABOR

A. Early detection of premature labor is the key to successful management. The symptoms are often so subtle that they may be ignored by the patient and the physician. Once labor is established, the use of tocolytic agents is seldom effective in delaying delivery for a significant amount of time or in improving survival. To achieve early detection:

1. The patient should be educated to recognize the early signs of premature labor, including:
  a. Menstrual-like cramping
  b. Low backache
  c. Pelvic pressure
  d. Increased vaginal discharge
  e. Increased frequency of urination

2. The patient should call her physician immediately if she sees vaginal bleeding, which can result from cervical dilation or rupture of the membranes.

3. The physician should perform weekly cervical examinations in patients at risk to detect subtle changes that may herald the onset of labor, including:
  a. Dilation of the internal and external os
  b. Cervical effacement or softening
  c. Direction of the cervix (anterior or posterior)
  d. Station of the presenting part

4. If a cervical change or uterine irritability with cramping is noted, then hospitalization should be considered.

5. If preterm labor is suspected, the patient should be evaluated according to the scheme illustrated in Figure 10-1.

B. Cervical incompetence

1. A history of a midtrimester loss preceded by the absence of perceived uterine contractions is the best evidence for cervical incompetence.

2. Hysterosalpingography (x-ray of the uterus) before pregnancy may show abnormal widening of the cervical canal and possibly an abnormally shaped uterine cavity, such as that seen in daughters of women who took DES.

3. When intrauterine pressure exceeds the strength of the cervix, the cervix will open *without* contractions.
  a. An incompetent cervix usually begins to open in the second trimester.
  b. A cervix that dilates past 3–4 cm may stimulate premature labor by the Ferguson reflex.

4. Cervical change without cramping in a pregnancy of less than 24 weeks indicates a need for cervical cerclage and bed rest. A cervical cerclage, however, is of no value as prophylaxis against premature labor and the use of tocolysis. Placement of a pessary for cervical incompetence is advocated if surgery would threaten the pregnancy (i.e., if the cervix is more than 80% effaced at 16 weeks). Complications of cervical cerclage include the following:
  a. Mother
    (1) Anesthesia risks, such as spinal headache or aspiration of gastric contents after general anesthesia
    (2) Cervical bleeding from cervical dilation or usually from placement of the suture into the cervical mucosa
    (3) Cervical deformity or autoamputation, if contractions cause the stitch to tear the cervix

MANAGEMENT OF PRETERM LABOR

Confirm the diagnosis of preterm labor
- (20–37 weeks gestation)

Determine the presence of
- Regular uterine contractions
- Rupture of membranes
- Cervical change
Dilation more than or equal to 2 cm
Effacement more than or equal to 80%

↓

Evaluate cervix

Rule out premature rupture of membranes
- Culture for group B *Streptococcus*, gonorrhea, and *Chlamydia*
- Document position, dilation, effacement, and station
- Evaluate urinary tract to rule out infection or calculi
Rule out early abruption

↓

Start intravenous line and hydrate with 1 L of normal saline

↓

Document fetal well-being

- Perform a nonstress or contraction stress test if regular contractions are present

↓

Ultrasound

Estimate gestational age and fetal weight
- Rule out intrauterine growth retardation
- Rule out anomalies, hydramnios, or multiple gestation
- Rule out placental abruption or placenta previa
Perform a biophysical profile
Consider amniocentesis to evaluate lung maturity

↓

Tocolysis

- Subcutaneous terbutaline

Response	No response
Place on oral terbutaline	Intravenous tocolysis

If successful and if gestation is at 26–32 weeks, steroids should be considered

Figure 10-1

(4) Chronic vaginal discharge from chronic inflammation because of a foreign body (suture)

(5) Increased incidence of amnionitis and postpartum endometriosis if prolonged rupture of the membranes occurs

(6) Increased prostaglandin release from surgical manipulation of the cervix

b. Fetus

(1) Rupture of the membranes

(2) Chorioamnionitis, possibly resulting from overwhelming sepsis from vaginal bacteria

V. THERAPY FOR PREMATURE LABOR

A. Major tenets of therapy

1. Maintain a high-risk index of suspicion.

2. Prescribe prolonged bed rest in the left lateral position and good hydration to enhance uterine blood flow.

3. Test for asymptomatic bacteriuria, which occurs in 3%–5% of all pregnancies.
   a. Ameliorate with a 7-day course of antibiotics.
   b. Test for recurrent infection with a urine culture every 6–8 weeks.

4. Recommend the reduction or abolition of cigarette smoking.

5. Suggest consultations with social workers, psychologists, and psychiatrists to reduce the psychological stress associated with preterm labor.

6. Perform therapeutic amniocentesis to remove 500 ml of fluid if hydramnios causes overdistension and contractions.

7. Recommend cessation of coitus between 20 and 36 weeks gestation in those patients at high risk for premature delivery.

8. Consider the use of home contraction monitoring.

B. Drug therapy

1. Pharmacologic agents that are no longer used include:
   a. Sedatives and analgesics, which have not proven to be effective
   b. Vasodilators, such as epinephrine and amyl nitrite, which are used only to break tetanic contractions
   c. Inhalation anesthetic agents, which are not safe for long-term use
   d. Diazoxide, which has marked hypotension as an untoward side effect

2. Pharmacologic agents that are in the early stages of study include:
   a. Inhibitors of prostaglandin synthesis, such as ibuprofen or indomethacin, which may cause premature narrowing of the fetal patent ductus arteriosus
   b. Calcium antagonists, such as verapamil and nifedipine.

3. Intravenous tocolysis for preterm labor
   a. Ethanol, which acts as a posterior pituitary inhibitor, thereby inhibiting oxytocin letdown, is rarely used today because of maternal side effects, including inebriation, vomiting, gastritis, aspiration, lactic acidosis, and fetal depression.
   b. Magnesium sulfate, which competes with free calcium ions, has been an effective pharmacologic agent at a dose of 1–3 g/hr after a loading dose of 4 g. The side effects are numerous, but obstetricians are familiar with this drug, and it has a good antidote, that is, calcium gluconate.
   c. The family of β_2-adrenergic agents are the most popular drugs used for arresting preterm labor.
   (1) The mechanism of action of β_2 mimetics is stimulation of the β_2 receptors in uterine smooth muscle, causing relaxation of the muscle and cessation of contractions.
   (2) The most commonly used agents are ritodrine and terbutaline (isoxsuprine is no longer used). Although only ritodrine is approved for use in pregnancy in the United States, many institutions use terbutaline exclusively. Terbutaline has the advantage of being used subcutaneously, whereas ritodrine is administered intravenously.
   (a) Terbutaline is given in a dosage of 0.25 mg subcutaneously every 30 minutes to a maximum of six doses followed by oral maintenance of 5.0 mg every 4–6 hours.
   (b) Intravenous administration of ritodrine, on the other hand, should be continued for 6–24 hours after contractions cease after a titration dose of a maximum of 0.35 mg/min. This may be followed by oral ritodrine, 10 mg every 2–6 hours.

(3) Maternal side effects include tachycardia with palpitations, hypertension with widening of the pulse pressure, tremor, nausea, irritability, hyperglycemia, hypokalemia, hyperuricemia, metabolic acidosis, and pulmonary edema.

(4) Contraindications to the use of β_2-adrenergic agents include maternal cardiac disease, severe eclampsia, significant hypertension, undiagnosed uterine bleeding, bleeding from a placenta previa or placental abruption, intrauterine infection, fetal demise, severe intrauterine growth retardation, maternal hyperthyroidism, uncontrolled maternal diabetes, or any condition that mandates termination of the pregnancy.

(5) Maternal complications include hyperglycemia secondary to hepatic glycogenolysis with consequent hyperinsulinemia and hypokalemia. A more significant but less common complication is pulmonary edema, which is thought to be secondary to overhydration and complicated cardiovascular, pulmonary, and renal mechanisms inherent to the gravid woman exposed to β_2 medications.

(6) Neonatal hypoglycemia, hypocalcemia, and hypotension have been reported after use of β_2-adrenergic drugs, especially if given within 2 or 3 days of delivery. Long-term (7 years) follow-up studies of children exposed to ritodrine in utero have not reported deleterious side effects on growth or development.

4. **Maternal corticosteroids** have potential value in decreasing the incidence of respiratory distress syndrome when administered between 28 and 32 weeks and 24 hours prior to delivery.

STUDY QUESTIONS

Directions: Each question below contains five suggested answers. Choose the **one best** response to each question.

1. The percentage of patients with a history of prematurity who will have another premature infant is

(A) 0%–10%
(B) 20%–30%
(C) 40%–50%
(D) 60%–70%
(E) 80%–90%

2. A 16-year-old primigravida reports that she is experiencing regular menstrual cramping every 2 minutes. She is 28 weeks pregnant. After taking a history, the *first* thing that the physician should do is

(A) send her to the labor floor immediately
(B) confirm the frequency of contractions by abdominal palpation
(C) evaluate fetal well-being with a fetal monitor
(D) evaluate the cervix by speculum examination
(E) order an ultrasound to confirm the pregnancy dating

3. The most common cause of vaginal bleeding complicating premature labor is

(A) a vaginal laceration
(B) an endocervical polyp
(C) cervical dilation
(D) placenta previa
(E) placental abruption

4. Inhibitors of prostaglandin synthesis are not generally used for tocolysis because

(A) they are ineffective
(B) they produce marked hypertension
(C) they may cause premature closure of the fetal ductus arteriosus
(D) they are too expensive
(E) they are associated with lactic acidosis

Directions: Each question below contains four suggested answers of which **one or more** is correct. Choose the answer

A   if **1, 2, and 3** are correct
B   if **1 and 3** are correct
C   if **2 and 4** are correct
D   if **4** is correct
E   if **1, 2, 3, and 4** are correct

5. Correct statements about a 2330 g infant born at 38 weeks gestation include which of the following?

(1) The low birth weight of the infant indicates prematurity
(2) The low birth weight of the infant indicates growth retardation
(3) The gestational age of the infant indicates prematurity
(4) The low birth weight places the infant at risk for neonatal complications

6. A 39-year-old former Olympic athlete (gravida 5, para 0311) comes for her first prenatal visit. At 8 weeks gestation, after a discussion of prenatal genetic counseling, she asks about current recommendations that would help her not have a premature infant. The physician should explain that

(1) she is at no increased risk for premature delivery
(2) she can continue her plans for running a marathon in 1 month
(3) her age has no bearing on this pregnancy
(4) you would like to see her more often to perform cervical examinations

---

SUMMARY OF DIRECTIONS

A	B	C	D	E
1, 2, 3 only	1, 3 only	2, 4 only	4 only	All are correct

---

7. Predisposing factors for prematurity include all of the following EXCEPT

(1) maternal age over 30 years
(2) smoking more than 10 cigarettes per day
(3) exposure to diethylstilbestrol in utero with a documented uterine structural abnormality
(4) multiparity with more than four previous deliveries

8. The onset of spontaneous labor at term involves which of the following factors?

(1) Maternal progesterone and estrogen
(2) Fetal oxytocin
(3) Maternal prostaglandins
(4) Fetal corticosteroids

9. A 24-year-old woman (gravida 1, para 0) presents to the labor and delivery floor at 26 weeks gestation, complaining of frequent abdominal cramps and vaginal spotting. The fetal membranes are intact, she is contracting every 10 minutes, and her cervix is 3 cm dilated and 80% effaced. The plan of management should include

(1) intravenous tocolysis with magnesium sulfate
(2) urine culture
(3) ultrasound for estimated fetal weight
(4) cervical cerclage

10. A 17-year-old girl (gravida 2, para 0100) has been treated for premature labor at 28 weeks gestation with multiple tocolytic agents. After 48 hours in labor, she is sent to the antepartum unit. At 3:00 a.m., the physician is called because the patient is having difficulty breathing. The physician should

(1) administer corticosteroids, sensing imminent delivery
(2) obtain a chest x-ray, electrocardiogram, arterial blood gases, a complete blood count, and coagulation profile
(3) increase her intravenous fluids to 150 cm/hr
(4) administer oxygen and elevate the head of the bed

ANSWERS AND EXPLANATIONS

1. The answer is B. (*I B; II*) Unfortunately, a premature birth in one pregnancy increases the risk of a premature birth in the next pregnancy by approximately 20%–30%. This is three times the rate of prematurity in the general population (7.5%), which has remained constant for the past 10 years. Even without apparent risk factors, it is necessary to warn patients who have had a premature birth that they are at a significant risk of having the same problem in future pregnancies.

2. The answer is B. (*IV A 1 a–e, 2–4; Figure 10-1*) The subtle signs of premature labor—low back pain, increase in vaginal discharge, pelvic pressure, and frequent urination—should arouse the suspicions of the physician. However, the 16-year-old described in the question is experiencing regular menstrual cramping, which *is* an early sign of premature labor. It is important to first palpate the uterus, a maneuver that may cause an irritable uterus to contract. Once the fetal heart rate has been auscultated, a sterile speculum should be inserted into the vagina to obtain a cervical culture for gonorrhea, *Chlamydia*, and group B *Streptococcus*; to exclude premature rupture of the membranes; and to evaluate cervical dilation. If no rupture of the membranes has occurred, a digital pelvic examination may be performed. After this, a urine specimen should be obtained to rule out asymptomatic bacteriuria, which occurs in 3%–5% of pregnant women.

3. The answer is C. (*IV A 2*) During premature labor when the cervix begins to dilate and efface, the separation of the placenta and membranes may produce vaginal bleeding. A placenta previa should be excluded before the pelvic examination is performed. A placental abruption often causes preterm labor that is not inhibited with tocolytic agents. Vaginal lacerations from vaginal trauma (i.e., intercourse) usually produce vaginal bleeding without uterine contractions.

4. The answer is C. (*V B 2 a*) The inhibitors of prostaglandin synthesis, the commonest being indomethacin, act by blocking the endogenous production of prostaglandins. Although prostaglandin inhibitors have been used to prevent spontaneous labor, there is significant concern that this class of drugs may produce premature closure of the fetal ductus arteriosus and eventually fetal death. Other potential serious side effects include thrombocytopenia, ulceration of the gastrointestinal tract, and allergic reactions. Because of these side effects, some clinicians use this drug only before 28 weeks of gestation when the fetal ductus is more resistant to closure. Other investigators have found that indomethacin may be used safely prior to 32 weeks. However, it may cause decreased fetal renal perfusion, resulting in oligohydramnios.

5. The answer is C (2, 4). (*I A*) A 2330 g infant born at 38 weeks gestation indicates intrauterine growth retardation of a term fetus. At any gestational age, a fetus that is less than the tenth percentile by weight is considered small for gestational age or is prenatally designated to have intrauterine fetal growth retardation. The neonatal outlook for growth and mental development is directly dependent on the etiology of the problem causing the growth retardation. The term prematurity denotes underdevelopment, which is clinically expressed by low birth weight and physical evidence of immaturity.

6. The answer is D (4). (*II A 1–5*) The woman described in the question has a number of risk factors for premature labor, including a previous premature delivery, maternal age greater than 30 years, and possibly increased physical stress. The key to preventing a premature delivery is to counsel this patient about her risk factors, recommend increased rest periods, and perform frequent cervical examinations. Should the cervix reveal signs of dilation or effacement, tocolytic measures must be taken.

7. The answer is A (1, 2, 3). (*II A 1–8*) There are multiple predisposing factors for prematurity that have been outlined in the text, including advanced maternal age, cigarette smoking, and exposure to diethylstilbestrol in utero. Usually more than one factor is operating at the same time. Unfortunately, over 50% of patients who deliver prematurely have no apparent risk factors.

8. The answer is E (all). (*III B 1, 2, C, D*) Maternal progesterone levels from beneath the placental implantation site may have a role in maintaining pregnancy. An increasing estrogen–progesterone level in late pregnancy may remove a local hormonal block of myometrial activity. Although the role of maternal oxytocin release in the onset of labor in humans is negligible, fetal oxytocin release may be a very important mechanism. The levels of oxytocin found at delivery are significantly higher in umbilical cord blood than in maternal blood. In addition, oxytocin levels are higher in the umbilical artery than in the umbilical vein, supporting evidence for a fetal source of oxytocin. The contractile properties of the prostaglandins and their appearance in amniotic fluid and maternal blood with the onset of labor strongly support their role in the mechanism of labor onset. These contractile properties are most likely mediated through changes in myometrial cell calcium flux. Additionally, fetal adrenal function appears to be significant in the mechanism of labor onset.

9. The answer is A (1, 2, 3). *(IV B 1–4; V A 3; Figure 10-1)* In the evaluation of preterm labor, a urinary tract infection should be ruled out, an ultrasound to determine fetal weight would be useful for future management decisions, and tocolysis with magnesium sulfate or a β-agonist should be used to attempt to arrest the preterm labor. The pregnancy of the woman described in the question would be placed in jeopardy by a cervical cerclage. Not only is this her first pregnancy, so there is no history of cervical incompetence, but she is contracting regularly and her cervix is very effaced. In this situation, a cervical cerclage would be very dangerous, possible leading to maternal morbidity and fetal morbidity or mortality.

10. The answer is C (2, 4). [V B 3 c (5)] The patient described in the question is most likely suffering from a rare but serious side effect of tocolytic therapy, that is, pulmonary edema. Given an increase in maternal blood volume, increased fluid administration, increased sodium absorption in pregnancy, and β$_2$-mimetic effects on pulmonary vessels, this condition is more common in the pregnant than the nonpregnant patient. Therapy must be centered on diagnosis, oxygenation, termination of tocolytic therapy, diuresis, and fluid restriction. Corticosteroids will actually exacerbate this condition.

11

Rh Isoimmunization

Nancy S. Roberts

Rh negative %
white American " 13%
black " 7%
American Indians & Asians 1%

I. INTRODUCTION

A. **Definition.** Any human who lacks a red blood cell antigen produces an antibody when exposed to that antigen. Rh isoimmunization is caused by maternal antibody production in response to exposure to fetal red blood cell antigens of the Rh group, including C, D, and E (the Rh alleles). The antibody response may potentially destroy fetal red blood cells, causing anemia, and may result in erythroblastosis fetalis. All of the Rh alleles on the surface of the red blood cell stimulate an IgG antibody response in the mother.

B. **Incidence.** Approximately 1.5% of all pregnancies are complicated by red blood cell sensitization. The incidence of Rh isoimmunization in the United States has fallen since the 1960s because of the widespread use of Rh_o (anti-D) immune globulin (RhoGAM).

C. **Epidemiology.** There are important racial differences in the distribution of the Rh antigens. American Indians and Asians are almost all (99%) Rh positive. Seven percent of black Americans are Rh negative, and thirteen percent of white Americans are Rh negative.

II. IMMUNOLOGY OF Rh DISEASE. The initial exposure to a foreign antigen results in the production of maternal immunoglobulin M (IgM), a 19s immunoglobulin. The subsequent exposures (anamnestic response) result in the production of maternal IgG, a 7s immunoglobulin. Other immunoglobulins—IgG, IgD, and IgA— are produced in response to foreign antigens, but only IgG is capable of placental transfer to the fetus because of its small size. The severity of fetal involvement with Rh isoimmunization in the mother is not directly proportional to the severity of maternal disease. This may be due to several factors, such as:

A. **The degree of sensitization**, which depends on factors other than the occurrence of fetal cells reaching the maternal circulation and stimulating foreign antigen production. These include:

1. The rates of occurrence, which vary from one individual to another, with one person affected and the other unaffected, regardless of a prior risk.

2. The difference in immunogenicity of the offending antigen (e.g., c and E produce more of an antigenic response than the Kidd antigens).

3. The low rate of transfer of the antigen from fetus to mother, possibly reducing the incidence and severity of the antibody response.

4. The low rate of transfer of antibody from mother to fetus, possibly reducing the fetal effects of maternal antibody production.

5. The variability of maternal response due to different degrees of incompatibility and other interfering antibodies (e.g., ABO incompatibility).

6. Differences in binding of the maternal antibody to the fetal red cell antigens.

B. **ABO incompatibility**, which has a protective effect for an Rh-negative mother carrying an Rh-positive fetus for the following reasons:

1. A and B antigens are capable of mounting a strong immunogenic response.

2. Because the A or B cells are cleared so quickly from the maternal circulation, the full antibody response is blunted.

3. Risk of Rh sensitization developing as a result of an ABO *incompatible* Rh-positive pregnancy is 10%–20% of the risk with ABO *compatibility*.

III. PATHOLOGY OF ERYTHROBLASTOSIS FETALIS

A. Fetal red blood cell destruction. Rh-positive fetal red blood cells are hemolyzed by maternal Rh antibody (IgG anti-D). The hemolysis produces high levels of bilirubin, a breakdown product of hemoglobin. Red blood cell fragments are cleared by the fetal phagocytosis, and fetal anemia develops. This stimulates erythropoietin production. When the bone marrow red cell production cannot overcome red blood cell destruction, then extramedullary hematopoiesis begins in the liver, spleen, adrenal gland, kidneys, placenta, and intestinal mucosa, causing:

1. Portal and umbilical vein obstruction, simulating portal hypertension

2. Cessation of normal hepatic function, which in turn causes:
   a. Decreased protein synthesis
   b. Hypoalbuminemia
   c. Decreased colloid osmotic pressure in blood vessels, resulting in edema

3. Fetal anemia, the severity of which depends on:
   a. The amount of circulating maternal IgG
   b. The avidity of maternal IgG for the fetal red blood cell
   c. The fetal compensation for the anemia. The severity of fetal anemia is **not** necessarily proportional to the presence of fetal hydrops. Some fetuses with very low hemoglobins are not very edematous.

B. Hemolytic disease of the fetus and newborn is synonymous with erythroblastosis fetalis. There are three classifications, which depend on the severity of the hemolysis and the ability of the fetus to compensate for its hemolytic anemia without developing hepatocellular damage, portal obstruction, and total body edema. All infants with hemolytic disease have a positive direct Coombs' test of their umbilical cord blood.

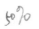

1. **Mild hemolytic disease**
   a. Half of all affected infants are classified as mild cases.
   b. No prenatal or neonatal treatment is required.
   c. Infants are mildly anemic at birth. Cord hemoglobin is 12 g/dl or higher, and cord bilirubin is not dangerously high (less than 3.5 mg/dl)
   d. In the neonatal period, the serum indirect bilirubin level rarely exceeds 20 mg/dl, and hemoglobin rarely falls below 8 g/dl.

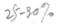

2. **Moderate hemolytic disease**
   a. Twenty-five to thirty percent of affected infants are classified as moderate.
   b. Prenatal treatment may include transfusions, but usually only one neonatal transfusion is required.
   c. Moderate anemia with hemoglobin levels from 7–12 mg/dl are found.
   d. In the neonatal period, treatment with exchange transfusions and phototherapy for hyperbilirubinemia is essential. This should prevent:
      (1) High blood levels of indirect bilirubin
      (2) Accumulation of bilirubin in the neurons
      (3) Profound neural damage, leading to:
         (a) Bilirubin encephalopathy (kernicterus)
         (b) Deafness

3. **Severe hemolytic disease**
   a. The remaining 20%–25% of affected fetuses become severely anemic.
   b. Prenatal treatment by transfusion is usually necessary to prolong the pregnancy until fetal viability (26 weeks) or preferably fetal maturity (32 weeks gestation).
   c. Severe anemia with cord hemoglobin levels of less than 7 mg/dl are found.
   d. In utero, total body edema (hydrops fetalis) occurs if the fetus is not transfused. Hydrops fetalis occurs when the hemoglobin falls by more than 7 mg/dl below the normal hemoglobin level. Hydrops is characterized by:
      (1) Generalized edema, which manifests as:
         (a) Scalp edema
         (b) Limb edema
         (c) Pleural and pericardial effusions
         (d) Ascites
      (2) Hepatosplenomegaly and hepatocellular damage—the most likely causes of hydrops fetalis. The hepatic circulation is distorted by islets of erythropoiesis; portal and umbilical venous obstruction lead to portal hypertension.
      (3) Congestive heart failure, which may or may not be present. However, it contributes to

anasarca (total body edema) but is not the usual cause of hydrops fetalis.

(4) Extramedullary hematopoiesis in many organ systems. Control of erythroid maturation is poor, so many immature forms of red blood cells appear in the fetal circulation.

(5) Enlarged, edematous placental villi with poor placental perfusion.

C. Bilirubin excretion

1. Amniotic fluid is stained with bilirubin in proportion to the degree of fetal red blood cell hemolysis.

2. Although the maternal liver can metabolize the excess bilirubin products, transfer across the placenta from the fetus to the mother is slow, allowing the fetal blood and urine bilirubin levels to rise.

3. Excess bilirubin deposition does not usually occur in utero—that is, there is no kernicterus until the neonatal period. Autopsy findings may show red blood cell breakdown products (pigment) in the brain of stillborn infants.

IV. CLINICAL MANAGEMENT OF THE IMMUNIZED PATIENT

A. The history and physical examination can help to predict the severity of Rh hemolytic disease. A detailed history should include information about:

1. **The maternal blood type and antibody screen**; if the mother is Rh negative, the blood type of the father of her infant must be determined
   a. If both the mother and father are Rh negative, there is no need to obtain further antibody screens for Rh disease.
      (1) A repeat screen at 28 weeks would be useful to exclude other antibodies that developed during the pregnancy.
      (2) Nonpaternity would explain fetal anemia from Rh disease in an Rh-negative couple.
   b. If the Rh-negative mother has an Rh-positive partner and has a positive antibody screen, then the antibody should be identified.
      (1) An IgM antibody does not place the pregnancy at risk for erythroblastosis fetalis (i.e., Lewis antigen).
      (2) An IgG antibody may cause erythroblastosis fetalis; so once it is identified, it should be titered to determine the antibody level.

2. **Previous episodes of possible sensitization** (Table 11-1), such as:
   a. Ectopic pregnancy
   b. Spontaneous abortion of more that 32 days gestation (46 days from the last menstrual period)
   c. Inadequate Rh_0 (anti-D) immune globulin dosage. If more than 30 ml of fetal blood (15 ml of fetal red cells) passed into the mother, than sensitization may have occurred.
   d. Previous blood transfusions with Rh-positive blood
   e. Sensitization in utero ("grandmother theory"). The pregnant women who is Rh negative may have been sensitized if she was exposed to her mother's Rh-positive cells at delivery. This is a very rare event, occurring in less than 2% of cases of Rh sensitization.

3. **Previously affected fetuses**
   a. Since Rh disease either remains at the same level of severity from infant to infant or becomes more severe with each successive pregnancy, it is important to document the severity of hemolytic disease of *previously* affected fetuses by the following cord blood studies:
      (1) Hemoglobin
      (2) Hematocrit
      (3) Direct Coombs' test

Table 11-1. Risks of Isoimmunization

Obstetric Event	Chance of Sensitization
Spontaneous abortion	3%–4%
Induced abortion	5%–6%
Ectopic pregnancy	<1%
Full-term pregnancy (before delivery)	1%–2%
Full-term delivery (ABO compatible or ABO incompatible)	14%–17%
Amniocentesis	1%–3%
Mismatched blood transfusion	90%–95%

  (4) Reticulocyte count
  (5) Bilirubin level
 b. Information about the delivery of previously affected infants is also important, including:
   (1) The gestational age at which delivery was accomplished and hydrops fetalis occurred. Generally, but not always, hydrops develops in a subsequent pregnancy at the same time or earlier than in a previous pregnancy.
   (2) The type of delivery and events surrounding delivery that may increase the risk of Rh isoimmunization, such as:
    (a) Cesarean section
    (b) Placental abruption
    (c) Preeclampsia and eclampsia
    (d) Manual placental removal
    (e) Amniocentesis, especially across an anterior placenta
    (f) External version
 c. It is important to determine the type of therapy that was indicated to combat hyperbilirubinemia and anemia, prenatally (e.g., intrauterine transfusion) and neonatally (e.g., double-exchange transfusions or phototherapy).
 d. Knowledge of previous titers helps to determine whether or not they have been carried from a previous pregnancy or are new events.

4. Maternal antibody titers and obstetric history, which help to predict the severity of erythroblastosis fetalis in the current pregnancy in approximately 62% of the cases. If amniocentesis and ultrasound are added to the regimen, then the predictability is increased to 89%. A critical titer is that antibody level above which the possibility of stillbirth is significant.
 a. Once the titer of maternal antibody measured in albumin reaches a level greater then 1:16, the fetus has a 10% risk of dying in utero. A titer of 1:32 carries a 25% risk, 1:64, a 50% risk, and 1:128, a 75% risk.
 b. An indirect Coombs' titer greater than 1:32 in most laboratories is significant. The critical titer for each laboratory must be determined.
 c. Amniocentesis should also be performed to determine the severity of the fetal anemia if the titer:
   (1) Equals or exceeds the critical titer
   (2) Rises by fourfold (two tube increase)
 d. Antibody titers should be repeated monthly, until serial amniocentesis is begun.

B. Amniocentesis. Amniotic fluid from a fetus suffering from hemolytic anemia has elevated levels of bilirubin. Since the fetus swallows amniotic fluid and urinates into it, fetal tracheal and pulmonary secretions are the most likely sources of bilirubin. Amniotic fluid bilirubin reflects the degree of hemolysis.

1. Real-time ultrasonography. The most accurate method of obtaining amniotic fluid is by using real-time ultrasonography to guide amniocentesis. However, special care must be taken to avoid the placenta and the umbilical cord and to note the fetal position and parts when choosing a site for needle insertion.
 a. Traversing the placenta with a needle has been shown to increase the likelihood of fetomaternal hemorrhage, producing a maternal anamnestic response, that is, elevation of maternal antibody titers, creating a worse hemolysis of fetal cells in the current or future pregnancies.
 b. When 10–20 ml of fluid are obtained, the fluid is quickly transferred to an opaque cylinder to avoid light-induced changes in bilirubin absorption.

2. Spectrophotometry is employed to measure the optical density (OD) reading at 450 nm (wavelength).
 a. Absorption of amniotic fluid in an unsensitized pregnancy follows a smooth curve with peak absorption in the lower wave lengths.
 b. Since bilirubin products show maximal deviation from the curve at 450 nm, the difference between test fluid and the control is measured as the ΔOD_{450} (Fig. 11-1).
 c. In a normal uncomplicated pregnancy, amniotic fluid bilirubin decreases as the gestation progresses. The bilirubin concentration is an indirect measure of fetal red blood cell hemolysis and anemia.
 d. Various systems for measuring bilirubin and plotting $\Delta 450$ versus gestational age have been employed (e.g., the Liley curve). They assess the severity of the disease and the timing for intervention, such as early delivery or fetal blood transfusion. The amniotic fluid ΔOD_{450} from pregnancies not complicated by fetal hemolysis usually fall in zone I or low zone II (see section IV B 3).
 e. Contaminants cause small peaks and can render the curve inaccurate.

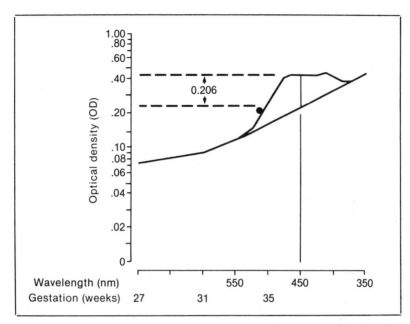

Figure 11-1. Amniotic fluid spectrophotometric reading (ΔOD_{450}) is 0.206 in this example, indicating impending fetal death. See this plotted on the Liley curve in Figure 11-2. (Reprinted with permission from Creasy R, Resnick R: *Maternal-Fetal Medicine: Principles in Practice*. Philadelphia, WB Saunders, 1984, p 576.)

     (1) Blood causes sharp peaks at 415 nm, 540 nm, and 580 nm.
     (2) Meconium causes a peak at 412 nm.

  3. The Liley curve was designed to provide a means by which to predict the severity of hemolytic disease in the third trimester only. The curve is divided into three prognostic zones (Fig. 11-2).
    a. Zone I (lowest zone) fetuses are usually unaffected and will be born with a hemoglobin greater than 12 g/100 ml. Normal hemoglobin at term is 16.5 mg/100 ml. Patients with zone I fetuses are usually allowed to deliver at term.
    b. Zone II (midzone) fetuses may be carried in utero until the amniotic fluid bilirubin level increases or until they are more than 32 weeks when delivery is advised. The hemoglobin is usually 8–12 g/100 ml. Early delivery is indicated if:
      (1) The lecithin/sphingomyelin (L/S) ratio is mature and phosphatidylglycerol is present.
      (2) A previous intrauterine demise occurred at about the same time.
      (3) The upward trend of OD_{450} is drastic.
    c. Zone III (highest zone) fetuses are in jeopardy of dying in utero within 7–10 days.
      (1) They must be transfused or delivered.
      (2) Hemoglobin is usually less than 8 g/100 ml.

  4. Timing of amniocentesis depends on the antibody titers and the history of previously affected fetuses.
    a. Since intrauterine transfusions are usually unsuccessful before 18–20 weeks gestation, there is rarely a need for amniocentesis until 18 weeks gestation, if the critical titer is reached before that time. However, if there is a history of a fetal or neonatal death, fetal transfusion, or birth of a severely affected infant, the first amniocentesis is generally performed 10 weeks prior to the time of the expected ominous event.
    b. If the critical titer is reached after 18 weeks gestation, then the initial amniocentesis is performed immediately after that titer is reached.
    c. Amniocentesis is repeated at 1–4-week intervals, depending on the previous values and past history of hydrops fetalis or stillbirths (see Fig. 11-3).
    d. The downward trend in the ΔOD_{450}, after a second or third amniotic fluid determination, is a good prognostic sign. If the ΔOD_{450} falls into zone I, no further intervention is required.

C. Percutaneous umbilical blood sampling (PUBS) [or cordocentesis]

  1. Sampling blood from the umbilical cord is performed, using fetoscopy (direct visualization) or

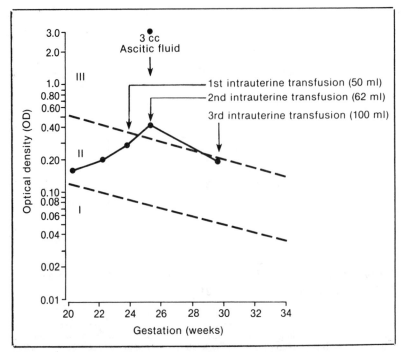

Figure 11-2. Liley curve showing readings from serial amniocenteses in a patient who eventually had three intrauterine transfusions. (Reprinted with permission from Creasy R, Resnick R: *Maternal-Fetal Medicine: Principles in Practice.* Philadelphia, WB Saunders, 1984, p 576.)

ultrasound-directed needle aspiration (indirect visualization). This provides information about fetal blood including:
  a. Hemoglobin and hematocrit
  b. Blood type
  c. Direct Coombs' titer (antibodies attached to fetal red cells)
  d. Bilirubin level
  e. Reticulocyte count

  2. During the second trimester, obtaining fetal blood for the hematocrit may be preferable to using the Liley curve to *estimate* the degree of fetal anemia because:
  a. The Liley curve is more predictive in the third trimester than in the second trimester, and it is not always predictive of the degree of erythroblastosis fetalis. Infants in zone I or II may be severely anemic.
  b. The duration of time that an infant's ΔOD_{450} is in zone III is not directly correlated to the severity of the fetal anemia.

D. Intrauterine transfusions (Fig. 11-3)

  1. Timing. After 34 weeks gestation, when the ΔOD_{450} falls in the highest zone (zone III), the patient should be delivered. If too premature (less than 34 weeks), an intrauterine transfusion should be performed since the risk from a transfusion is less than the risk of prematurity. Transfusions may be started as early as 18 weeks gestation.

  2. Approaches
    a. Intraperitoneal transfusion
      (1) Technique. Intraperitoneal transfusion is the classic approach, guided by real-time ultrasound. Following maternal sedation and analgesia, local anesthesia is infiltrated into the maternal abdomen and a 16-gauge Tuohey needle is inserted through the maternal abdomen and uterine wall into the amniotic fluid and, finally, into the fetal abdomen. Packed red blood cells deposited into the fetal peritoneal cavity are absorbed by the lymphatic system and enter the fetal vascular system.
      (2) Complications
        (a) Pregnancy loss rate is 3%–10%.
        (b) Laceration of a fetal organ, such as liver, bowel, bladder, may occur.
        (c) Premature labor may begin.

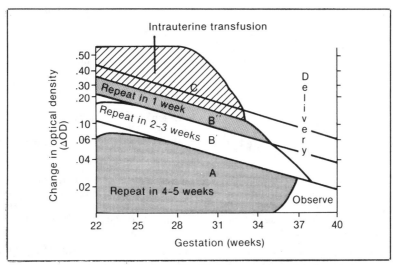

Figure 11-3. Suggested management scheme for repeat amniocentesis, intrauterine trans-fusions, and delivery according to ΔOD_{450} versus weeks of gestation. Maternal history and antibody titers and especially ultrasound findings should also be considered. (Reprinted with permission from Bolognese RJ, Schwarz RH, Schneider J: *Perinatal Medicine*: *Management of the High Risk Fetus and Neonate*, 2nd ed. Baltimore, Williams & Wilkins, 1982, p 273.)

    (d) Premature rupture of the membranes may occur.
    (e) Chorioamnionitis may be a complication.
  b. Intravascular transfusion
    (1) Technique. After locating the fetal lie and the site of the cord insertion, the patient is given a narcotic, tranquilizer, antiemetic, tocolytic agent, and an antibiotic. The 20- or 22-guage Tuohey needle is advanced through the maternal abdominal wall, entering the umbilical vein lumen shortly after it inserts into the placenta. The needle stylet is removed, and a pretransfusion fetal hematocrit is obtained. Packed red cells are inserted through the needle, and another sample of blood is aspirated to check the final fetal hematocrit and assess the adequacy of therapy. Curare is given either intravenously (through the umbilical vein) or intramuscularly to the fetus to deter movement that may dislodge the needle from the umbilical vein.
    (2) Complications
      (a) Pregnancy loss rate from hemorrhage, blood clot in the umbilical vein, or chorio-amnionitis is 1%.
      (b) Premature labor may begin.
      (c) Premature rupture of the membranes may occur.
      (d) Placental bleeding at the site of cord puncture may occur.
      (e) Fetal bradycardia may result but usually spontaneously resolves in 45–60 seconds.

E. Real-time ultrasonography

  1. Real-time ultrasonography enables the clinician to detect many of the pathologic features of early (a and b) and advanced (c–j) hydrops fetalis, including:
    a. Polyhydramnios (increased quantities of amniotic fluid)
    b. Fetal hepatosplenomegaly, resulting from extramedullary hematopoiesis in the liver and spleen
    c. Increased bowel echogenicity from edema in the bowel wall
    d. Cardiomegaly and pericardial effusion
    e. Ascites and hydrothorax
    f. Scalp and limb edema
    g. Abnormal fetal posturing, known as the "Buddha" stance of a fetus whose spine and extremities are deflexed around a swollen abdomen
    h. Sluggish limb movements and overall decreased fetal movement characteristic of a fetus suffering from severe hemolytic disease
    i. Placental hypertrophy and thickening from edema
    j. Poor contractility and wall thickening of the fetal cardiac ventricles

  2. Specific measurements of organs involved in erythroblastosis by real-time ultrasonography may allow the clinician to quantify the degree of fetal disease, including:

   a. Umbilical vein diameter (dilated values are more than 10 mm)

   b. Vertical liver length. Over 45 mm is abnormal.

   c. Placental thickness. Over 5 cm is a late sign of disease.

   d. Increased velocity of blood flow in the fetal descending aorta. The velocity is inversely proportional to fetal hemoglobin.

3. Real-time ultrasonography may replace or serve as an adjunct to amniocentesis when there is:

   a. Premature rupture of the membranes in which case there is not enough amniotic fluid left in the uterus to perform a safe procedure

   b. A multiple gestation where only one sac might be sampled. The other fetus may be examined with ultrasound.

   c. Contamination of the amniotic fluid with blood meconium

   d. A large, thick, anterior placenta with no safe site for amniocentesis or cordocentesis

   e. Patient noncompliance—that is, refusal to allow amniocentesis or cordocentesis

   f. A need to identify or exclude hydropic fetuses. Ultrasound increases the sensitivity of the elevated ΔOD_{450} measurements in detecting severely anemic fetuses and identifies those infants who are anemic but have ΔOD_{450} values in zone I or II.

4. Ultrasonography should be performed weekly unless the fetal condition deteriorates at which point daily or every other day scanning may be necessary.

5. The progression or regression of fetal hydrops can be followed by real-time ultrasonography. It can help to determine when the next transfusion is needed. Amniocentesis is of little value after intrauterine transfusions have been performed as the amniotic fluid is usually stained with blood from the procedure. This would falsely elevate the amniotic fluid bilirubin levels, indicating a greater degree of fetal red blood cell hemolysis than is actually present.

F. Delivery should be entertained:

1. When maturity is documented by a lecithin/sphingomyelin ratio of more than 2:1 and the presence of phosphatidylglycerol. Many perinatologists give the mother corticosteroids at the time of the first fetal transfusion to mature the fetal lung since they anticipate a premature delivery.

2. When the risks of prematurity are less than the risk of an intrauterine transfusion. This is usually after 32–34 weeks gestation.

3. With the help of the neonatal team. The neonatal group and blood crossmatched and available for transfusion should be in the delivery room. Cesarean section is usually the best alternative for deliveries before 34 weeks. Severely anemic infants rarely tolerate active labor since the oxygen–carrying capacity of their red blood cells is lowered. This produces fetal distress and the need for cesarean delivery.

V. PREVENTION OF Rh ISOIMMUNIZATION

A. Mechanism of action. In 1909, it was demonstrated in laboratory animals that when an antigen and its antibody are injected together, there is no immunologic response, provided the dose of antibody is adequate. By this same principle, Rh immune globulin (the antibody) protects against an immunologic reaction when an Rh-negative woman is exposed to Rh-positive (D positive) fetal cells (the antigen). Rh immune globulin will **not** protect against sensitization from the other Rh-positive alleles—that is, *c, C, e,* and *E.*

B. Indications for protection. Rh immune globulin (350 µg) should be given:

1. At 28 weeks gestation to an Rh-negative, nonimmunized woman (negative anti-D titer) who has an Rh-positive husband (partner)

2. Postpartum if the woman remains unimmunized and delivers an Rh-positive fetus. A Du-positive fetus who is D negative should be treated as D positive since the Du antigen is capable of immunizing an Rh-negative woman.

3. Following amniocentesis or chorionic villus sampling

4. Following evacuation of a molar pregnancy

5. Following an ectopic pregnancy

6. After a postpartum tubal ligation or pregnancy termination

   7. After an accidental transfusion of Rh-positive blood to an Rh-negative mother

   8. After a platelet transfusion

   9. After a clinical situation associated with a spill of fetal cells into the maternal circulation, such as:
      a. Placental abruption or undiagnosed uterine bleeding
      b. Maternal trauma (e.g., automobile accident)

C. Administration of Rh immune globulin

   1. Standard dose. A 300 mg dose of Rh immune globulin covers a fetomaternal hemorrhage of 30 ml fetal whole blood or 15 ml red cells.

   2. Determination of the correct dose
      a. Kleihauer-Betke test estimates the quantity of fetal red blood cells that have entered the maternal circulation. This is especially helpful in suspected large fetomaternal hemorrhage or after the administration of mismatched blood.
      b. Indirect Coombs' test measures free circulating anti-D (or Rh immune globulin). If an appropriate amount of Rh immune globulin has been given, there should be a positive indirect Coombs' (excess free antibody) measured a day after the dose.

D. Failure of Rh immune globulin prophylaxis may result from the following:

   1. The dose given may have been too small.

   2. The dose may have been given too late. Rh immune globulin is most effective if given within 72 hours of delivery or exposure to Rh-positive cells.

   3. The patient may already be immunized, but the level of antibody is lower than can be measured by the laboratory.

   4. The Rh immune globulin may have been defective or contain a substandard dose.

STUDY QUESTIONS

Directions: Each question below contains five suggested answers. Choose the **one best** response to each question.

1. The incidence of Rh isoimmunization following a full-term delivery (no Rh immune globulin prophylaxis) in a D-positive infant to an Rh-negative mother is

(A) 1%
(B) 5%
(C) 17%
(D) 40%
(E) 90%

2. The ΔOD_{450} is 0.04 at 30 weeks in a 30-year-old woman. This corresponds to which of the following Liley curve zones?

(A) Below zone I
(B) I
(C) II
(D) III
(E) None of the above

Directions: Each question below contains four suggested answers of which **one or more** is correct. Choose the answer

A   if **1, 2, and 3** are correct
B   if **1 and 3** are correct
C   if **2 and 4** are correct
D   if **4** is correct
E   if **1, 2, 3, and 4** are correct

3. Correct statements about certain classes of immunoglobulins that cross the placenta include which of the following?

(1) Only particles of a small enough size cross the placenta
(2) Immunoglobulins 19s are too large to cross the placenta
(3) The configuration and ionization of a molecule affect placental passage
(4) Immunoglobulins pass more readily if they are not clumped in immune complexes

4. Which of the following maternal antibodies may cause erythroblastosis fetalis in the fetus?

(1) Anti-C
(2) Anti-E
(3) Anti-D
(4) Anti-Lewis

5. Events occurring during pregnancy and delivery known to increase the risk of sensitization include

(1) type of delivery
(2) vaginal bleeding
(3) preeclampsia
(4) maternal age

6. Which of the following signs of erythroblastosis fetalis can be detected by ultrasound?

(1) A head measurement that is small for gestational age
(2) Fetal ascites
(3) Bowing of the fetal femur
(4) Thickening of the placenta

Directions: The group of questions below consists of lettered choices followed by several numbered items. For each numbered item select the **one** lettered choice with which it is **most** closely associated. Each lettered choice may be used once, more than once, or not at all.

Questions 7–10

For each clinical presentation that follows, select the antibody titer that would most apt to be associated with it.

(A) Indirect Coombs' 1:8
(B) Indirect Coombs' negative
(C) Indirect Coombs' 1:64
(D) Indirect Coombs' 1:128
(E) Indirect Coombs' 1:2048

7. An Rh-negative woman had six pregnancies. The fifth and sixth infants needed three intrauterine transfusions each.

8. An Rh-negative woman is pregnant for the first time.

9. An Rh-negative woman received Rh_o (anti-D) immune globulin 2 weeks previously after amniocentesis. She is now 40 weeks pregnant.

10. An Rh-negative woman is seen 72 hours after receiving an inadequate dose of postpartum Rh_o (anti-D) immune globulin.

ANSWERS AND EXPLANATIONS

1. The answer is C. (*II B 3*) There is a significant risk of sensitization following a term delivery since a large fetomaternal hemorrhage occurs during the actual delivery process. Antibodies may appear either postpartum or following exposure to the Rh antigen in the next pregnancy. ABO incompatibility between the mother and infant confers very mild protection against Rh sensitization.

2. The answer is B. (*IV B 2, 3*) An optical density value of 0.04 is in zone I. If the *repeat* value is also found in zone I, it probably indicates an unaffected fetus.

3. The answer is E (all). (*II A 1–6*) There are many factors that contribute to placental passage. Since a particle with a sediment coefficient of 7s will cross the placenta but a particle, such as IgM, with a 19s sedimentation coefficient will not, we know that large molecule size inhibits passage. A highly ionized compound will not cross the placenta as readily as a nonionized molecule.

4. The answer is A (1, 2, 3). (*I A; II; III A, B*) Only IgG antibodies are able to cross the placenta and attack fetal red blood cells. This produces red cell destruction from hemolysis as well as increased red blood cell production in the fetal bone marrow initially, followed by production in extramedullary sites. All of the Rh alleles (*C, D,* and *E*) on the surface of the red blood cell stimulate an IgG antibody response in the mother. However, only IgM is produced against the Lewis antigen. Therefore, the fetus of a mother with anti-Lewis antibodies is not at risk for anemia.

5. The answer is A (1, 2, 3). (*IV A 2 a–e, 3 a–d; V B 1–9*) There are several events that occur during pregnancy and delivery that are known to increase the risk of more severe transplacental hemorrhage, resulting in maternal sensitization. These include antepartum hemorrhage, preeclampsia, eclampsia, cesarean section, manual removal of the placenta, and external version. The incidence and amount of transplacental hemorrhage increase as the pregnancy progresses. By the third trimester, 10%–15% of women may have evidence of fetomaternal hemorrhage. At least 0.1 ml of fetal blood must enter the maternal circulation for sensitization to occur. Following either spontaneous or therapeutic abortion, there is a 5%–25% incidence of transplacental hemorrhage. If the abortion occurs after 30 days gestation, the Rh (D) antigen has been well enough developed to result in sensitization.

6. The answer is C (2, 4). (*IV E 1 a–j*) Ultrasound is a reliable tool for detecting fetal compensation for a hemolytic anemia. Usually the head circumference and the biparietal diameter are as large or larger than the anticipated gestational age since there may be fluid retention, which manifests as scalp edema. Fetal ascites also may be present as a manifestation of the edema. In addition, the placenta is often thickened due to hypertrophy and extramedullary hematopoiesis (a normal placenta measures less than 5 cm in its widest diameter). Serial measurements of the placenta at the same site, (e.g., at the cord insertion) enable the clinician to follow a progression of thickening due to erythroblastosis fetalis. Bowing of the fetal femur is a sign of skeletal dysplasia, not Rh disease.

7–10. The answers are: 7-E, 8-B, 9-A, 10-B. (*IV A 1–4; V C 2 b*) Rh (D) antibody titrations, when carried out in the same laboratory, may be of some value in predicting the severity of Rh hemolytic disease. However, Rh (D) antibody measurement determines only whether the fetus is at risk. It cannot predict accurately the severity of Rh disease. The Rh-negative woman who had six pregnancies is likely to have a high antibody titer (1:2048) since there is a history of hydropic fetuses.

In an Rh-negative woman who is pregnant for the first time, it is unlikely that the indirect Coombs' titer will be positive. However, if the woman was sensitized while *she* was in utero, if she had a previous undiagnosed pregnancy that resulted in miscarriage after 30 days gestation, or if she received a blood transfusion, she could possibly have an indirect Coombs' titer that is significant.

In an Rh-negative woman who received an appropriate dose of Rh_0 (anti-D) immune globulin, the indirect Coombs' titer is generally low but present. The titer is usually less than 1:16 since, in some laboratories, a titer of 1:32 or greater may carry a significant risk of erythroblastosis fetalis.

If an Rh-negative woman received an inadequate dose of postpartum Rh_0 (anti-D) immune globulin, then the Rh-positive fetal red cells have bound an inadequate quantity of anti-D in the immune globulin. All of the Rh_0 (anti-D) immune globulin would be bound by Rh fetal cells, and there would be no circulating unbound Rh_0 (anti-D) immune globulin to be measured by the indirect Coombs' test. This scenario might occur after massive transplacental hemorrhage. This occurs sometimes during the latter part of pregnancy but is more common at the time of delivery. Routine screening of fetal cells at the time of delivery, performed by the Kleihauer-Betke test, is recommended. Information obtained from these tests would predict the exact dosage of Rh_0 (anti-D) immune globulin that the patient should receive to prevent maternal sensitization.

12
Prenatal Diagnosis
PonJola Coney

I. INTRODUCTION

A. **Genetic counseling** determines the parental risk of having a child with a genetic or congenital birth defect, interprets the risk, and assists the parents in making a decision regarding contraception, sterilization, adoption, artificial insemination, carrier detection, referrals to agencies concerned with handicapped children, prenatal diagnosis, and options for terminating the pregnancy.

B. **Prenatal diagnosis** is indicated in **8% of all pregnancies.** The diagnostic procedures currently available, including **ultrasound, amniocentesis, maternal blood studies, fetoscopy, chorion and trophoblast sampling, and percutaneous umbilical blood sampling**, are the subject of this chapter.

II. ULTRASOUND

A. **Basic physics.** Any sound greater than 20 kHz is ultrasound, but higher frequencies are used in obstetrics (2.25–5.0 mHz) for greater tissue differentiation. As ultrasound passes through the body, it encounters multiple reflecting surfaces separated by areas with varying capacity to reflect echoes displayed in the form of x-ray photography. **Anechoic** describes tissues with few or no echoes, such as the bladder, brain, cavities, and amniotic fluid. **Echogenic** describes tissues with great capacity to reflect ultrasound.

   1. **Specular echoes** are flat or smooth with well-defined surfaces whose dimensions are large in relation to the wavelength of sound that reaches them (vault of fetal skull, spine, and chorionic plate of placenta).

   2. **Scattered echoes** are interfaces that are small in relation to the wavelength of the ultrasound or large surfaces with an irregular or ill-defined outline. These echoes are dispersed in a number of directions (placenta, fetal viscera, and myometrium).

B. **Basic components of ultrasonic equipment**

   1. **The B-scan** is composed of an **A-mode** and a **M-mode**, which provide precise measurements, and a **time position scan** with a permanent record of cinephotography. The **grey scale** displays each echo in a shade of grey that corresponds to its intensity. The B-scan is not portable, has a large number of controls, and requires a great deal of experience to operate. It is unsuitable to study most types of fetal movement.

   2. **Real-time** is a portable scanner, which is ideal for demonstrating motion of solid structures within fluid contents. It does not require a great deal of time or experience to operate, and it provides the easiest, most immediate, and most definitive demonstration of fetal life. The **transducer** is made from specially treated ceramic, which generates ultrasound via the piezoelectric effect.* The **scan converter** reproduces the record in a television compact form.

C. **Clinical indications for ultrasound.** Ultrasound is regarded as a noninvasive procedure that can be used at anytime during pregnancy with a high degree of accuracy. There are no data to suggest that it is hazardous to the fetus or mother. The most common obstetric indications include **pregnancy dating, diagnosis of multiple pregnancy, fetal growth, placental localization**, pre-

---

*When crystalline substances (i.e., quartz, Rochelle salt, and lithium sulfate) are subjected to forcible alterations in shape, small but appreciable voltages are generated between their surfaces. In the case of ultrasound, man-made ceramic crystals specially treated become strongly piezoelectric. Strong electrical voltages passed across the crystals result in shape changes, and the vibrations as pressure waves pass out as ultrasound.

sentation, position and lie of the fetus, amniocentesis for prior knowledge of placental site and position of fetal parts, and detection of congenital anomalies. Congenital malformations and abnormal conditions detectable by ultrasound include the following:

1. **Central nervous system disorders**
   a. Anencephaly
   b. Spina bifida
   c. Encephalocoele
   d. Hydrocephalus
   e. Microcephaly
   f. Iniencephaly

2. **Gastrointestinal disorders**
   a. Ascites
   b. Duodenal atresia
   c. Diaphragmatic hernia
   d. Abdominal wall defects (gastroschisis and exomphalos)

3. **Renal disorders**
   a. Renal agenesis
   b. Congenital hydronephrosis–hydroureter
   c. Polycystic kidneys

4. **Cardiopulmonary disorders**
   a. Pleural effusions
   b. Cardiac anomalies
   c. Thoracic cysts

5. **Miscellaneous disorders**
   a. Cystic hygroma
   b. Conjoined twins
   c. Phocomelia
   d. Congenital lymphangiectasia

III. AMNIOCENTESIS is a transabdominal, fine needle aspiration of amniotic fluid. The amniotic fluid contains fetal cells, which can be cultured and evaluated for chromosomal abnormalities. Amniocentesis should be performed at 16 weeks gestation, at which time ample fluid is present, diagnostic tests can be performed, and elective abortion, if indicated, is still possible.

A. **Indications.** The risk for a major chromosomal abnormality in a live-born child is 1.5%; however, this risk increases in **women over 35 years of age,** for whom 70% of antenatal studies for chromosomal anomalies are performed. Although amniocentesis can also detect many inborn errors of metabolism and neural tube defects, it may not always be indicated as the *first* procedure for diagnosis. Prenatal detection should be considered as a diagnostic tool when:

1. **A woman is over 35 years of age.** There is an increased risk in this age group of meiotic nondisjunction, leading to the birth of a trisomic infant.

2. **There is a previous child with a chromosomal anomaly.**

3. **One parent is known to carry a balanced translocation.** Translocation is the transfer of part of one chromosome to a nonhomologous chromosome. A balanced translocation in one parent should be suspected in the following circumstances:
   a. When a child is born with an unbalanced translocation.
   b. When mental retardation is present in a child with or without other congenital anomalies.
   c. If there is a maternal history of three or more spontaneous abortions.

4. **One parent is known to carry an inversion.** Inversion is the fragmentation of a chromosome followed by reconstitution with inversion of the section of the chromosome between the breaks. The abnormal conceptuses can abort early in pregnancy or go to term.

5. **There is a family history of neural tube defect.**

6. **One or both of the parents are known carriers of sex-linked or autosomal recessive traits.**

B. **Complications.** The risk of the procedure (1.5%) should be less than the risk of the offspring having the disorder to be diagnosed. **Penetration of the placenta** can be associated with untoward effects, but this is rare. Rh-negative women who are not sensitized should receive Rh_o (anti-D) immune globulin (RhoGAM) after the procedure. Other complications of the procedure include the following:

1. Premature rupture of membranes PROM

2. Premature labor

3. Spontaneous abortion

4. Fetal puncture

5. Bloody tap

6. Missed tap

C. Chromosomal abnormalities and congenital malformations detected by amniocentesis

1. **Down's syndrome (trisomy 21)** is the most prevalent cytogenic abnormality, occurring in about 1 in 600 live-births to mothers under 35 years of age. Of all children with trisomy 21, 95% have an extra chromosome 21, 4% have unbalanced translocations, and the remaining 1% are mosaics. Down's syndrome children may live to 50 years of age, but all (100%) are mentally retarded with an intelligence quotient (IQ) range of 25–60, and 50% also have congenital heart defects. The risks for having a child with trisomy 21 are listed in Table 12-1.

2. **Neural tube defect.** Neural tube defects (i.e., spina bifida, meningomyelocele, and anencephaly) result from polygenic/multifactorial inheritance with a general incidence of 1–2/1000 live-births (6000/yr in the United States). The highest incidence is in Ireland (9.7%), and the lowest incidence is in Japan (0.9%). Most cases of neural tube defect occur in families not known to be at risk and carry a high incidence of perinatal morbidity, mortality, and long-term disability.

   a. **Diagnosis**
      (1) **Open neural tubes.** α-Fetoprotein, a glycoprotein that is synthesized in the embryonic fetal yolk sac, developing gastrointestinal tract, and liver, is elevated three to five times in amniotic fluid secondary to leakage from the open neural tube. It crosses the placenta and appears in lower concentration in maternal serum than in amniotic fluid. Fetal serum concentration, maternal serum concentration, and amniotic fluid concentration are highest at 15–16 weeks gestation and decline during the remainder of pregnancy.
      (2) **Closed myeloceles** may not have increased α-fetoprotein levels in the amniotic fluid and maternal serum and are associated with fewer neurologic defects and a good prognosis.
      (3) **Spina bifida occulta**, the mildest form, is found in 20% of the general population.
   b. **Screening** for neural tube defects should begin with **measurement of α-fetoprotein levels in maternal serum.** (The incidence of false–positive α-fetoprotein levels is 0.1%–0.2%.) If elevated 2.5 times normal, the following protocol should be followed:
      (1) Ultrasound should be performed to verify gestational age, fetal life, and singleton pregnancy and to localize the placenta for a "free window" through which to aspirate amniotic fluid.
      (2) The entire spinal column of the fetus should be evaluated for widening of the canal, abnormal vertebrae, ventricular/head size, and size and defects of the abdomen.
      (3) The gel electrophoresis assay of acetylcholinesterase in amniotic fluid is not specific for neural tube defect but is less influenced by fetal blood admixture and is a valuable adjunct in the diagnosis.
   c. **Individual or recurrence risks for neural tube defect**
      (1) One affected parent (5%)
      (2) Prior affected child with unaffected parents (5%)

Table 12-1. Risk Factors for Trisomy 21

Risk Factors	Incidence/Live Births
Maternal Age*	
29	1/935
30–34†	1/600
35	1/365
35–39	1/300–1/100
40–44	1/60–1/50
45+	1/40

*Of children with trisomy 21, 50% are born to mothers over 35 years of age.
†Risks for offspring with trisomy 21 if there is a previous child with trisomy 21 and maternal age is less than 35 is 1%–2%.

Table 12-2. Conditions in Which the α-Fetoprotein Concentration Is Elevated

Missed abortion	Cystic hygroma
Congenital nephrosis	Trisomy 30
Multiple pregnancy	Fetal bowel obstruction
Sacrococcygeal teratoma	Incorrectly dated pregnancy
Turner's syndrome	Intrauterine growth retardation
Omphalocele	

        (3) Two previously affected children (10%)
        (4) Three previously affected children (21%)
        (5) One affected parent with affected child (13%)
        (6) Defect in second-degree relative (1%)

  3. Other conditions characterized by elevated α-fetoprotein levels are listed in Table 12-2.

  4. Low α-**fetoprotein levels.** When the α-fetoprotein level is 0.5 times normal or less, an amniocentesis for chromosomal evaluation must be performed.
    a. Fifteen to twenty percent of trisomy 21 (Down's syndrome) fetuses have a low α-fetoprotein value.
    b. Less than 5% of the subsequent amniocenteses will reveal the trisomy 21 fetus after the low α-fetoprotein measurement.

D. Inborn errors of metabolism (Table 12-3) are abnormalities of lipid, amino acid, carbohydrate, and mucopolysaccharide metabolism. Most are inherited as X-linked recessive or autosomal recessive traits and are compatible with severe mental retardation, severe disability, and death in early childhood.

  1. Diagnosis is possible by enzyme, amino acid, hormone, and abnormal metabolic product estimation on cell-free amniotic (cultivated or uncultivated) fluid. If the enzyme in question can be demonstrated in cultivated skin fibroblasts, it may be demonstrated in cultivated amniotic fluid.

  2. Three genetic lethals represent the disorders of this group:
    a. Tay-Sachs disease is a disorder of lipid metabolism that is common among Ashkenazi Jews. There is a marked deficiency of β-D-hexosaminidase A in maternal serum and in cultured amniotic fluid cells. Carrier incidence is 1/30.
    b. Lesch-Nyhan syndrome is a rare X-linked disorder of protein synthesis with absence of the enzyme hypoxanthineguanine phosphoribosyl transferase (HGPRT).
      (1) There is overproduction of purines.
      (2) The onset is very early in life.
      (3) It is characterized by aggressive behavior that leads to self-mutilation.
    c. Duchenne muscular dystrophy is another X-linked recessive disorder, a primary myopathy, that is rapidly progressive and debilitating. Death usually occurs before age 20.

E. Rh sensitization occurs in 1.5% of all pregnancies. Amniocentesis is performed in the second and third trimesters for diagnosis and therapy (see Chapter 11).

F. The lecithin-sphingomyelin (L/S) ratio and the presence of phosphatidylglycerol in amniotic fluid are measured in the third trimester of pregnancy to assess pulmonary maturity of the fetus.

Table 12-3. Inherited Errors of Metabolism That Can Be Diagnosed Prenatally

Disorder	Deficient Enzyme or Metabolic Defect
Acid phosphatase deficiency	Acid phosphatase
Adrenogenital syndrome	C-21 hydroxylase
Argininosuccinic aciduria	Argininosuccinase
Aspartylglycosaminuria	Specific hydroxylase (AADG)
Ataxia, intermittent	Pyruvate decarboxylase
Cholesteryl ester storage disease	Cholesteryl ester hydrolase
Citrullinemia	Argininosuccinic acid synthetase
Combined immunodeficiency	Adenosine deaminase

Table 12-3. Continued

Disorder	Deficient Enzyme or Metabolic Defect
Cystinosis	Cystine accumulation
Ehlers-Danlos type IV	Type III collagen
Ehlers-Danlos type VI	Collagen lysyl hydroxylase
Ehlers-Danlos type VII	Procollagen peptidase
Fabry's disease (X-linked)	Ceramide trihexosidase
Farber's disease	Ceramidase
Fucosidosis	α-Fucosidase
Galactokinase deficiency	Galatokinase
Galactosemia	D-Galactose-1-phosphate uridyl transferase
Gangliosidosis GM_1, type I	β-Galactosidase A, B, C
Gangliosidosis GM_2, type II	β-Galactosidase B, C
Gangliosidosis GM_2, type I (Tay-Sachs)	Hexosaminidase A
Gangliosidosis GM_2, type II (Sandhoff's)	Hexosaminidase A, B
Gaucher's disease	β-Glucocerebrosidase
Glucose-6-phosphate dehydrogenase deficiency (X-linked)	Glucose-6-phosphate dehydrogenase
Glycogen storage disease type II (Pompe's)	α-4-Glucosidase
Glycogen storage disease type III	Amylo-1, 6-glucosidase
Glycogen storage disease type IV	Amylo-1,4 to 1,6-transglucosidase
Homocystinuria	Cystathionine synthase
Hyperlipoproteinemia type II	Impaired regulation of 3-hydroxy-3-methylglutaryl CoA reductase
Hyperlysinemia	Lysine-ketoglutarate reductase
Hypophosphatasia	Alkaline phosphatase
Isovaleric acidemia	Isovaleric acid CoA dehydrogenase
Krabbe's disease	Galactocerebroside-β galactosidase
Lactosyl ceramidosis	Lactosyl ceramidase
Lesch-Nyhan disease (X-linked)	Hypoxanthineguanine phosphoribosyl transferase
Mannosidosis	α-Mannosidase
Maple syrup urine disease	Keto acid decarboxylase
Menkes' syndrome	Abnormal copper uptake
Metachromatic leukodystrophy	Arylsulfatase A
Methylmalonic aciduria I	Methylmalonic CoA mutase
Mucolipidosis type II (I-cell disease)	Lysosomal enyzme leakage
Mucolipidosis type III (pseudo-Hurler's polydystrophy)	Lysosomal enyzme leakage
Mucopolysaccharidosis I (Hurler's and Scheie's)	α-L-Iduronidase
Mucopolysaccharidosis II (Hunter's, X-linked)	Sulfo-iduronide sulfatase
Mucopolysaccharidosis III (Sanfilippo A)	Heparan sulfate sulfatase
Mucopolysaccharidosis III (Sanfilippo B)	N-Acetyl-D glucosaminidase
Mucopolysaccharidosis IV (Morquio's)	N-Acetylhexosamine-6-sulfate sulfatase
Mucopolysaccharidosis VI (Maroteaux-Lamy)	Arylsulfatase
Mucopolysaccharidosis VII	β-Glucuronidase
Niemann-Pick disease	Sphingomyelinase
Ornithinemia	Ornithine keto acid amino transferase
Oroticaciduria I	Orotidylic pyrophosphorylase and orotidylic decarboxylase
Oroticaciduria II	Orotidylic decarboxylase
Osteogenesis imperfecta congenita	Type I collagen
Phosphohexose isomerase deficiency	Phosphohexose isomerase
Porphyria, congenital erythropoietic	Uroporphyrinogen III cosynthetase
Porphyria, acute intermittent	Porphobilinogen deaminase
Propionic acidemia	Propionyl CoA carboxylase
Refsum's disease	Phytanic acid oxidase
Testicular feminization syndrome (X-linked)	Androgen binding protein
Valinemia	Valine transaminase
Wolman's disease	Acid lipase
Xeroderma pigmentosum	Ultraviolet specific endonuclease

Note.—Reprinted with permission from Siggers DC: *Prenatal Diagnosis of Genetic Disease.* Oxford, Blackwell Scientific, 1978, p 20.

IV. CHORION AND TROPHOBLAST SAMPLING, OR CHORIONIC VILLI SAMPLING (CVS), provides an early source of DNA.

A. Sampling is transcervical or transabdominal and can be performed at 6–11 weeks gestation, thereby reducing the waiting period and making earlier and safer abortion possible.

B. This procedure has been successful for the diagnosis of fetal sex and the hemoglobinopathies (i.e., sickle cell disease and β-thalassemia).

C. The amniotic sac is not penetrated, but potential complications include bleeding from the biopsy site, compromise of fetal membranes, and infection. There is a 1%–3% spontaneous abortion rate associated with CVS.

V. FETAL BLOOD SAMPLING

A. Percutaneous umbilical blood sampling (PUBS) is a new technique for prenatal diagnosis. It is used for sampling fetal blood and for direct intravascular transfusion of blood into the fetus. Ultrasound is used to select the aspiration site. The risk, like other new techniques, is not clear.

B. Fetoscopy is direct visualization of the fetus and intrauterine environment. Fetal blood sampling from the cord or chorionic plate can be performed for the diagnosis of many disorders, such as thalassemia, sickle cell anemia, hemophilia, von Willebrand's disease, and diseases of immunodeficiency. Skin biopsy can be performed for diagnosis of ichthyosis and certain types of muscular dystrophy. Extra digits and major cleft defects can also be visualized. Diagnostic benefit must outweigh potential fetal/maternal risks. Pregnancy wastage can be as high as 12% from this procedure.

BIBLIOGRAPHY

American College of Obstetrics and Gynecology: Technical Bulletin, no. 67, October 1982

Gosden JR, et al: Direct vision chorion biopsy and chromosome-specific DNA probes for determination of fetal sex in first trimester diagnosis. *Lancet* 1:1416, 1982

Law RG: *Ultrasound in Clinical Obstetrics.* Bristol, John Wright, 1980

Milunsky A: Prenatal detection of NTD. VI. Experience with 20,000 pregnancies. *JAMA* 244:2731, 1980

Milunsky A, et al: Prenatal diagnosis of NTD. IV. Maternal serum alpha-fetoprotein screening. *Obstet Gynecol* 55:60, 1980

Siggers DC: *Prenatal Diagnosis of Genetic Disease.* Oxford, Blackwell Scientific, 1978, p 20

Thompson J, Thompson M: *Genetics in Medicine,* 2nd ed. Philadelphia, WB Saunders, 1973, p 151

STUDY QUESTIONS

Directions: Each question below contains five suggested answers. Choose the **one best** response to each question.

1. The most accurate and definitive documentation of fetal life is made by

(A) fetoscope
(B) Leopold maneuver
(C) B-scanner
(D) Real-time scanner
(E) Doppler ultrasound

2. An α-fetoprotein of 0.44 times normal would predict the possibility of which of the following conditions?

(A) Omphalocele
(B) Trisomy 21
(C) Multiple pregnancies
(D) Trisomy 30
(E) Turner's syndrome

3. Fetoscopy is a valuable diagnostic tool in obstetrics because of

(A) the ease of test performance and safety to mother and fetus
(B) its ability to diagnose more disabling disorders than amniocentesis
(C) its ability to collect large quantities of fetal blood
(D) the reduced risk of Rh sensitization during the procedure
(E) the benefit of direct visualization of the fetus and blood sampling at the same time

Directions: Each question below contains four suggested answers of which **one or more** is correct. Choose the answer

A   if **1, 2, and 3** are correct
B   if **1 and 3** are correct
C   if **2 and 4** are correct
D   if **4** is correct
E   if **1, 2, 3, and 4** are correct

4. Fetal blood sampling is possible with which of the following procedures?

(1) Fetoscopy
(2) Chorionic villi sampling
(3) Percutaneous umbilical blood sampling
(4) Amniocentesis

5. Correct statements about amniocentesis include which of the following?

(1) The procedure is relatively safe and diagnostically useful
(2) The procedure can be performed without ultrasound
(3) The procedure can be performed via penetration of the placenta
(4) The procedure is not recommended after the second trimester

Directions: The group of questions below consists of lettered choices followed by several numbered items. For each numbered item select the **one** lettered choice with which it is **most** closely associated. Each lettered choice may be used once, more than once, or not at all.

Questions 6–10

Match the following.

(A) 1–2/1000
(B) 5%
(C) 1/365
(D) 9%
(E) 1.5%

6. Incidence of neural tube defect in Ireland

7. Risk of neural tube defect after one previously affected child

8. Incidence of neural tube defect in the general population

9. Risk of trisomy 21 in women 35 years of age

10. Risk of a chromosomal abnormality in a live-born child in women less than 35 years old

ANSWERS AND EXPLANATIONS

1. The answer is D. (*II B 2*) Real-time ultrasound provides an excellent display of fetal movement, particularly the heart, and, therefore, is of immense value in demonstrating fetal life. It is a portable scanner that does not require a great deal of time or experience to operate.

2. The answer is B. (*III C 4*) An α-fetoprotein of 0.44 times normal suggests the possibility of a Down's syndrome (trisomy 21) fetus as 15%–20% of Down's fetuses have a low α-fetoprotein value. Values are considered low if the α-fetoprotein is 0.5 times normal or less. The other possibilities are conditions in which the α-fetoprotein concentration is elevated.

3. The answer is E. (*V B*) Fetoscopy is direct visualization of the fetus and intrauterine environment. However, the additional benefit of visualizing intrauterine contents and fetal blood sampling are achieved at greater expense than with any other diagnostic procedure in obstetrics. Fetoscopy requires expertise far greater than amniocentesis and should be performed in major high-risk care centers to minimize fetal loss.

4. The answer is B (1, 3). (*III–V*) Fetal blood is sampled in procedures that can actually tap a source of fetal blood, either in the umbilical cord or on the placenta. Both fetoscopy, where there is direct visualization of the fetal vessels, and percutaneous umbilical blood sampling, where the vessels are identified via ultrasound, provide opportunities for fetal blood sampling. Amniocentesis harvests amniotic fluid and fetal cells for evaluation. Chorionic villi sampling takes a small portion of the trophoblastic tissue; it does not sample blood.

5. The answer is A (1, 2, 3). (*III*) Amniocentesis has become a routine procedure for the majority of obstetric services. The risks are low, and although ultrasonic guidance for needle placement is preferable, it can be performed without ultrasound with penetration of the placenta if necessary with few untoward effects. Amniocentesis can be performed at any time in a pregnancy from 14–16 weeks on, for example, for prenatal diagnosis, fetal lung maturity studies (during the third trimester), and maternal/fetal sensitization studies.

6–10. The answers are: 6-D, 7-B, 8-A, 9-C, 10-E. (*III A, C 1, 2 a, c; Table 12-1*) The highest incidence of neural tube defect is in Ireland (9.7%), and the lowest incidence is in Japan (0.9%). Incidence in the general population is 1–2/1000 live-births. Most cases occur in families not known to be at risk. There is a 5% risk of neural tube defect after having one previously affected child. Trisomy 21 (Down's syndrome) is the most prevalent cytogenetic abnormality, occurring in about 1 in 365 live-births to mothers 35 years of age. The risk for a major chromosomal abnormality in a live-born child in women less than 35 years of age is 1.5%.

13
Ultrasound in Pregnancy
Nancy S. Roberts

I. PHYSICS OF ULTRASOUND. The ultrasound used in clinical practice is limited to frequencies in the range of 1–10 million cycles per second (1–10 million Hertz). In obstetric ultrasound, the most commonly used frequencies are 3.5 mHz and 5 mHz. The 3.5 mHz beam penetrates deeper into the body than the 5 mHz.

A. Ultrasonograms. An ultrasonogram is produced when transmitted pulses of sound from the transducer cross body structures and reflect energy back to the transducer from the interfaces of organs, from vessel walls, or from differences in tissue density and structure of an organ. About 1000 pulses of sound are emitted from the transducer each second. The same transducer transmits and receives sound waves; in general, 999/1000 of each second is spent receiving and 1/1000 of each second in transmitting.

B. Acoustic properties of tissue determine the fate of sound waves as they traverse the tissues.

1. Reflection
   a. Echogenic tissues are tissues that are very reflective.
   b. Anechoic (without echoes) tissues are tissues that are not reflective.

2. Attenuation
   a. Attenuating tissues are solid tissues that reduce the intensity of sound waves as they pass through.
   b. Sonolucent tissues are tissues that allow total transmission of sound waves.

3. Examples
   a. The first-trimester placenta has no echoes within, so it is anechoic, but it will attenuate sound waves, so it is mildly attenuating.
   b. Amniotic fluid is usually clear early in pregnancy and thus is anechoic and sonolucent. Later in pregnancy, it becomes echogenic and sonolucent.

C. Types of ultrasound

1. A-mode (amplitude modulation). The echoes of A-mode ultrasound are displayed as vertical spikes on a screen. This is rarely used in clinical practice except possibly as a guide for amniocentesis, especially when it is necessary to measure distances.

2. B-mode (brightness modulation). The amplitude of B-mode ultrasound is represented by a spot of light on a cathode ray tube; when the spots are combined, it produces a slice or tomogram of the body. The two types of B-mode are:
   a. Static B-scanner. An image is produced by moving the transducer over the body surface. It is useful for visualizing the entire uterus.
   b. Real-time B-scanner. An image is produced that appears to be continuous as long as the frame rate is rapid. These images are generally produced by the following transducers:
      (1) Linear array
      (2) Sector scanner

3. M-mode (motion modulation). The spots of light of M-mode ultrasound are represented in time–motion and produce a wave-form representation reflected from moving structures. This type of ultrasound is used almost exclusively in the evaluation of cardiac structure and function (i.e., the prenatal diagnosis of congenital heart disease).

II. **ULTRASOUND IN OBSTETRICS.** The major indications for sonographic evaluation are listed below.

    A. **Confirmation of an intrauterine pregnancy.** If a woman's last menstrual period was at least 5 weeks ago, the gestational sac visualized on ultrasound confirms an intrauterine pregnancy. A gestational sac should be seen in all pregnancies once the β-subunit of human chorionic gonadotropin (HCG) has risen above 6500 mIU/ml.

    B. **Exclusion of an ectopic pregnancy.** An ectopic pregnancy may have a decidual cast lining the uterus (pseudosac) that mimics an intrauterine pregnancy. However, a pseudosac does not have the same shape or wall thickness on ultrasound as an intrauterine sac.

    C. **Assessment of an intrauterine pregnancy.** Fetal heart motion should be visualized in all pregnancies after 8 weeks from the last menstrual period. If heart motion is not present, either the date of conception is in error or the pregnancy is not viable. After fetal heart motion has been recorded, there is only a 2% chance of spontaneous abortion.

    D. **Determination of gestational age.** The size of the gestational sac on ultrasound can accurately predict the due date (within $+ 3$ days) and should be used with women who:

        1. Are uncertain of the date of conception because they:
           a. Recently stopped using oral contraceptives
           b. Conceived while breastfeeding
           c. Have irregular menses
           d. Are uncertain of the date of their last menstrual period

        2. Are at high risk for:
           a. A repeat cesarean section
           b. Red blood cell isoimmunization
           c. Complications related to:
               (1) Insulin-dependent diabetes
               (2) Hypertension
               (3) Renal disease
           d. Conditions that predispose to intrauterine growth retardation
           e. Premature delivery
           f. Ectopic pregnancy

    E. **Discrepancies between gestational age and uterine size**

        1. If the uterus is **large for dates**, ultrasound can help to diagnose:
           a. Leiomyoma (fibroids)
           b. Multiple gestation
           c. Hydatidiform mole
           d. Bicornuate uterus
           e. Polyhydramnios
           f. An adnexal mass
           g. A normal pregnancy more advanced than expected

        2. If the uterus is **small for dates**, ultrasound can help to diagnose:
           a. Missed abortion
           b. Blighted ovum
           c. Fetal demise
           d. Oligohydramnios
           e. Intrauterine growth retardation
           f. A normal pregnancy that is not as far advanced as expected

    F. **Investigation of uterine bleeding.** Ultrasound can pinpoint the etiology of uterine bleeding by determining:

        1. The location of the placenta

        2. If the membranes have been lifted off the uterine wall by a blood clot

        3. The presence of a retroplacental clot

        4. Increased echogenicity of placental cotyledons

G. Visualization for high-risk procedures

  1. Amniocentesis, which is performed for:
   a. Genetic studies
   b. α-Fetoprotein levels
   c. Bilirubin levels in Rh isoimmunization
   d. Fetal maturity studies [lecithin/sphingomylin (L/S) ratio and phosphatidylglycerol levels]
   e. Presence of blood or meconium in amniotic fluid

  2. Chorionic villi sampling (CVS). In this procedure, villi are aspirated either vaginally, using a thin catheter, or abdominally, using a needle, between the ninth and eleventh weeks of gestation. Although this technique affords a diagnosis and options for termination earlier in the pregnancy than amniocentesis, the drawbacks include:
   a. A 1%–3% miscarriage rate from the procedure
   b. No information about neural tube defects until 16 weeks when a maternal serum α-fetoprotein level is measured
   c. Detection of a chromosomal abnormality of the placental cells that is not confirmed on follow-up CVS or amniocentesis (rare)

  3. Percutaneous umbilical blood sampling is performed after 18 weeks of gestation. With ultrasound guidance under sterile conditions, a 22–25-gauge needle is inserted into the umbilical vein. The preferred site for sampling is at the insertion of the umbilical cord in the placenta. The fetal loss rate is around 1%. Fetal blood is aspirated and may be used to determine:
   a. Hematocrit
   b. Hemoglobin
   c. Blood group
   d. Platelet count
   e. Blood gases
   f. Culture (e.g., for toxoplasmosis)
   g. Chromosomal analysis
   h. Hemoglobin electrophoresis to exclude a hemoglobinopathy

  4. Intrauterine transfusion (see Chapter 11, Rh Isoimmunization)

  5. Insertion of shunts for a hydrocephalic fetus or a fetus with a bladder outlet obstruction

  6. Drainage of a fetal cystic mass, ascites, or pleural effusion

H. Evaluation of fetal well-being

  1. Ultrasound can help to distinguish congenital malformations by:
   a. Examining fetal organ systems
   b. Plotting the growth of a particular organ (e.g., serial limb length studies in a fetus at risk for achondroplastic dwarfism)

  2. Occasionally, ultrasound is performed to reassure the mother and to encourage bonding between the parents and their unborn child.

  3. The biophysical profile (nonstress testing and real-time ultrasound) is used to study the intrauterine behavior of the fetus (see section VII for details).

III. FIRST TRIMESTER

A. Normal development in the first trimester is suggested if a gestational sac and a fetal pole are visualized on ultrasound. The maternal bladder should be filled but not overdistended, lest compression and flattening of the gestational sac occur.

  1. The gestational sac may be measured by taking a sagittal and cross-sectional view and measuring the mean diameter. **Gestational sac mean diameter** is + 10% of the value obtained, which is accurate to within 4–5 days. The sac has a highly echogenic border from the decidual reaction and trophoblastic layer.
   a. At 5 weeks, the gestational sac occupies 25% of the uterine volume. This is the earliest point at which a sac may be seen, and the fetal heart beat may be visualized.
   b. At 6 weeks, the gestational sac occupies 35% of the uterine volume. The fetal pole, which measures about 5 mm, can usually be identified at this time.
   c. At 8 weeks, the gestational sac occupies 50% of the uterine volume. The fetal pole is identified easily, and in all pregnancies, fetal heart motion should be seen. The placenta is usually identified as an echogenic thickening of the gestational sac. The yolk sac is cystic, located adjacent to the fetus, and is usually seen until 11 weeks.

    d. At 10 weeks, the gestational sac occupies the entire uterine cavity; thus, the endometrial cavity has been obliterated. The fetal head, body, and limbs can be identified. The placenta is located by:
      (1) Its crescent shape
      (2) Its echogenicity
      (3) The site of the umbilical cord insertion
    e. At 12 weeks, the amnion fuses with the chorion.

  2. The crown–rump length is a linear measurement of the longest axis. It is most accurate (to within 3–4 days) between 8 and 12 weeks gestation, which makes it **the most accurate method for dating a pregnancy**. Usually three images are taken, and the maximum length is used as the final measurement. Errors in measurement occur after 12 weeks gestation (Fig. 13-1).

  3. Vaginal sonography is a new technique performed mostly in the first trimester with a sector probe called the **endovaginal probe**. The advantages of the endovaginal approach over the standard abdominal technique include:
    a. Greater patient comfort since the urinary bladder does *not* have to be full to afford adequate visualization.
    b. Earlier recognition of the gestational sac. With endovaginal scanning, the gestational sac is usually identified by 5 weeks from the last menstrual period, thereby excluding an ectopic pregnancy.
    c. Earlier and more accurate identification of adnexal pathology, including ectopic pregnancies.
    d. Earlier identification of a fetal heart beat. After the gestational sac reaches 8 mm in diameter, fetal heart motion is usually seen.

B. Abnormal development

  1. Impending abortion. The sonographic features of an impending abortion include:
    a. A poorly formed sac that is collapsed or demonstrates poor growth over a period of 7–14 days. A collapsed, crescent-shaped sac or an angular sac that is abnormally implanted close to the cervix may also be seen. The echogenic trophoblastic rim is usually irregular in thickness with areas in which no trophoblast is seen. However, poorly formed sacs may still develop normally, so every woman should be given the benefit of the doubt.
    b. A clot between the sac and internal os
    c. Absence of a fetal pole after the time at which it should be seen or a fetal pole without cardiac motion

  2. Ectopic pregnancy. The sonographic features of an ectopic pregnancy include:
    a. An incomplete mantle of myometrium over the entire gestational sac
    b. Absence of the endometrial cavity echo next to the gestational sac
    c. Endometrial cavity echoes that are linear, such as those found in the nonpregnant uterus
    d. A uterus of normal size or slighty enlarged
    e. Round or ovoid fluid collection surrounded by an echogenic ring (pseudosac). This ring is actually blood surrounded by a decidual cast.
    f. An adnexal mass
      (1) Sometimes a sac with fetal parts and fetal heart motion is evident.
      (2) Often there is a mass on the opposite side, representing either the corpus luteum of pregnancy or a hematoma.
      (3) A solid or cystic mass may be seen in either adnexa, consisting of blood or a chronic ectopic with overlying bowel.

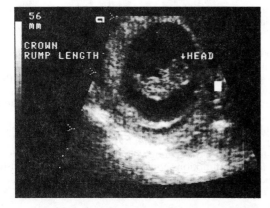

Figure 13-1. An ultrasound of the fetal crown–rump length. The fetus is surrounded by amniotic fluid (*dark shadow*).

g. Free fluid in the cul-de-sac. This may be anechoic if the ectopic pregnancy has recently ruptured.

3. Molar pregnancy (hydatidiform mole). The uterus of a molar pregnancy is larger than expected for gestational age in 50% of cases. There is a typical sonographic appearance from many fluid-filled vesicles of different sizes. Ovarian theca-lutein cysts may be found in about half the cases. The physician should rule out a co-existent fetus since management of such cases is controversial.

4. Uterine abnormalities that can be detected by ultrasound include:
  a. A bicornuate uterus in which a decidual cast is often seen in the nonpregnant cornua
  b. Leiomyoma uteri, which may present as:
    (1) An anechoic solid mass
    (2) An echogenic mass with calcification that causes shadows
    (3) A solid mass with an anechoic center from degeneration
    (4) A well-circumscribed thickening of the uterine wall

5. Ovarian abnormalities that can be detected by ultrasound include:
  a. A corpus luteum cyst of pregnancy
  b. A cystadenoma
  c. A dermoid cyst, consisting of teeth, hair, or sebaceous material, which produce echoes

6. An intact intrauterine device (IUD) will be brightly echogenic. Implantation may occur next to the IUD.

7. Multiple gestations are seen in the first trimester as multiple gestational sacs, each containing a fetus. After 10 weeks gestation, the amniotic membrane separating the fetuses should be seen unless it is a monoamniotic pregnancy. In up to 15% of twin pregnancies, one fetus will be lost in the first trimester. This is known as "the vanishing twin syndrome." The amniotic fluid, placenta, and fetal tissue are slowly reabsorbed until the remaining twin is seen as a single intrauterine pregnancy.

IV. SECOND AND THIRD TRIMESTERS. Ultrasound performed during the second and third trimesters should include measurement or evaluation of the following structures.

  A. The biparietal diameter is measured after 12 weeks gestation at the level of the triangular-shaped thalamus and the box-shaped cavum septi pellucidi. Of all the second-trimester measurements possible, the biparietal diameter reflects gestational age most closely and is reproducible to within 2 mm (standard error + or − 2 mm). The reliability of the biparietal diameter measurement to gestational age decreases as the pregnancy advances (after 26 weeks) because the biologic variability of fetal head size increases dramatically. Normal intracranial structures as well as absence of gross abnormalities, such as hydrocephaly, anencephaly, cystic structures, and meningoencephalocele, should be noted (Fig. 13-2).

  B. The abdominal circumference or transtrunk abdominal diameter may be used to evaluate the head:abdomen ratio and follow the progression of abdominal enlargement. It is taken at the level of the umbilical vein entering the liver.

    1. Fetal weight may be predicted by using the biparietal diameter, femur length, and the abdominal circumference and referring to a standardized table; it is accurate to within 10%.

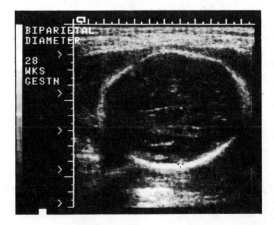

Figure 13-2. An ultrasound of a biparietal diameter measured between the calipers.

2. **The fetal head:abdominal circumference** ratio begins at a maximal value of 1.29 at 12 weeks gestation, falls to 1.00 at about 36 weeks, and is less than 1.00 after 37 weeks.
   a. **Conditions that would decrease the ratio** include:
      (1) Microcephaly
      (2) Anencephaly
      (3) Fetal abdominal enlargement associated with:
         (a) Fetal ascites
         (b) Infants of diabetic mothers
         (c) Infants with congenital anomalies, such as:
            (i) Hydronephrosis
            (ii) Intestinal obstruction

   b. **Conditions that would increase the ratio** include:
      (1) Hydrocephaly
      (2) Asymmetric intrauterine growth retardation in which the abdominal circumference is small but the head circumference is normal
      (3) Chromosomal disorders, such as triploidy
      (4) Intracranial masses or cysts
      (5) Abdominal pathology, such as diaphragmatic hernia in which the stomach contents, bowel, and liver may be in the fetal chest, rendering the abdomen small

3. **Serial measurements of the abdominal circumference** are valuable in following the progression of conditions that might enlarge the fetal abdomen, such as:
   a. Erythroblastosis fetalis with or without ascites
   b. Infants of diabetic mothers
   c. Abdominal masses, such as renal or gallbladder cysts and gastric or intestinal obstruction

C. **Fetal thorax.** Examination of the fetal thorax should include:

1. **Demonstration of fetal heart motion, a four chambered fetal heart, the side on which the fetal heart rests in the chest (exclude dextrocardia), and the fetal heart rate.** Between 16 and 24 weeks gestation, a transient but profound slowing of the fetal heart rate to 60–80 beats per minute has been observed in normal hearts.

2. **Demonstration of the fetal lung and breathing motion.** The fetal lung is fluid filled and collapsed so it has an echogenicity that is similar to other organs, such as liver and spleen. Fetal breathing includes expansion and relaxation of the chest wall and diaphragm excursions. Fetal breathing movements should be distinguished from hiccups, which are regular, forceful, and slow.

D. **Fetal abdomen.** Examination of the fetal abdomen should include the:

1. **Stomach,** which is seen as a C-shaped, fluid-filled structure caudad to the fetal heart. Sometimes fluid-filled loops of nondilated bowel are seen in the normal fetus. At term, the bowel may contain meconium, causing the bowel to be more echogenic and prominent.

2. **Liver,** which fills the upper abdomen and includes many vascular structures

3. **Umbilical vein.** In a true transverse cut of the fetal abdomen, the umbilical vein is rectangular and is not seen in its entirety. The abdominal circumference or diameter measurements are taken from a transverse section at the level where the intrahepatic umbilical vein is one-third of the way across the abdomen.

4. **Kidneys.** It is very important to visualize the fetal kidneys since many congenital anomalies involve the renal system. The kidneys are best visualized in a transverse cut, below the liver, as two relatively sonolucent circular structures on either side of the fetal spine. They are usually not seen until after 15 weeks gestation.

5. **Bladder.** This is a fluid-filled cystic structure in the pelvis. It should not be confused with amniotic fluid that is between the fetal thighs. Visualization of a fetal bladder is important to document renal function. The bladder should be seen routinely after 20 weeks gestation.

E. **Fetal limbs.** Examination of the fetal limbs should include documentation of:

1. **Four extremities**

2. **Limb motion**

3. **The length of the fetal femur or the tibia.** The lengths of the femur and humerus are usually identical before 22 weeks gestation. Femur length is accurate to within 14 days.

F. Amniotic fluid. Evaluation of the amniotic fluid should include:

1. **The amniotic fluid volume**, which is usually a subjective measurement; however, the total intrauterine volume can be calculated using the static scanner. At term, two pockets of fluid can be measured vertically from 2–8 cm in height. Over 8 cm may represent hydramnios, and under 1–2 cm may indicate oligohydramnios (see section VII). Either increased or decreased amniotic fluid volume may be an early sign of congenital anomalies.

2. **The umbilical cord**, which is usually seen in the second or third trimester unless there is oligohydramnios. Two small arteries surround the large umbilical vein where the cord is seen in cross section. A two vessel cord (single umbilical artery and vein) may be associated with:
   a. Congenital anomalies of the cardiovascular or genitourinary systems
   b. Maternal diabetes mellitus
   c. Twin gestation
   d. Increased neonatal mortality

3. **Particulate matter** that appears as bright reflections moving through the amniotic fluid. This is usually vernix, but in the third trimester, it may be meconium.

G. Fetal spine. Evaluation of the fetal spine should include:

1. **Longitudinal scans of the spine**, which show two parallel lines (posterolateral laminae) with mild normal cervical widening and gradual sacral tapering. The vertebral bodies can be identified after 14 weeks gestation. With a meningomyelocele, there is irregularity in the parallelism of the lines.

2. **Transverse scans of the spine**, which demonstrate rounded individual vertebrae without splaying of the posterolateral sections (the laminae). This projection of the spine is best visualized with a sector scanner.

V. SONOGRAPHIC DIAGNOSIS OF CONGENITAL ANOMALIES.
Ultrasound has proven to be an invaluable tool in the antenatal diagnosis of congenital anomalies. Very few infants with anomalies are heralded by a maternal history. Therefore, every prenatal examination with ultrasound should include a systematic search for congenital anomalies. Management protocols range from pregnancy termination at the time of diagnosis, to interventional procedures in utero, to early delivery, depending on the type of anomaly and stage of gestation.

A. Excessive amniotic fluid. This may be the sign heralding a problem pregnancy. Overall, 2% of pregnancies are complicated by hydramnios, while 20% of those pregnancies are due to anomalous fetuses. Polyhydramnios may be associated with malformations of the central nervous system, gastrointestinal system, and a few skeletal dysplasias.

B. Nervous system abnormalities

1. **Hydrocephaly**, a condition marked by dilation of the occipital horns of the lateral ventricles and dilation of the frontal horns, is rarely diagnosed before the eighteenth week of gestation. Generally, the ventricles begin to dilate before the biparietal diameter becomes abnormally enlarged. In utero shunts from the ventricles to the amniotic fluid have been used with varying degrees of success and uncertain benefit to long-term neurologic function.

2. **Anencephaly**, a condition marked by the absence of the cranial vault, is clearly seen early in the second trimester. The fetal head appears to stop at the top of prominent orbits, and the biparietal diameter is difficult to measure. If the head is low in the maternal pelvis, anencephaly may be mistakenly diagnosed.

3. **Microcephaly**, a condition marked by abnormal smallness of the head, is usually diagnosed after 20 or 24 weeks gestation in a fetus that had demonstrated normal head growth, followed by falling incremental head measurements. The head:body ratio is low for the gestational age. Because of the unfortunate long-term implications, a search for causes of microcephaly, such as fetal alcohol syndrome, chromosomal abnormalities, inherited syndromes, and in utero infections, should be pursued at the time of diagnosis.

4. **Defects of the neural axis** that can be diagnosed with ultrasound include:
   a. **Hydranencephaly**, which is the congenital absence of the cerebral hemispheres
   b. **Holoprosencephaly**, which is a defect in the development of midline cranial structures. Associated facial defects include cleft lip and cyclopia.
   c. **Posterior fossa cysts.** These resemble the cysts found in the Dandy-Walker syndrome (dilation of the fourth ventricle) and subarachnoid cysts.
   d. **Intracranial hemorrhage**

5. **Encephaloceles** are identified by sacular structures protruding from the bony calvarium in a frontal or occipital location. They occur in 1 in 2000 pregnancies, and should be distinguished from cystic hygromas and hemangiomas. Absence of brain tissue in the sac is the single most optimistic feature for survival that can be identified with ultrasound.

6. **Meningomyelocele (spina bifida cystica)** results from failure of fusion along the spine. In the United States the incidence is 1 in 1000 births. It may be associated with other anomalies, such as hydrocephaly and encephalocele. Movement of the fetal extremities in utero and spina bifida cystica are not mutually exclusive.

C. **Abnormalities of the thorax and abdomen**

1. The thorax may be abnormally shaped in the following clinical situations:
   a. Skeletal dysplasias
   b. Rib fractures (osteogenesis imperfecta)
   c. Oligohydramnios from renal dysplasia

2. The prenatal diagnosis of pulmonary problems, such as pleural effusions, tumors, or thoracic cysts, have been reported. Elevation of intrathoracic pressure may result in obstruction of venous return (preload) and heart failure or failure of normal lung maturation secondary to compression of normal lung tissue. Figure 13-3 is a sagittal view of a fetus with ascites and a large pleural effusion.

3. The antenatal diagnosis of cardiac problems is made with both real-time and M-mode fetal echocardiography. Both structural and functional disorders, such as arrhythmias, may be identified. Certain disorders are associated with chromosomal defects, such as endocardial cushion defects and trisomy 21.

4. Disorders of the gastrointestinal tract include:
   a. Diaphragmatic hernia
   b. Esophageal atresia
   c. Bowel obstruction
   d. Defects of the anterior abdominal wall, such as gastroschisis and omphalocele
      (1) In gastroschisis, the abdominal contents have herniated into the amniotic cavity, and a normal insertion of the umbilical cord may be identified.
      (2) In omphalocele, there is a covering membrane around the abdominal contents, and often there are associated congenital anomalies, especially of the cardiac system.

D. **Genitourinary abnormalities**

1. Two kidneys and a bladder should be recognized in every fetus after 16–20 weeks gestation, or a renal disorder should be suspected.

2. Infantile polycystic kidneys may be recognized in utero after 20 weeks gestation by enlarged kidneys filled with microscopic cysts. The adult form of polycystic kidneys has been seen antenatally.

3. Multicystic kidney disease, a condition marked by large cysts in the periphery of the kidney, is usually unilateral.

4. Several obstructive disorders have been recognized on ultrasound.
   a. Obstruction at the ureteropelvic junction is usually unilateral and associated with dilation of the renal calyces and pelves.

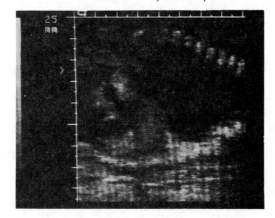

Figure 13-3. An ultrasound of a fetus at 33 weeks gestation shows the thorax on the right and the abdomen on the left. There is a large pleural effusion (only fluid is seen below the echogenic rib cage), and on the left side of the picture, there is bowel floating in ascitic fluid. Nonimmune hydrops due to a chylothorax from a thoracic duct obstruction is causing the pleural effusion.

b. Obstruction from a posterior urethral valve, found only in males, sometimes produces massive dilation of the bladder and bilateral hydroureters and hydronephrosis.

5. Renal agenesis or dysplasia should be suspected when there is decreased amniotic fluid volume. Decreased urine production and urinary output is the mechanism for low fluid volume.

E. Skeletal abnormalities

1. The short-limbed bone dysplasias, such as achondroplasia, chondroectodermal dysplasia (Ellis-van Creveld syndrome), achondrogenesis, and thanatophoric dysplasia, have been diagnosed before 22 weeks gestation in offspring of families at risk. Serial measurements of femoral and more distal bones, such as the radius, ulna, tibia, and fibula, are important. In certain syndromes, such as heterozygous achondroplasia, bone growth may not fall off until late in the second trimester.

2. Limb reduction abnormalities are found in many inherited syndromes. These include missing bones, deformed bones, and extra digits (i.e., polydactyly).

3. Fractures in utero or hypomineralization of the bony structures result from several bony disorders; the classic example of fractures is found in osteogenesis imperfecta. The hypomineralized bones in hypophosphatasia fail to produce a normal reflection and acoustic shadow of normal bone.

VI. PLACENTAL DEVELOPMENT

A. Placental localization should be performed during each ultrasound examination. As pregnancy progresses, the placenta matures, taking on different sonographic appearances. By the ninth week of gestation, the placenta is easily identified. Three basic areas of the placenta are:

1. The chorionic plate

2. The basal plate

3. The placental substance

B. Placental thickness increases linearly until 32 weeks gestation, after which time it may actually decrease. Thickness greater than 4 cm is unusual. Disorders known to increase thickness include:

1. Maternal diabetes

2. Syphilis

3. Erythroblastosis fetalis

4. Nonimmune hydrops fetalis

5. Congenital anomalies

C. Placenta previa. The diagnosis of placenta previa is easily made by ultrasound unless the posterior placenta is in the shadow of a fetus whose head is low and cannot be lifted by pelvic examination. Normally, the placenta migrates cephalad toward the fundus. Most second-trimester placenta previas are above the cervix at term unless they are accompanied by vaginal bleeding.

D. Placental abruption can sometimes be diagnosed by ultrasound. Associated findings include:

1. Increased echogenicity of one placental lobe due to fresh bleeding

2. Elevation of the chorioamniotic membrane from retroplacental blood

3. Clotted blood adjacent to the placenta

VII. THE BIOPHYSICAL PROFILE is a combination of nonstress testing and real-time ultrasound examination used to study the dynamic, intrauterine behavior of the fetus. Research has shown that normal intrauterine activities describe a functional level of the central nervous system as it relates to the environment and indicate adequate fetal oxygenation.

A. The biophysical profile consists of five variables that are scored by either 0 or 2. The maximal score for a biophysical profile is 10, and the minimal score is 0. In general, a score of 6 or more is acceptable. A score of 2 is given if the following criteria are met:

1. **Fetal breathing movement**—30 seconds of sustained breathing during a 30-minute observation

2. **Fetal movement**—three or more gross body movements in a 30-minute observation (simultaneous limb and trunk movements are counted as a single movement)

3. **Fetal tone**—at least one episode of motion of a limb from a position of flexion to extension and a rapid return to flexion

4. **Fetal reactivity**—two or more fetal heart rate accelerations of at least 15 beats/min, lasting at least 15 seconds, and associated with fetal movement in a 10–20-minute observation

5. **Qualitative amniotic fluid volume**—the presence of a pocket of amniotic fluid that measures at least 2 cm in two perpendicular planes with fluid evident throughout the uterine cavity

B. The utility of the biophysical profile is extensive. In some centers, it is being used as the primary mode of antepartum surveillance, while in others, it is only used if there is a positive or suspicious contraction stress test. For example, the biophysical profile has been employed in cases of premature rupture of the membranes. Chorioamnionitis is a known complication of premature rupture and has rarely been found in cases where the biophysical profile is good. In general, the earliest part of the profile to disappear in chorioamnionitis is the reactive nonstress test.

VIII. DOPPLER FLOW EVALUATION

A. **Introduction.** Pulsed or continuous wave Doppler has been used to evaluate blood flow in several anatomic locations within the maternal pelvis. Vessels studied so far include (Fig. 13-4):

1. External iliac artery

2. Uterine artery

3. Carotid artery

4. Umbilical artery

5. Fetal descending aorta

B. **Principles**

1. During a normal pregnancy, development of a normal placenta includes a secondary wave of trophoblastic invasion into the maternal vessels during the early second trimester. The end result is maximal dilation of the spiral arterioles (terminal branches of the uterine artery feeding the placenta), which are free from maternal autoregulation.

2. The placental blood flow is high volume with extensive flow in diastole. Uterine blood flow increases from 50 ml/min after conception to 500–700 ml/min at term.

3. During a normal pregnancy, the amount of diastolic flow increases. Placental pathology, such as a reduced number of vessels, causing fetal growth retardation, has been found in cases when the diastolic flow fails to increase as a pregnancy progresses.

C. **Artery waveforms**

1. The normal waveforms show a peak velocity in systole and a smaller amount of flow in diastole. Several different formulas have been employed to compare the systolic to diastolic (S/D) flow during one cardiac cycle (i.e., S/D ratios, S-D/S ratios, S-D/mean).

2. There is a characteristic waveform for each vessel studied (see Fig. 13-4).

3. Absence of flow in diastolic, reverse flow (toward the transducer), or notching of the waveform at the end of systole are abnormal findings and are clear indicators for intensive fetal surveillance since there is a strong association with fetal death in utero (Fig. 13-5A and B). In the umbilical circulation, when there is increased resistance in the placental vessels, there is such great back pressure during diastole that forward flow (from the fetus to the placenta) ceases. When placental resistance is most severe, the direction of flow in the umbilical artery may actually be reversed—that is, it may flow from the placenta to the fetus. In other vessels, such as the uterine artery, absent diastolic flow may occur due to spasm of the vessel. This is commonly associated with maternal hypertension.

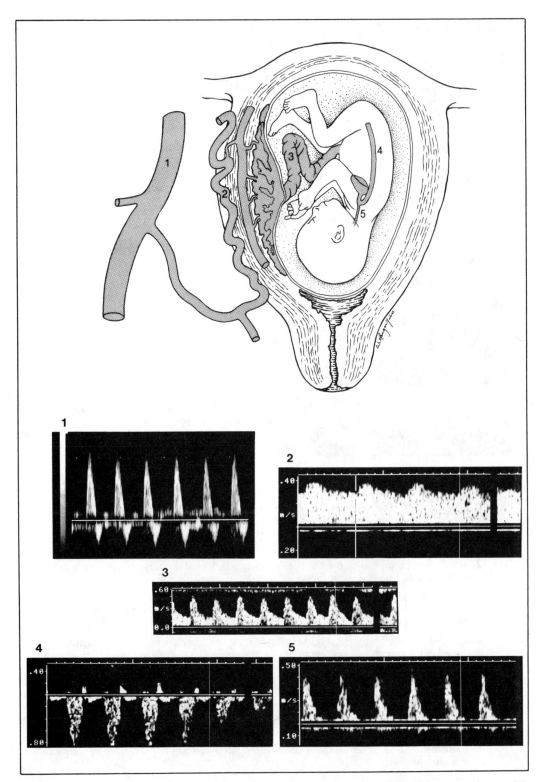

Figure 13-4. Doppler waveforms from a normal pregnancy. Shown are waveforms from (*1*) the maternal external iliac artery, (*2*) uterine artery, (*3*) umbilical artery, (*4*) descending aorta, and (*5*) carotid artery. (Reprinted with permission from Copel JA, et al: Doppler ultrasound in obstetrics. In *Williams Obstetrics*, 17th ed, Supplement, no. 16, edited by Pritchard JA, MacDonald PC, Gant NF, Appleton and Lange, Norwalk, CT, 1988.)

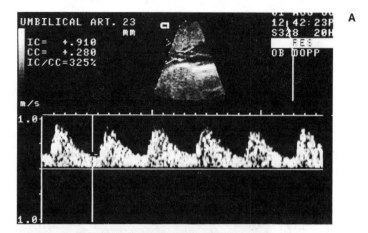

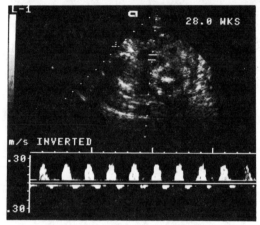

Figure 13-5. A, A normal umbilical artery waveform. The + (cross) is on the maximal velocity in diastole. B, A severely growth retarded infant at 28 weeks gestation (only the size of a 22-week gestation). The normal umbilical artery waveform in A is contrasted with an abnormal waveform, characterized by reverse diastolic flow in B.

D. Clinical applications

1. Intrauterine fetal growth retardation has been detected 60%–80% of the time in cases where the umbilical artery waveforms are abnormal. The growth retardation is usually due to uteroplacental insufficiency from a placental abnormality or maternal disorder, such as hypertension.

2. The incidence of fetal distress and a complicated neonatal course are higher in pregnancies with abnormal uterine artery waveforms than in normal pregnancies.

3. Umbilical vein blood flow velocity may be increased in maternal uterine bleeding and fetal anemia from isoimmunization. A direct correlation between velocity and hematocrit has not been observed.

4. Blood flow through the fetal aorta, mainly representing right ventricular output, may be reduced in intrauterine growth retardation. After chronic oxygen treatment to the mother, one study showed a return toward normal of aortic blood velocity.

5. Doppler has also been helpful in identifying fetal cardiac arrhythmias.

6. In twin gestations, Doppler has correctly predicted discordant growth, either from a difference in placentation or from twin–twin transfusion syndrome with placental vascular anastomosis.

7. If normal, the Doppler study is usually repeated at monthly intervals. If abnormal, it is repeated weekly.

STUDY QUESTIONS

Directions: Each question below contains four suggested answers of which **one or more** is correct. Choose the answer

    A if **1, 2, and 3** are correct
    B if **1 and 3** are correct
    C if **2 and 4** are correct
    D if **4** is correct
    E if **1, 2, 3, and 4** are correct

1. A patient has suffered from chronic hypertension for 3 years. Her blood pressure throughout the pregnancy has been well controlled. Which of the following tests should a physician order during the pregnancy?

(1) Ultrasound at 10 weeks
(2) Ultrasound at 28 weeks
(3) Doppler flow study at 32 weeks
(4) Nonstress test at 18 weeks

2. Which of the following congenital anomalies are associated with increased quantities of amniotic fluid?

(1) Duodenal atresia
(2) Anencephaly
(3) Hydrocephaly
(4) Renal agenesis

Directions: The group of questions below consists of lettered choices followed by several numbered items. For each numbered item select the **one** lettered choice with which it is **most** closely associated. Each lettered choice may be used once, more than once, or not at all.

Questions 3–7

For each fetal complication listed below, select the head:body ratio that is most likely to be associated with it.

(A) Ratio is normal for gestational age
(B) Ratio is increased for gestational age
(C) Ratio is decreased for gestational age
(D) Ratio is insignificant
(E) None of the above

3. Asymmetric intrauterine fetal growth retardation

4. Macrosomia in an infant of a diabetic mother

5. Hydrocephaly in an infant at 38 weeks gestation

6. Trisomy 21 in an infant with duodenal atresia

7. Diaphragmatic hernia in a term infant

ANSWERS AND EXPLANATIONS

1. The answer is A (1, 2, 3). [*II D 2 c (2), E 2 e; VIII B 3, D 1*] In maternal hypertension, there is a significant risk of placental insufficiency due to poor blood flow to the uterus. Since growth retardation may result from this, important testing should include a scan at 10 weeks to confirm the estimated date of conception, since it would be hard at 30 weeks to tell if the infant is small or if the due date is wrong; a scan at 28 weeks to evaluate fetal growth and amniotic fluid volume; and a Doppler at 32 weeks to test resistance and supply from placental vessels. Eighteen weeks is too early for a nonstress test.

2. The answer is A (1, 2, 3). (*IV F 1; V A, B 1, 2, D 1, 4*) Excessive quantities of amniotic fluid (polyhydramnios) are often associated with congenital anomalies of the gastrointestinal tract, nervous system, or skeletal system. The pathophysiologic mechanism may be due to impaired swallowing of amniotic fluid, such as in an anencephalic fetus, obstruction of fluid through the bowel, such as in an obstruction, or from unknown causes, such as with skeletal dysplasias. In renal agenesis, because of poor or absent kidney function, there are usually low quantities of amniotic fluid (oligohydramnios).

3–7. The answers are: 3-B, 4-C, 5-B, 6-C, 7-B. (*IV B 1–3*) The head:abdomen ratio measured as the ratio of circumferences or diameters has been used as one of the many parameters for following fetal growth. The classic example is the fetus who suffers from intrauterine malnutrition in the third trimester. This fetus may exhibit signs of head-sparing intrauterine fetal growth retardation because most blood and nutrients are sent to vital organs, such as the brain, leaching from such areas as the liver, skin, and muscle. In such instances, the head size might remain normal, but the abdominal size would be low, elevating the ratio.

In the infant of a diabetic mother, extra glucose may be stored as glycogen in the liver, rendering the abdomen larger than normal and the head:body ratio low.

In hydrocephaly, the head may be unusually large compared to the remainder of the body, rendering the ratio high.

Infants with gastrointestinal obstruction may have enlarged abdominal cavities from bowel distension. This would lower the head:abdomen ratio.

Abdominal pathology, such as diaphragmatic hernia in which the stomach contents, bowel, and liver may be in the fetal chest, may render the abdomen small and the head:abdomen ratio high.

14

Antepartum Bleeding

William W. Beck, Jr.

[拔]

产前

I. PLACENTA PREVIA

A. **DEFINITION.** In placenta previa the placenta is implanted in the lower pole of the uterus instead of high up in the fundus; it is located either over or very near the internal os. There are four degrees of placenta previa.

(中央性前置) **1. Total placenta previa.** The placenta completely covers the internal os.

部分 **2. Partial placenta previa.** The placenta partially covers the internal os.

边缘性 **3. Marginal placenta previa.** The edge of the placenta is palpable at the margin of the internal os.

低置 **4. Low-lying placenta previa.** The placenta is implanted near the internal os so that the edge of the placenta can be palpated through the cervix by the examining finger.

B. **Incidence.** Placenta previa is an infrequent complication of pregnancy, occurring in 1 out of 200 term pregnancies.

C. **Etiology**

1. While little is known about the cause of placenta previa, the following factors are thought to play a role:
   a. It is more common in multiparous women: About 20% of all cases of placenta previa occur in primigravidas.
   b. Women over 35, regardless of parity, are more likely to have placenta previa than women under 25.
   c. A previous history of placenta previa is rare.

2. Placenta previa is fundamentally an abnormality in the implantation of the placenta. Several factors that contribute to this abnormal placentation are associated with advanced maternal age and parity.
   a. Defective vascularization of the decidua as a result of atrophic changes or inflammation
   b. Scarring of the endometrium with advanced maternal age as a result of repeated pregnancies
   c. Changes in vessels at the placental site that decrease the blood supply to the endometrium and necessitate a greater surface area for placental attachment to provide adequate maternal blood flow
   d. Multiple pregnancies (twins or triplets), which increase the surface area of placental implantation so that the lower portion of the placenta approaches the region of the internal os
   e. Erythroblastosis, which is often accompanied by a large placenta
   f. Alterations of the blood supply to the endometrium and changes in the quality and depth of the endometrium as a result of a previous incision in the lower uterine segment (i.e., myomectomy, cesarean section, or hysterotomy)

D. **Clinical presentation**

1. **Painless vaginal bleeding** in the third trimester is the most characteristic sign of placenta previa.
   a. This bleeding can occur:
      (1) During rest or activity
      (2) Suddenly and without warning

(3) After trauma, coitus, or a pelvic examination
b. Bleeding usually occurs for the first time early in the third trimester when the lower uterine segment begins to change, causing the cervix to efface and dilate. Bleeding results from the tearing of the placental attachments at or near the internal os as the cervix changes. The bleeding continues because the stretched fibers of the lower uterine segment are unable to contract (because of the undelivered pregnancy) and compress the torn vessels.
2. Maternal blood loss and fetal morbidity are problems encountered with placenta previa.
　a. Maternal bleeding can be made worse by a pelvic examination, if the diagnosis is not suspected, resulting in maternal shock due to acute blood loss.
　b. Fetal distress can result if the mother is in shock.
　c. If delivery becomes necessary at less than 34 weeks gestation because of maternal bleeding, the infant may experience the complications of prematurity.

E. Diagnosis

1. Placenta previa should always be suspected in the presence of painless vaginal bleeding in the third trimester. The index of suspicion is heightened if any of the following clinical findings accompany vaginal bleeding:
　a. Malposition of the fetus (breech or transverse lie)
　b. Multiple gestation
　c. Multiparity or advanced maternal age

2. Women suspected of having placenta previa should be examined to rule out other causes of third-trimester bleeding; the examination should always be performed in a hospital.

3. Indirect methods of diagnosing placenta previa at any time in the third trimester include:
　a. Ultrasound scanning, which is 90%–95% accurate
　b. Isotope scanning, amniography, and arteriography, which are invasive methods that are potentially dangerous to the mother and fetus because they involve radiation, amniocentesis, and arterial puncture

4. Definitive diagnosis of placenta previa is made by passing a finger through the cervix and palpating the placenta or the edge of the placenta. Since this can precipitate hemorrhage, such an examination should never be undertaken unless:
　a. Delivery is contemplated at the time of the examination.
　b. The examination is performed in the delivery room with the patient prepared for a cesarean section, meaning that blood is crossmatched and anesthesia is available.
　c. The pregnancy is at or near term with or without ongoing bleeding.
　d. The bleeding is continuous and dangerous at any time during the third trimester.

F. Management

1. Management of placenta previa is based on three principles.
　a. The initial hemorrhage in placenta previa, in the absence of digital manipulation of the cervix, **is rarely fatal**.
　b. Vaginal or rectal examination often precipitates severe bleeding.
　c. The major cause of perinatal loss in placenta previa **is prematurity**.

2. Expectant management. Watchful waiting is justifiable in placenta previa if the fetus is premature and can benefit from further intrauterine development. However, an expectant attitude is appropriate only if labor has not begun, the fetus is stable, and the bleeding is not severe. Expectant therapy should proceed in the following steps:
　a. Hospitalization
　b. Careful speculum examination to rule out local lesions of the cervix and vagina
　c. Careful evaluation of the fetal monitoring strip to rule out the possibility of abruptio placentae
　d. Placental localization and determination of the type of placenta previa
　e. Close observation either in the hospital or at home; in the latter case, with careful instructions to restrict activity, to refrain from sexual intercourse, and to return to the hospital if bleeding recurs

3. Decisions concerning delivery are based on the gestational age of the fetus and the amount of maternal bleeding. Delivery of the infant in a woman with placenta previa is accomplished by cesarean section with the following guidelines:
　a. The delivery is performed electively when the fetus weighs more than 2500 g and the gestational age is 37 weeks or more as determined by ultrasound, the amniotic fluid lecithin/sphingomyelin (L/S) ratio, and the presence of phosphatidylglycerol.
　b. The delivery is performed acutely when the amount of bleeding presents a threat to the mother, regardless of fetal size or gestational age.

G. Complications

1. Cerebral problems (Sheehan's syndrome) or renal damage (acute tubular necrosis) may result from excessive blood loss and prolonged hypotension.

2. Severe postpartum hemorrhage can result because the site of placental implantation is in the lower uterine segment, which has diminished muscle content; thus, muscle contraction to control bleeding may be less effective.

3. Placenta accreta (the growth of placental tissue into the myometrium) may appear in patients with placenta previa as a result of the thinner endometrium in the lower uterine segment and an inability to control the invasive properties of the trophoblast.

II. ABRUPTIO PLACENTAE

A. Definition. In abruptio placentae, or placental abruption, the normally implanted placenta (not a placenta previa) prematurely separates from the uterus before the delivery of the fetus. The hemorrhage involved in placental abruption includes:

1. External hemorrhage. With this type of bleeding, there is:
 a. Peripheral detachment of the placenta and membranes
 b. Escape of blood through the cervix
 c. External bleeding

2. Concealed hemorrhage. Less frequently, there is bleeding between the placenta and the uterus with the periphery of the placenta and the membranes still adherent to the uterus. The blood is trapped behind the placenta and does not escape.

B. Incidence. Placental abruption occurs in approximately 1 out of 100–120 deliveries.

C. Etiology. The pathophysiology of abruptio placentae involves the spontaneous rupture of blood vessels at the placental bed, the inability of the uterus to contract and thus close off torn vessels, and the formation of a retroplacental clot.

1. Maternal hypertension has been associated with about one-half of the cases of severe placental abruption. **Chronic vascular disease** and **pregnancy-induced hypertension** are equally responsible.

2. Less frequent associations include:
 a. Trauma in the form of a direct blow to the uterus, forceful external version, or needle puncture at the time of amniocentesis—a rare etiologic cause for placental abruption
 b. Sudden decompression of the uterus, with rupture of membranes in polyhydramnios or the delivery of the first infant in a twin gestation, which leads to a shearing effect on the placenta as the uterus contracts

D. Clinical presentation. The clinical signs of placental abruption vary with the type and degree of placental detachment. Peripheral detachment and bleeding are usually less severe than central detachment with concealed bleeding. Abruptio placentae is designated as mild, moderate, or severe, depending on both the maternal and the fetal condition.

1. Mild abruptio placentae is characterized by:
 a. Scant to moderate dark vaginal bleeding
 b. Absence of fetal distress
 c. Minimal blood loss with stable maternal vital signs
 d. Lower abdominal discomfort
 e. Incomplete relaxation of the uterus with each contraction

2. Moderate abruptio placentae is characterized by:
 a. Separation of one-fourth to one-half of the placental surface
 b. Gradual or abrupt onset of symptoms with the appearance of continuous uterine pain and moderate vaginal bleeding
 c. Uterine tenderness with the maintenance of a sustained firm or partial contraction
 d. Fetal distress

3. Severe abruptio placentae is characterized by:
 a. Separation of over one-half of the placental surface
 b. Abrupt onset, usually without warning
 c. Continuous knife-like, tearing uterine pain with a board-like, unrelaxed uterus
 d. Moderate or absent (because of concealed hemorrhage) external bleeding
 e. Severe fetal distress or demise
 f. Occasional association with shock, consumption coagulopathy, or oliguria

E. Diagnosis

1. Placental abruption is basically a clinical diagnosis that depends on **signs and symptoms** and a **high index of suspicion**.

2. The **fetal monitor** may reveal a loss of **variability** or **late decelerations**. The **contraction monitor** may show **coupled contractions** without the return of uterine relaxation to baseline resting tone and an increased frequency of contractions.

3. **Premature uterine contractions that cannot be controlled with tocolytic agents** suggest a small or chronic abruption.

4. The demonstration of a **retroplacental clot** by ultrasound scan is occasionally helpful in making the diagnosis of placental abruption.

5. Clotting studies may reveal thrombocytopenia, hypofibrinogenemia, and fibrin-split products.

F. Management. The course of action is dependent on the condition of the mother and fetus and on the estimated degree of placental abruption. No matter what clinical course is followed, there must be a constant awareness of the potential for the development of hypovolemia secondary to blood loss with the need for adequate replacement of intravenous fluids and whole blood.

1. **Immediate delivery is not necessary if the fetus is alive and not distressed**, as in the case of mild placental abruption. However, there must be close fetal monitoring for fetal distress and a good progression of labor. Cesarean section is indicated whenever distress is detected or maternal hemorrhage becomes a factor.

2. **A rapid delivery must be accomplished if the fetus is alive and distressed** with the following factors being considered:
   a. The decision between vaginal delivery versus cesarean section is determined by the cervical dilation, the parity of the woman, and the labor pattern.
   b. A vaginal delivery is acceptable if the cervix is widely dilated, if the woman is in a good labor pattern, and if the vaginal delivery can be accomplished within a short period of time.
   c. For moderate to severe placental abruption, cesarean section should be chosen for the sake of the fetus. Because the extent of the placental abruption can always progress, a cesarean section is indicated if the fetus cannot quickly be delivered vaginally.

3. **Vaginal delivery is preferred if the fetus is dead** unless the hemorrhage is so brisk that it cannot be controlled by blood replacement. Amniotomy and oxytocin are helpful in hastening the vaginal delivery of a dead fetus.

G. Complications

1. **Hemorrhagic shock** from blood loss can occur with either concealed or external bleeding.

2. **Consumption coagulopathy**
   a. This bleeding diathesis occurs in 30% of cases of severe placental abruption with fetal demise. The disseminated intravascular coagulation occurs because of thromboplastin that enters the circulation from the retroplacental clot. Abnormal laboratory values include thrombocytopenia, hypofibrinogenemia, abnormal clot formation, and elevated fibrin-split products.
   b. Consumption coagulopathy is treated with:
      (1) Vigorous hydration with intravenous fluids
      (2) Fibrinogen replacement when hypofibrinogenemia is severe and surgery is contemplated
      (3) Avoidance of the use of heparin as a method of interrupting the disseminated intravascular coagulation
      (4) Prompt termination of the pregnancy, which causes the coagulation defects to repair spontaneously within 24 hours

3. **Renal failure** in the form of acute tubular necrosis and cortical necrosis is rare. Renal failure in severe abruption is due to intrarenal vasospasm as the consequence of massive hemorrhage and hypovolemia.

4. **Couvelaire uterus** is caused by widespread extravasation of blood into the uterine musculature and beneath the serosa of the uterus. These myometrial hematomas seldom interfere with uterine contractions and respond well to intravenous oxytocin. A Couvelaire uterus is not an indication for a hysterectomy.

III. OTHER CAUSES OF THIRD-TRIMESTER BLEEDING

A. Obstetric. Although much less common than placenta previa and abruptio placentae, entities such as bloody show, ruptured uterus, and ruptured vasa previa can present as worrisome third-trimester bleeding.

1. Bloody show usually has an admixture of mucus and is associated with labor.

2. Ruptured vasa previa is very serious because the fetus can bleed to death; this extremely rare condition should be considered when fetal distress accompanies **painless vaginal bleeding (no uterine contractions)**. The problem is caused by the rupture of a placental vessel, which allows the fetus to lose blood.

3. A ruptured uterus must be considered when there is excessive blood loss in a well-contracted uterus after the removal of the placenta.

B. Nonobstetric. Local factors in the vagina and on the cervix can cause bleeding and should be ruled out by visual inspection so that unnecessary cesarean sections are not performed. These include:

1. Vaginal lacerations or condyloma acuminatum

2. Erosions, polyps, or condyloma acuminatum of the cervix

3. Carcinoma of the cervix

STUDY QUESTIONS

Directions: Each question below contains five suggested answers. Choose the **one best** response to each question.

1. All of the following signs or symptoms characterize placenta previa EXCEPT

(A) painless vaginal bleeding
(B) increased uterine tone
(C) thinning of the lower uterine segment
(D) early third-trimester bleeding
(E) erythroblastosis

2. With painless vaginal bleeding at 37 weeks gestation, which of the following measures is immediately indicated?

(A) Cesarean section delivery
(B) Induction of labor
(C) Coagulation profile
(D) Rupture of membranes
(E) Speculum examination of the vagina

3. All of the following signs or symptoms characterize severe placental abruption EXCEPT

(A) fetal demise
(B) tetanic uterine contractions
(C) retroplacental clot
(D) extensive external bleeding
(E) severe abdominal pain

4. Severe placental abruption has been associated with all of the following conditions EXCEPT

(A) fetal demise
(B) renal failure
(C) thrombocytopenia
(D) Rh sensitization
(E) hypertension

Directions: Each question below contains four suggested answers of which **one or more** is correct. Choose the answer

A   if **1, 2, and 3** are correct
B   if **1 and 3** are correct
C   if **2 and 4** are correct
D   if **4** is correct
E   if **1, 2, 3, and 4** are correct

5. Clinical situations that may lead to the formation of placenta previa include

(1) defective vascularization of the decidua
(2) maternal hypertension
(3) multiple pregnancies
(4) trauma

6. Postpartum hemorrhage following placenta previa may be complicated by

(1) implantation in the lower uterine segment
(2) acute tubular necrosis
(3) ineffective uterine muscular control
(4) retained placental fragments

7. Management of suspected abruptio placentae should include

(1) a coagulation profile
(2) fetal monitoring
(3) measurement of urinary output
(4) intravenous heparin

Directions: The group of questions below consists of lettered choices followed by several numbered items. For each numbered item select the **one** lettered choice with which it is **most** closely associated. Each lettered choice may be used once, more than once, or not at all.

Questions 8 and 9

For each clinical presentation listed below, select the condition that it is most likely to represent.

(A) Ruptured vasa previa
(B) Placenta previa
(C) Ruptured uterus
(D) Bloody show
(E) Cervical cancer

8.   A woman presents in active labor with significant vaginal bleeding. She is incoherent but does say that she had had a previous cesarean section. Fetal heart tones are heard at 60/min.

9.   A 39-year-old patient who has had no previous obstetric care presents to the labor floor at term with heavy vaginal bleeding. Her last pregnancy was 12 years ago. Examination of the abdomen with ultrasound reveals a fetal heart rate of 145/min and a fundal placenta.

ANSWERS AND EXPLANATIONS

1. The answer is B. *(I C 2 c, e, D 1)* Increased uterine tone is one of the cardinal signs of abruptio placentae and is due to the bleeding behind the placenta as it prematurely separates from the uterus. Placenta previa appears first early in the third trimester when changes begin to take place in the lower uterine segment. As that segment starts to thin out, the vascular connections of the overlying placenta are broken, leading to painless bleeding. Erythroblastosis is frequently associated with placenta previa because of the characteristic large placenta, which can cover much of the uterine cavity, including the lower uterine segment.

2. The answer is E. *(I E, F)* With painless vaginal bleeding at 37 weeks gestation, there is no longer a danger of delivering a premature infant, but there may be a question about the diagnosis. Rupture of the membranes, induction of labor, and cesarean section all imply that the diagnosis of placenta previa is without question and that delivery is indicated. Both induction of labor and rupture of membranes could lead to excessive bleeding if placenta previa were present. There is no need to do an immediate coagulation profile with suspected placenta previa, as changes in coagulation occur in abruptio placentae. The most important aspect of painless vaginal bleeding is its cause, which may not be placenta previa; therefore, a speculum examination of the vagina is immediately indicated to rule out cervical and vaginal causes of the bleeding.

3. The answer is D. *(II C, D 1–3)* Severe placental abruption is characterized by a central detachment of the placenta so that there is bleeding between the uterine wall and the placenta without any external bleeding. The blood is trapped behind the placenta, forming a retroplacental clot, which leads to tetanic uterine contractions and severe abdominal pain. In this situation, the fetus usually dies. There is very little, if any, external bleeding because the placental separation is central and not peripheral.

4. The answer is D. *(II C 1, D 1–3, E 5, G 2)* By definition, severe placental abruption means that over half of the placenta has separated. Because of that extensive separation, the fetus often dies from lack of blood and oxygen. Associated with severe placental abruption are both acute tubular necrosis and consumption coagulopathy with thrombocytopenia. Hypertension is a common association with abruptio placentae in general. On the other hand, Rh sensitization and erythroblastosis with its large placenta are often accompanied by placenta previa.

5. The answer is B (1, 3). *(I C 2; II C 1, 2)* Conditions that encourage the growth of the placenta over large areas lead to placenta previa and implantation in the lower uterine segment. Defective vascularization of the decidua and the large placentas of multiple gestations are good examples. Other factors that may encourage abnormal placentation include scarring of the endometrium as a result of repeated pregnancies, erythroblastosis, and alterations of the blood supply to the endometrium. Maternal hypertension and trauma are associated with placental abruption.

6. The answer is E (all). *(I G 1–3)* Postpartum hemorrhage is always a possibility following a delivery complicated by placenta previa. Because the placenta is implanted in the lower uterine segment where there is less muscle than in the fundus, the postpartum muscular contractions may be ineffective, allowing for continuous bleeding from the placental site. With heavy bleeding and hypotension, renal damage with acute tubular necrosis can occur. Because of the association of placenta previa with placenta accreta, small pieces of placenta may adhere to the uterus, remain in situ, and prevent the uterus from contracting down enough to close off vessels bleeding from the placental site.

7. The answer is A (1, 2, 3). *(II F, G)* Abruptio placentae may be mild, moderate, or severe. There is always the danger of severe fetal distress, so there must be constant fetal monitoring. In the severe form of abruption, the complications may be consumption coagulopathy and acute tubular necrosis, and so the coagulation picture and the urinary output must be monitored. Heparin therapy is not indicated in the management of abruption; prompt delivery should correct the consumption coagulopathy and obviate the need for heparin.

8 and 9. The answers are: 8-C, 9-E. *(III B 3)* The key to the diagnosis of the woman in active labor is the previous cesarean section and her moribund condition. Such a picture is not typical of either placenta previa or vasa previa. There is usually not enough blood loss with placenta previa to affect both the patient and the fetus, and only the fetus is affected with vasa previa. This patient had a previous cesarean section, and the scar represents a potential weak spot. With a ruptured uterus, there can be a great deal of blood loss, much of it hidden if the bleeding is intra-abdominal. If the placenta is involved with the rupture, the fetus can become distressed very quickly. The hypotension by itself can lead to fetal distress.

The woman who presents with heavy vaginal bleeding does not have a placenta previa or vasa previa because of the ultrasound findings, that is, a normal fetal heart rate and a fundal placenta. There is no historical reason to suggest a ruptured uterus, and the bleeding is too heavy for bloody show. This patient has a previously unattended advanced cervical cancer, which has locally eroded into a blood vessel and caused the bleeding. She had not been seen for a number of years, including during this pregnancy and has had no Pap smear for over 10 years.

15
Teratology
Nancy S. Roberts

I. INTRODUCTION. A teratogenic agent is any chemical (drug), infection, or physical or deficiency state that can alter fetal morphology or subsequent function if the fetus is exposed during a critical stage of development. Teratogenicity appears to be related to genetic predisposition (both maternal and embryonic), the developmental stage of the fetus at the time of exposure, and the route and length of administration of the teratogen. Women in their reproductive years, who may be pregnant, should not be given *any* medication unless it is absolutely necessary. If drugs are medically indicated, the women should be warned of their teratogenic potential (Table 15-1).

A. Genetic susceptibility. Species differences in response to teratogens have been demonstrated. Human newborns exposed to the tranquilizer thalidomide in utero demonstrated major malformation of the arms (phocomelia), whereas laboratory animals (rats) showed no effect at similar doses.

B. Developmental stage at time of exposure (Fig. 15-1). Susceptibility of the conceptus to teratogenic agents depends on the developmental stage at the time of exposure.

1. **Resistant period.** From day 0 to day 7 of gestation (postovulation), the fetus exhibits the "all or none" phenomenon—that is, it will either be killed by the insult or will survive unaffected. This is the period of predifferentiation when the aggregate of totipotential cells can recover from an injury and continue to multiply.

2. **Maximum susceptibility (embryonic period).** From day 7 to day 57 of gestation, the fetus is undergoing organ differentiation and, at this time, is *most susceptible* to the adverse effects of teratogens. The particular malformation is dependent on the time of exposure. After a certain time in organogenesis, it is felt that abnormal embryogenesis can no longer occur. For example, since the neural tube closes between day 22–28 postconception (5 weeks after the last menstrual period), a teratogen must be active before or during this period to initiate development of a neural tube defect (e.g., spina bifida or anencephaly).

3. **Lowered susceptibility (fetal period).** After 57 days (8 weeks) of gestation, the organs have formed and are increasing in size. A teratogen at this stage may cause a reduction in cell size and number, which is manifested by:
   a. Growth retardation
   b. Reduction of organ size
   c. Functional derangements of organ systems

Table 15-1. Causes of Congenital Anomalies

Cause	Percent of Total
Multifactorial or unknown	65%–75%
Genetic	20%–25%
Environmental	
Intrauterine infections	3%
Maternal metabolic disorders	4%
Environmental chemicals	4%
Drugs and medications	< 1%
Ionizing radiation	1%–2%

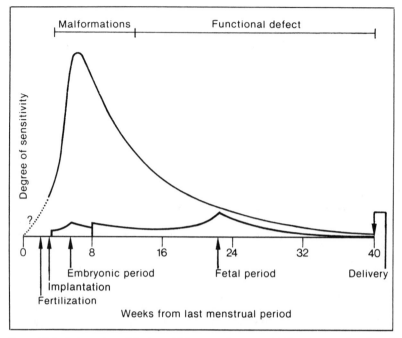

Figure 15-1. Embryonic and fetal sensitivity to environmental influences as a function of developmental stage. (Reprinted with permission from Creasy RK, Resnik R: *Maternal-Fetal Medicine: Principles and Practice.* Philadelphia, WB Saunders, 1984, p 95.)

C. The route and length of administration of a teratogen alter the type and severity of the malformation produced. Abnormal developments increase in frequency and degree as the dosage increases. Agents may be less teratogenic if systemic blood levels are reduced by the route of administration (e.g., poor gastrointestinal antibiotic absorption may account for lower blood levels in pregnancy).

D. Teratogenicity of an agent or factor is defined by the following criteria:

1. Presence during the critical period of development when the anomaly was likely to appear

2. Production of the anomaly in experimental animals when administered during a stage of organogenesis similar to that of humans. Teratogenicity may not become apparent for several years; for example, in utero exposure to diethylstilbestrol is known to cause genital tract abnormalities, such as adenosis and carcinoma, but these abnormalities may not become apparent until the reproductive years.

3. The ability to act on the embryo or fetus either directly or indirectly through the placenta [e.g., heparin is not teratogenic because, unlike warfarin (Coumadin), it cannot cross the placenta because of its large molecular weight]

II. TERATOGENIC AGENTS

A. Ionizing radiation

1. **Acute high dose** (over 250 rads). The dose of radiation as well as the gestational age during exposure are predictive of the adverse neonatal effects: microcephaly, mental retardation, and growth retardation. For example, the in utero victims of the atomic explosions in Hiroshima and Nagasaki have suffered from both birth defects and leukemia. However, follow-up studies have shown that the largest number of children with these adverse effects were those exposed *before* 15 weeks gestation, during the period of organogenesis, while most of the children exposed during the third trimester had growth retardation but normal intelligence.

   a. Time of exposure. Fetal effects are dependent on the gestational age (postovulation) at the time of exposure.

   (1) At 2–4 weeks, either the fetus is normal or a spontaneous abortion occurs.

   (2) At 4–12 weeks, the fetus may have microcephaly, mental retardation, cataracts, growth retardation, or microphthalmia.

    (3) At 12–16 weeks, there is mental retardation or growth retardation.
    (4) After 20 weeks, the effects are the same as with postnatal exposure:
        (a) Hair loss
        (b) Skin lesions
        (c) Bone marrow suppression
  b. Dose effect
    (1) After exposure to less than 5 rads, and probably less than 10 rads, an adverse fetal out-some is unlikely to result.
    (2) After exposure to 10–25 rads, there may be some adverse fetal effects.
    (3) After exposure to over 25 rads, classic fetal effects, including growth retardation, struc-tural malformations, and fetal resorption may be detected. At this level of exposure, termination of the pregnancy should be offered as an option.

2. Chronic low dose
  a. In diagnostic radiation, the dose to the conceptus should be calculated by the hospital's radiation biologist (Table 15-2). Rarely, does such a dose add up to significant exposure even if several x-ray studies are performed. Interpretation of the fetal effects should be based on the criteria stated above in section II A 1 b (1)–(3).
  b. Risks of teratogenicity
    (1) The mutagenic effects of radiation, if present, have proven to be very small. The esti-mated risk of leukemia for children exposed in utero to radiation during maternal x-ray pelvimetry increases from 1 in 3000 unexposed children to 1 in 2000.
    (2) The results of several studies provide no conclusive evidence that links preconceptual low-dose radiation with an increased risk of delivering an infant with a chromosomal abnormality.

3. Radioactive iodine. Radiation exposure from radioisotopes administered internally for organ visualization is roughly equal to that of x-ray procedures; however, after the tenth week of gestation, fetal thyroid development can be retarded in addition to any adverse effects of radi-ation. Iodine-containing cough preparations, antiseptic solutions, or x-ray adjuncts should be avoided throughout pregnancy.

B. Drugs and medications. In the United States, surveys show that 45%–95% of pregnant women ingest either over-the-counter or prescription drugs, other than iron and vitamins during their pregnancy. Many are taken before a woman realizes that she is pregnant or *without* the advice of a physician. The issue of whether a medication is harmful to the fetus is raised in most preg-nancies.

  1. Congenital malformations. Three to five precent of newborns have congenital malforma-tions caused by a host of environmental and genetic factors, most of which are unable to be identified. Drugs and medications comprise less than 1% of these factors (see Table 15-1).

  2. Access to the fetoplacental unit is critical in the causation of developmental anomalies. Fac-tors affecting access of the drug or medication to the fetus include:
    a. Maternal absorption
    b. Drug metabolism
    c. Protein binding and storage
    d. Molecular size
    e. Electrical charge
    f. Lipid solubility

  3. Animal research is helpful in identifying teratogenic potential, but results may be misleading because of species variation. The most striking example is the thalidomide debacle in which

Table 15-2. Uterine Exposure to Diagnostic Radiation

Examination	No. Films/ Examination	Average Radiation Dose to Uterus/ Examination
Chest	2.0	1–8 mR
Hip and pelvis	1.5	220 mR
Upper gastrointestinal series	4.2	558 mR
Barium enema	11.6	1080 mR
Kidney, ureters, and bladder	1.9	140 mR
Intravenous pyelogram	5.0	308 mR

exposure failed to produce limb defects in the animals tested (mice and rats) but caused severe limb reduction defects in humans, monkeys, and rabbits. Of the 1600 drugs that have been tested in *animals*, about one-half cause congenital anomalies; however, there are only 30 documented *human* teratogens.

4. **Risk factors for adverse fetal effects** have been assigned to all drugs based on the teratogenic risk that the drug poses to the fetus. Below is an outline that has been proposed by the Food and Drug Administration, which is generally accepted by manufacturers and authors.

   a. **Category A**: Controlled studies fail to demonstrate a risk to the fetus (e.g., prenatal vitamins).

   b. **Category B**: Animal studies have not demonstrated a fetal risk, but there are no controlled studies in pregnant women. Also, in this category, there are drugs that may have shown an adverse effect in animals that was not reproduced in human subjects (e.g., penicillins, digoxin, epinephrine, and terbutaline).

   c. **Category C**: Animal studies have shown either teratogenic or embryocidal effects on the fetus, but there have been no human studies. These drugs should be administered only when their benefit outweighs the potential fetal harm (e.g., furosemide, quinidine, verapamil, and β-blockers)

   d. **Category D**: There is evidence of fetal risk in humans. The benefit may outweigh the fetal risk in certain extenuating circumstances (e.g., phenytoin).

   e. **Category X**: Studies in animals or humans have demonstrated clear fetal risk. The drugs in this category are contraindicated in women who are or may become pregnant [e.g., isotretinoin (Accutane)].

5. **Known teratogenic drugs.** There is a surprisingly short list of proven teratogens. Certain commonly used agents should be avoided even while a patient is trying to conceive. These include the vitamin A isomer isotretinoin or doses of vitamin A over 8000 IU daily, alcohol, caffeine, and some of the sex steroids. The live-virus vaccines, such as rubella, should *never* be prescribed if a patient is possibly pregnant or planning to conceive within 3 months. However, if the aforementioned drugs are inadvertently given, the outcome is still usually favorable. The most common drugs and environmental chemicals known to cause congenital anomalies are listed in Table 15-3.

6. **"Recreational" drugs.** The problem of recreational drugs has become epidemic over the past 5 years. Since most recreational drugs are taken with other agents, such as alcohol or tranquilizers, the precise effect is difficult to ascertain. Listed below are commonly used drugs and their potential effects.

   a. **Alcohol.** Consumption of alcohol in pregnancy is the most common known teratogenic cause of mental retardation. Both abortion and stillbirth are increased in heavy drinkers. The **fetal alcohol syndrome**, which manifests as mental retardation, growth retardation, abnormal facies, ocular and joint anomalies, and cardiac defects, has been associated with the ingestion of 1 oz or more of absolute alcohol per day.

      (1) **The threshold dose of alcohol** at which point congenital anomalies are induced is unknown, so alcohol consumption in pregnancy can never be regarded as "safe."

      (2) **Early exposure.** The critical period for facial dysmorphology has been found to be around the time of conception.

      (3) **Late exposure.** Exposure late in gestation or in small quantities may result in isolated effects, such as learning or behavioral disorders.

      (4) **Heavy alcohol consumption** (over 3 oz of absolute alcohol or six drinks) is associated with some of the features of the fetal alcohol syndrome or the full-blown syndrome, consisting of:

         (a) **Prenatal or postnatal growth retardation.** Growth retardation is usually prenatal in onset, but postnatal catch-up generally does not occur. It is manifested by decreased birth weight, length, and head circumference.

         (b) **Central nervous system involvement** includes small brain size and brain malformations. Functional deficits, such as moderate mental retardation, delayed motor development, poor coordination, tremulousness, hyperactivity, and poor attention spans, have been noted.

         (c) **Characteristic facial dysmorphology** includes a shortened palpebral fissure (observed in over 90% of affected children), short upturned nose, hypoplastic maxilla, and a thinned upper lip. One study linked craniofacial abnormalities with prenatal alcohol exposure in a dose-response manner.

      (5) **Risk of the fetal alcohol syndrome.** A large number of children whose mothers drank moderately or heavily during pregnancy may exhibit features of prenatal alcohol exposure, such as developmental delay, but not the full-blown syndrome.

         (a) Thirty percent of children born to chronic alcoholic women will have the fetal alcohol syndrome.

Table 15-3. Drugs and Environmental Chemicals That Cause Congenital Defects

Substances	Defects
Alcohol	The principal features of the fetal alcohol syndrome include prenatal onset growth deficiency, developmental delay, short palpebral fissures, a long philtrum with a thin upper lip, multiple joint anomalies, and cardiac defects.
Androgenic hormones	
Testosterone	Masculinization of the female fetus
Progestins	Masculinization of the female fetus (clitorimegaly), genital deformities of male (hypospadias) and female (fusion of the labia majora) fetuses, and cardiac defects
Cancer chemotherapeutic agents	
Aminopterin and methyl aminopterin (folate antagonists)	Small stature; abnormal cranial ossification, leading to a malformed head, hypoplastic orbital ridges, ocular hypertelorism, small low-set ears, and micrognathia; cleft or arched palate; hydrocephaly; and myelomeningoceles
Busulfan (alkylating agents)	Cleft palate and eye defects, hydronephrosis, growth retardation, and unilateral renal agenesis (one case)
Chlorambucil	Unilateral renal and ureteral agenesis (one case)
Cyclophosphamide	Absence of toes and flattening of nasal bridge
Diethylstilbestrol	Both anatomic and functional defects in the female with cervical hood, T-shaped uterus, hypoplastic uterus, ovulatory disorders, infertility, premature labor, and cervical incompetence.
Diphenylhydantoin (Dilantin)	Intrauterine exposure was previously thought to comprise a specific pattern of malformations known as the fetal hydantoin syndrome, including growth and mental retardation, microcephaly, ridged metopic suture, inner epicanthal folds, eyelid ptosis, depressed nasal bridge, nail hypoplasia, and hernias. Thirty percent of infants exposed to phenytoin (Dilantin) in utero exhibit only minor craniofacial abnormalities and digital anomalies and not the full-blown syndrome. Anomalies appearing most frequently among infants exposed in utero to anticonvulsants are oral clefts and congenital heart defects.
Isotretinoin (Accutane)	Central nervous system defects, facial palsy, deafness, and congenital heart defects
Lead	Abortion from embryotoxicity, growth retardation, increased perinatal mortality, and developmental delay
Lithium	Cardiac defects, including Ebstein's anomaly and malformations of the great vessels
Organic mercury	Fetal neurologic damage including seizures, psychomotor retardation, cerebral palsy, blindness, and deafness
Polybrominated biphenyls (PBBs)	There are no good human studies, but in rats, PBBs were not teratogenic unless the dosage was high enough to cause maternal death.
Polychlorinated biphenyls (PCBs)	Intrauterine growth retardation, dark brown skin pigmentation, exophthalmos, gingival hyperplasia, skull calcification, low IQ, and neurobehavioral abnormalities
Streptomycin	Fetal ototoxicity due to eighth nerve damage

Table 15-3. Continued

Substances	Defects
Tetracycline	If tetracycline is given after the fourth month, it may result in deciduous teeth that are yellow, abnormally susceptible to decay, and have enamel hypoplasia. The permanent teeth are unaffected.
Thalidomide	Limb reduction, ear and nasal anomalies, cardiac and lung defects, pyloric or duodenal stenosis, and gastrointestinal atresia
Thiourea compounds	Inhibited thyroid function
Trimethadione	The features of a fetal trimethadione syndrome include prenatal onset growth delay, mental deficiency, cardiac septal defects, and typical facies, consisting of a short upturned nose with a broad and low nasal bridge, prominent forehead, upslanted eyebrows, and a poorly developed overlapping helix of the external ear.
Warfarin (Coumadin)	First-trimester exposure (between the sixth and ninth weeks) may result in a syndrome resembling the genetic disorder, Conradi's syndrome. There is a stippling of the uncalcified epiphyseal regions (chondrodysplasia punctata), primarily the axial skeleton, proximal femurs, and calcanei, and severe nasal hypoplasia. Probably central nervous system problems develop from drug exposure in the middle and last trimesters. These include mental deficiency, seizures, microcephaly, and optic atrophy.
Valproic acid	Neural tube defects, cleft lip, and renal defects

  (b) The risk of major or minor congenital anomalies in infants of mothers who ingest excessive amounts of alcohol but do not meet the criteria for chronic alcoholism is around 32%.
  (c) Intrauterine fetal growth retardation is increased 2.7 times in pregnant women who drink excessively.
 b. Marijuana. There is no evidence that smoking marijuana is teratogenic although the adverse effects of smoking in pregnancy should not be overlooked. Maternal smoking level correlates with:
  (1) Increased perinatal mortality
  (2) Preterm delivery
  (3) Premature rupture of the membranes
  (4) Bleeding during pregnancy
 c. Heroin has *not* been shown to cause birth defects. It is the drugs that are often taken with heroin that are associated with congenital anomalies. The principal adverse fetal effect in heroin addicts is severe neonatal withdrawal, causing death in 3%–5% of neonates. Methadone is used to replace heroin, and although it is not teratogenic, it is also associated with severe neonatal withdrawal, which is treated with paregoric, valium, or phenobarbital in the neonatal period.
 d. Phencyclidine (PCP), or "angel dust," is an hallucinogenic agent associated with facial abnormalities in a small percentage of exposed infants.
 e. Cocaine is rapidly becoming the most abused drug in pregnancy, second only to alcohol. One study showed an increased risk of congenital malformations, stillbirths, and low-birthweight infants in cocaine users. There is a clear causal relationship of cocaine and placental abruption due to its vasoconstrictive properties.
7. Cancer chemotherapy. Although there is a high incidence of fetal wastage, including abortion and stillbirth, the incidence of congenital malformations, with the exception of those agents listed in Table 15-3, is surprisingly low.
 a. There are varied and unpredictable effects, ranging from severe deformity to no abnormality, when cancer chemotherapy is administered during the first trimester of pregnancy.
 b. After the period of organogenesis, there is no teratogenic risk of chemotherapy in pregnancy.

C. Hyperthermia. Studies suggest that sustained maternal hyperthermia (body temperature above 38.9°C between 4 and 14 weeks gestation), not spiking fevers, is teratogenic. Malformations noted in infants of mothers who were febrile from infectious agents or who frequented saunas in the first trimester include the following:

1. Growth retardation

2. Central nervous system defects
  a. Mental deficiency
  b. Microcephaly
  c. Hypotonia

3. Facial anomalies, including midfacial hypoplasia, cleft lip and palate, microphthalmia, micrognathia, and external ear anomalies

4. Minor limb anomalies, such as syndactyly

D. Maternal medical disorders. Women with medical disorders should be counseled about the teratogenic risks from the condition being treated as well as the treatment. In some cases, the untreated medical disorder poses greater risks to the fetus than the teratogenic potential of the specific drug therapy.

  1. Diabetes mellitus. Infants of insulin-dependent diabetic mothers have a 6%–22% incidence of cardiac, renal, gastrointestinal, central nervous system, and skeletal malformations. Most of the malformations occur between the third and sixth week postconception and are increased if there is hyperglycemia during that stage of gestation.

  2. Phenylketonuria. This is a genetic disorder characterized by a deficiency of phenylalanine hydroxylase, a liver enzyme that catalyzes the conversion of phenylalanine to tyrosine. The resulting high levels of phenylalanine in maternal serum result in high levels in the fetus. A special diet low in phenylalanine beginning *before* conception can prevent the adverse effects (mental retardation) of this disorder.

  3. Virilizing tumors (arrhenoblastoma) can have masculinizing effects on the mother and pseudohermaphroditic changes in the female fetus, including fusion of the labia and clitorimegaly.

  4. Epilepsy is a classic example of a disease process and its treatment contributing to the increase in birth defects.
    a. Epileptics who take anticonvulsants throughout the pregnancy have a two- to threefold increased rate of malformed infants.
    b. Untreated epileptics are also at an increased risk of delivering infants with birth defects, perhaps due to hypoxia from seizures or from an unknown factor.

E. Infections. Exposure to viral infections during gestation has recently been recognized as a significant cause of birth defects. Most infants, if infected during the first trimester, will suffer from a syndrome of congenital malformations and will be small for gestational age.

  1. Rubella virus (German measles). When rubella infections occur in the first month of pregnancy, there is a 50% chance of anomalous development. This chance falls to 22% in the second month, and 6%–10% in the third to fourth month. If a mother is infected at the time of delivery, the newborn may develop pneumonitis or encephalitis. The congenital rubella syndrome includes the following:
    a. Neuropathologic changes
      (1) Microcephaly
      (2) Mental and motor retardation
      (3) Meningoencephalitis
    b. Cardiovascular lesions
      (1) Persistent patent ductus arteriosus
      (2) Pulmonary artery stenosis
      (3) Atrioventricular septal defects
    c. Ocular defects
      (1) Cataracts
      (2) Microphthalmia
      (3) Retinal changes
      (4) Blindness
    d. Inner ear problems, resulting in sensorineural deafness
    e. Symmetric intrauterine growth retardation

  2. Cytomegalovirus (CMV) is an ubiquitous virus that infects 1%–2% of all infants in utero. Between 1 in 5000 to 1 in 20,000 infants suffer severe problems that are recognizable at birth.

    a. The risk of severe complications is much higher for infants of mothers who had a primary infection in pregnancy compared to those who had a recurrent infection.

        (1) Seronegative mothers infected with primary CMV will transmit the infection to the fetus in 30%–40% of cases. Of those infected, 2%–4% will be severely symptomatic at birth.

        (2) Seropositive mothers who have a recurrent infection will transmit the infection to the fetus in only 1% of cases, and 99% of these infants will appear normal at birth. Later in life, these affected infants may suffer from delayed speech development and learning difficulties due to sensorineural hearing loss. A small group will have chorioretinitis.

    b. A specific relationship of time of exposure to subsequent deficit has not been demonstrated, although the most damage seems to occur early in pregnancy. Gestational age at the time of exposure does not appear to influence the *rate* of fetal infection. The neonatal effects of a fetal CMV infection include the following:

        (1) Microcephaly and hydrocephaly

        (2) Chorioretinitis

        (3) Hepatosplenomegaly

        (4) Cerebral calcification

        (5) Mental retardation

        (6) Heart block

        (7) Petechiae

3. Herpesvirus hominis type 2 (HSV-2). Although mucocutaneous herpetic infection is quite common, less than 1 in 7500 infants suffer from perinatal transmission of HSV-2. Fetal transmission occurs by hematogenous spread during a maternal viremia or by direct contact during passage through an infected birth canal, but congenital infection, causing fetal malformations is quite rare. It is thought that fetal infection during the first trimester results in miscarriage. In a few cases, a syndrome was described that resembled other infants with viral infections during the first trimester, including the following fetal anomalies:

    a. Growth retardation

    b. Microcephaly

    c. Chorioretinitis

    d. Cerebral calcification

    e. Microphthalmia encephalitis

4. Toxoplasmosis is caused by a protozoan, *Toxoplasma gondii*, and may be transmitted from mother to fetus antepartum. Although infection is most common outside the United States (i.e., in Sweden and Alaska), the incidence of congenital infection in the United States ranges from 1–6 cases/1000 live-births. About 30% of infected women will transmit the disease to their unborn children. In a French population of 550 women who acquired toxoplasmosis during pregnancy, 61% of the neonates had evidence of congenital infection; of these neonates, 6% died, 5% had severe clinical illness, 9% had mild disease, and 41% had subclinical disease.

    a. Fetal infection early in pregnancy increases the severity of infection.

        (1) The pregnancy may result in:

            (a) Abortion

            (b) Perinatal death

            (c) Severe congenital anomalies

            (d) Abnormal growth

            (e) Residual handicap

        (2) In severe disease, the characteristic triad of anomalies includes:

            (a) Chorioretinitis

            (b) Hydrocephaly or microcephaly

            (c) Cerebral calcification, resulting in psychomotor retardation

    b. Transmission to the fetus is more likely later in pregnancy, although the neonatal handicap is much more benign and, in fact, is often subclinical.

5. Syphilis (*Treponema pallidum*) cases increased by 30% in 1981. In the United States, the rise in congenital syphilis has paralleled the increase in primary and secondary syphilis in the adult. There are several hundred cases of congenital syphilis diagnosed each year; half of these infants are born to women with no prenatal care. *T. pallidum* appears to cross the placenta at any time during pregnancy. Due to an immature immune system, the fetus is rarely infected before 16–18 weeks gestation. Prior to this time, antibiotic therapy is highly successful.

    a. The incidence of congenital infection is inversely proportional to the duration of maternal infection and the degree of spirochetemia.

(1) Recent or secondary infection in the mother confers the greatest risk of fetal infection. All infants born to women with primary and secondary infection will be infected, but 50% will be asymptomatic.

(2) Only 40% of infants born to women with early latent disease will be infected, and the incidence drops to 5%–15% for late latent infection.

b. In utero infection may result in:

(1) Preterm delivery or miscarriage

(2) Stillbirth

(3) Neonatal death in up to 50% of affected infants

(4) Congenital infection

(a) Asymptomatic

(b) Symptomatic problems, including:

(i) Hepatosplenomegaly

(ii) Joint swelling

(iii) Skin rash

(iv) Anemia

(v) Jaundice

(vi) Snuffles

(vii) Metaphyseal dystrophy

(viii) Periostitis

(ix) Cerebrospinal fluid changes

c. Adequate antibiotic therapy for the pregnant woman is generally thought to provide adequate therapy for the unborn child. However, several case reports have described congenitally infected infants born to mothers treated with benzathene penicillin G. The risk of treatment failure appears to be greater for women who are treated for secondary syphilis or who are in the last trimester of pregnancy.

6. Varicella zoster (VZV, chickenpox) is an uncommon virus, occurring in 1–7 of 10,000 pregnancies. Infection in the adult is much more severe than in childhood, but pregnancy does not seem to alter this risk. Transplacental transmission of VZV is now well documented, and occurs in about 24% of cases following maternal *varicella* in the last month of pregnancy and 0% for maternal *zoster* (see section II E 6 c). Transmission in the first half of pregnancy is around 5%–10% at most.

a. Inconclusive reports have described an increased risk of leukemia in infants born with gestational varicella. There is also a description of chromosome breaks in the leukocytes of a child whose mother had varicella in pregnancy.

b. There are multiple cases of congenital malformations in the offspring of women who develop chickenpox during the first 20 weeks of pregnancy. These include abnormalities of several organ systems:

(1) Cutaneous

(a) Cicatricial skin scarring with denuded skin and limb hypoplasia

(b) Vesicular rash (hemorrhagic rash) if infection is in the last 3 weeks of pregnancy

(2) Musculoskeletal

(a) Limb hypoplasia (unilateral), involving the arm, mandible, or hemithorax

(b) Rudimentary digits

(c) Club foot

(3) Neurologic

(a) Microcephaly

(b) Cortical and cerebellar atrophy

(c) Seizures

(d) Psychomotor retardation

(e) Focal brain calcifications

(f) Autonomic dysfunction, such as loss of bowel and bladder control, dysphagia, and Horner's syndrome

(g) Ocular abnormalities, such as microphthalmia, optic atrophy, cataracts, and chorioretinitis

(4) Other

(a) Symmetric intrauterine growth retardation

(b) Fever, vesicular rash, pneumonia and widespread necrotic lesions of the viscera, leading to death, if infection occurs in the last 3 weeks of pregnancy

c. Herpes zoster. There is no good evidence proving that herpes zoster causes congenital anomalies. A few case reports have described microcephaly, microphthalmia, cataracts, and talipes equinovarus in infants born to mothers suffering from zoster during pregnancy, but these cases may represent chance occurrences.

7. **Mumps.** Mumps infection is not strictly teratogenic, but after maternal exposure neonates have been born with:
   a. Endocardial fibroelastosis
   b. Ear and eye malformations
   c. Urogenital abnormalities

8. **Enteroviruses (coxsackie B).** Serious or fatal illness (40%) in the fetus results from maternal exposure to coxsackie B virus. Surviving infants may exhibit the following:
   a. Cardiac malformations
   b. Hepatitis, pneumonitis, or pancreatitis
   c. Adrenal necrosis

STUDY QUESTIONS

Directions: Each question below contains four suggested answers of which **one or more** is correct. Choose the answer

A   if **1, 2, and 3** are correct
B   if **1 and 3** are correct
C   if **2 and 4** are correct
D   if **4** is correct
E   if **1, 2, 3, and 4** are correct

1.   Two 30-year-old women who have manic-depressive psychoses took lithium throughout their first pregnancies. One had a infant boy with no congenital anomalies, while the second had a infant boy with Ebstein's anomaly. The different neonatal outcomes may be explained by the fact that

(1) the lithium must have gained access in differing quantities during the period of cardiac development
(2) one mother may have had a lower blood lithium level during this pregnancy
(3) lithium may produce a wide spectrum of insults in the same species
(4) the affected infant may have a weaker genetic constitution and thus was more susceptible

2.   The spectrum of adverse outcomes that may result from insults during the course of development include which of the following?

(1) Death
(2) Malformation
(3) Growth retardation
(4) No effect

Directions: The groups of questions below consist of lettered choices followed by several numbered items. For each numbered item select the **one** lettered choice with which it is **most** closely associated. Each lettered choice may be used once, more than once, or not at all.

Questions 3–5

For each of the drugs listed below, select the malformation most commonly associated with it.

(A) Chondrodysplasia punctata
(B) Ototoxicity
(C) Absence of toes
(D) Hypospadias
(E) Limb reduction

3.   Synthetic progestins

4.   Thalidomide

5.   Streptomycin

Questions 6–9

Match each description listed below with the viral syndrome that is most appropriately described by it.

(A) Cytomegalovirus
(B) Toxoplasmosis
(C) Varicella zoster virus
(D) Syphilis
(E) Rubella virus

6.   Causes birth defects when a mother is infected with primary infection versus recurrent infection

7.   Congenital infection very rare before 16 weeks gestation

8.   Has a 24% incidence of congenital infection when maternal infection occurs in the last month of pregnancy

9.   Infects all infants, 50% of whom will be asymptomatic, born to women with recent infection

ANSWERS AND EXPLANATIONS

1. The answer is E (all). (I A, C; Table 15-3) This case study illustrates the great variation from one individual to another that must be considered when estimating the teratogenic effects of a medication. The different neonatal outcomes illustrate the principle that environmental influences on embryologic and fetal development result in a wide range of effects for a multitude of reasons. We can only *estimate* the risk of malformations for a teratogen, not *predict* the precise outcome for a developing human fetus.

2. The answer is E (all). (I A–D) There is a wide range of effects that occur from in utero exposure to a suspected teratogen. Depending on the stage of gestation, the effect of the teratogen may be minimal (no perceptible effect) or so serious as to result in death in utero. The fetus exposed before the seventh day of gestation or the twenty-first day from the last menstrual period may be either unaffected or killed by the insult. This is the period of predifferentiation. Malformations are most likely to occur during the embryonic period (7–57 days postconception) when the organ systems are forming and differentiating. For instance, congenital malformations found in infants of diabetic mothers can be pinpointed to the time of gestation in which they occurred. Caudal regression syndrome, a syndrome seen only in infants of diabetic mothers, which consists of severe congenital malformations, including agenesis of the sacrum and lumbar spine and hypoplasia of the lower extremities, occurs in the third week postconception. Anencephaly and other defects of neural tube closure occur before the fourth week postconception. In the fifth and sixth weeks, the common cardiac defects—transposition of the great vessels and ventricular and atrial septal defects—commonly develop. In the second and third trimesters, after the organ systems have differentiated but are continuing to develop, exposure to a specific chemical or toxic environmental agent may produce growth retardation.

3–5. The answers are: 3-D, 4-E, 5-B. (*Table 15-3*) There is continuing controversy about the teratogenicity of progestational agents. Indeed, if they are teratogenic, the risk is extremely small. Exposure during the first trimester is possibly related to a two- to threefold increase in cardiac defects (from 8/1000 to approximately 20/1000 live-births). Prenatal exposure to a progestin may double the incidence of hypospadias in the offspring. The resulting incidence of 140/10,000 male births is extremely low. Though uncommon, fusion of the labia majora and clitorimegaly have been observed in the female fetus.

It was not until the early 1960s that prenatal exposure to thalidomide was identified as a cause of serious defects in structural development. Thalidomide was used all over Europe as a very effective sleeping medication. Unfortunately, the pregnant animals that were used to test the safety of thalidomide in pregnancy rarely developed limb defects when exposed to teratogens. It was only after humans had been born with limb hypoplasia that repeat experimental studies in species similar to humans revealed devastating limb reduction defects, which serves to exemplify the variation of genetic susceptibility among species.

A high incidence of vestibular abnormalities has been reported among children born to women who received long-term treatment with streptomycin. However, no gross functional impairment has been reported.

6–9. The answers are: 6-A, 7-D, 8-C, 9-D. (II E 1, 2, 4–6) Both cytomegalovirus and *Herpesvirus hominis* are DNA viruses of the herpesvirus group, which may reinfect the same individual. Cytomegalovirus is now recognized as the most common cause of intrauterine infection. Children born to women with acute infection have neurologic sequelae in a small percentage of cases, and these cases are more frequent when a seronegative mother converts to seropositive during pregnancy rather than when a mother is seropositive before pregnancy and has a reactivation of the virus.

The incidence of congenital syphilis has paralleled the increase in primary and secondary syphilis in the adult. *Treponema pallidum*, the causative agent, appears to cross the placenta at anytime during pregnancy, but because of an immature immune system, the fetus is rarely infected before 16 weeks gestation. Recent or secondary infection confers the greatest risk of fetal infection. All infants born to women with primary and secondary infections are infected, although 50% will be asymptomatic.

Varicella zoster (chickenpox) is an uncommon virus in pregnant women, occurring in 1–7 of 10,000 pregnancies. Transplacental transmission of varicella zoster is now well documented, occurring in 24% of cases following infection in the *last* month of pregnancy. Congenital infection is very rare before 16 weeks gestation (5%–10% at most).

16
The High-Risk Neonate
Luciano Lizzi

I. INTRODUCTION. The threefold improvement in neonatal mortality in the United States over the past 15 years has been truly remarkable. Among the many factors responsible for this improvement are the development of the subspecialty of perinatology, the use of ultrasound in the management of pregnancy, and, most importantly, the advances in the field of neonatology. The greatest achievements have occurred in the management of preterm infants, particularly those who weigh less than 1500 g at birth. The cost of this care is enormous and will likely be what limits future advances. Most problems of the neonate can be anticipated by close monitoring of the mother prenatally and during labor and delivery.

II. RESUSCITATION OF THE NEWBORN

  A. Physiology of the fetal circulation

    1. Ninety percent of the fetal circulation bypasses the lung by flowing through the ductus arteriosus since the placenta rather than the lungs allows for gas exchange.

    2. Maintenance of the fetal circulation requires that the pressure relationship between right to left atria and pulmonary artery to aorta be sustained.
      a. The high pulmonary artery pressure is due to the constricted arterioles in an airless collapsed lung.
      b. The low resistance of the aorta is mostly due to the presence of the placental circulation.

    3. Deoxygenated blood passes through the branches of the arteries to the intervillous space of the placenta. Oxygenated blood returns via the umbilical vein through the ductus venosus, portal and hepatic veins, and then to the inferior vena cava. Blood enters the right atrium, and approximately 50% of this blood is directed to the foramen ovale where it mixes with pulmonary venous blood and enters the left ventricle. Along with blood from the superior vena cava, the remainder is directed to the pulmonary artery and then through the patent ductus arteriosus and descending aorta.

  B. Conversion to adult circulation

    1. The most important functions of the newborn infant are respiration and conversion of the circulation from the placenta to the lung as the organ of gas exchange. There are two events at delivery that initiate this conversion:
      a. Clamping of the umbilical cord
      b. Ventilation of the lung

    2. The sequence of events that changes the newborn circulation include the following:
      a. Aortic resistance increases when the umbilical cord is clamped.
      b. Aortic pressure increases.
      c. Blood flow is decreased through the ductus arteriosus.
      d. Pulmonary artery resistance is decreased with the onset of ventilation.
      e. Pulmonary artery pressure is decreased.
      f. Pulmonary blood flow is increased.
      g. Volume into and pressure of the left atrium increases.
      h. The foramen ovale closes.

    3. Neonatal resuscitation helps these circulatory changes to occur and helps to counteract medical conditions that threaten the infant's survival.

  C. The Apgar score, which is performed at 1 and 5 minutes after birth, assesses five characteristics of the newborn—heart rate, respiratory effort, skin color, muscle tone, and reflex response. It is used to determine which infants need resuscitation; it should not be used as a predictor of outcome. Moreover, attempts to correlate Apgar scores with fetal and newborn scalp pH values have shown wide discrepancies. To obtain the Apgar score, score 0, 1, or 2 for each of the following categories, then add them together.

1. Heart rate
   a. Absent (0)
   b. Less than 100 beats per minute (1)
   c. Over 100 beats per minute (2)

2. Respiratory effort
   a. Absent (0)
   b. Slow and irregular (1)
   c. Good cry (2)

3. Skin color
   a. Cyanosis (0)
   b. Acrocyanosis (1)
   c. Pink (entire body) (2)

4. Muscle tone
   a. Flaccid (0)
   b. Slight (1)
   c. Active (2)

5. Reflex response
   a. Absent (0)
   b. Slight (1)
   c. Active (2)

D. Transition from fetal to neonatal life

   1. A reassuring Apgar score is between 7 and 10, indicating no need for special resuscitative efforts. Infants must be kept warm as they can loose heat rapidly by the following four mechanisms and become cold stressed.
   a. Evaporation occurs as amniotic fluid changes from liquid to gas, decreasing the newborn's skin temperature. The infant should, thus, be dried off immediately to prevent heat loss from evaporation.
   b. Convection is the transmission of heat by air currents. Objects in a room have different temperatures, such as cold metal objects and warm electrical equipment. The air warmed by the warm objects rises and creates air currents, which cool other objects in a room including an infant. The warm isolated environment that an isolette provides can prevent this.
   c. Conduction is the direct transfer of heat from the infant to a cooler object; thus, keeping the infant against the mother's body, wrapped in blankets, or under a radiant heater helps to maintain its body temperature.
   d. Radiation. Heat is radiated from the surface of the infant and travels out into the room. Any warm object produces heat waves, which travel through the air to colder objects.

   2. Moderately depressed infants have Apgar scores between 4 and 6, requiring stimulation and possibly assisted ventilation.
   a. Temperature support is as important in the moderately depressed infant as in the normal infant.
   b. A clear airway must be assured and adequate ventilation provided.
      (1) Short (1–2 seconds) periods of suctioning of the upper airway may be needed to clear mucus and secretions. Oversuctioning can cause bradycardia and arrhythmias through vagal stimulation.
      (2) If gasping or apnea is present, stimulation may be needed. Gentle slapping of the back, buttocks, or feet may induce spontaneous respiration.
      (3) If the infant does not respond to stimulation after 30–60 seconds, bag and mask ventilation with supplemental oxygen at a rate of 30–40 times/min is indicated.
      (4) Successful ventilation is measured by an increase in heart rate, which occurs prior to a change of skin color from cyanosis to pink.

   3. Severely depressed infants have Apgar scores of 3 or less or do not respond to bag and mask ventilation. The infant is obtunded, has a heart rate less than 100, and has little if any respiratory effort. The infant usually requires endotracheal intubation, artificial ventilation, and possibly cardiac massage.

    a. Intubation and ventilation are needed immediately, using a nontapered endotracheal tube. Intubation should be performed by an experienced physician.

    b. An absent heart beat or a heart rate of less than 50 requires cardiac massage, using the thumbs at a rate of 100 times/min.

    c. If it is known that the mother is addicted to narcotics or if excessive narcotics have been administered during labor, naloxone (a narcotic antagonist) should be administered.

    d. Medications that may be used during resuscitation include the following:

        (1) Glucose infusion, 10%

        (2) Sodium bicarbonate, 2 mEq/kg

        (3) Epinephrine (1:10,000 dilution), 0.1–0.3 ml/kg

        (4) Calcium gluconate, 100 mg/kg

        (5) Atropine, 0.01 mg/kg

    e. Infants with arrhythmias need an immediate electrocardiogram to establish a diagnosis.

    f. Monitoring of blood gases should be done by umbilical artery catheterization. After stabilization, pulse oximetry may be used.

E. Special problems requiring resuscitation

  1. Meconium aspiration syndrome occurs when an infant breathes in meconium that was passed into the amniotic fluid.

    a. Meconium is present in 10% of all deliveries. Of these infants, 2% develop an aspiration syndrome, which is often associated with:

        (1) Placental insufficiency

        (2) Postdates pregnancy

        (3) Cord problems

        (4) Hypertension

        (5) High-risk situations

    b. When meconium is present in the infant's alveoli, the cardiopulmonary status can be compromised in the following ways:

        (1) Thick meconium plugs can block ventilation of sections of the lung and cause atelectasis.

        (2) Meconium causes spasm of the pulmonary arterioles, resulting in pulmonary hypertension and persistent fetal circulation with continued shunting of blood across the ductus arteriosus.

        (3) Meconium, although sterile, can act as a culture medium for the development of pneumonia.

    c. Intrapartum suctioning by the obstetric/neonatal team can result in a 75% reduction in the incidence of meconium aspiration.

        (1) The obstetrician should perform catheter suctioning of the infant's nasopharynx immediately after delivery of the head.

        (2) The mouth should be cleared of secretions concurrently with delivery of the chest and body.

        (3) The cord should be clamped immediately and the infant given to the pediatrician who intubates and suctions the trachea prior to the first breath.

        (4) Chest physiotherapy should be administered until meconium is no longer in the secretions.

  2. Congenital abnormalities

    a. Diaphragmatic hernia

        (1) This condition results from the failure of closure of the posterolateral pleuroperitoneal folds during the eighth to ninth week of gestation.

        (2) Herniation of the intestines into the chest occurs in 90% of cases.

        (3) Liver herniation occurs in 50% of cases.

        (4) The left side is affected 85% of the time, thus more commonly than the right.

        (5) Normal lung development is interrupted, and pulmonary hypoplasia can result.

        (6) Early detection is mandatory with cautious ventilation via endotracheal tube to avoid pneumothoraces in hypoplastic lungs.

        (7) A nasogastric tube is necessary to keep the stomach decompressed.

        (8) Once stabilized, the infant requires emergency surgery.

        (9) Death occurs in over 50% of cases due to pulmonary hypoplasia and hypoxia.

    b. Esophageal atresia and tracheoesophageal fistula

        (1) Any interruption in the normal division of the foregut during the fourth week of gestation into trachea and esophagus can result in esophageal atresia and tracheoesophageal fistula. The overall incidence is 1 in 3000 births.

        (2) These conditions can occur together or separately; the most common deformity is esophageal atresia with distal tracheoesophageal fistula.

    (3) Excess neonatal mucus is a warning sign of this disorder, and inability to pass a nasogastric tube is highly suggestive of esophageal atresia.

    (4) Head elevation and nasogastric suction of the upper esophagus are important until surgical repair can be performed on a stable infant.

c. Myelomeningocele and encephalocoele

    (1) These neural tube defects are characterized by herniation of the meninges, medulla, and spinal cord.

    (2) It is important to prevent infection of exposed meninges, using sterile technique with wet to dry dressings.

    (3) Position infant on the abdomen at all times until surgical repair can be performed on a stable infant.

d. Choanal atresia

    (1) Since infants are obligate nose breathers, the infant is cyanotic at rest, which resolves with crying.

    (2) If a catheter cannot be passed through each nostril, tape an oral airway in place.

e. Gastroschisis and omphalocele

    (1) These are ventral wall defects that are characterized by intestinal herniation.

    (2) To minimize heat loss, management includes handling with sterile gloves and wrapping the sac or bowel in wet saline dressings until surgical repair can be performed.

3. Drug-depressed infants

a. If a narcotic analgesic, such as meperidine, has been given to the mother within several hours of delivery, narcotic depression can occur.

b. Immediate treatment with intramuscular or intravenous naloxone, 0.01 mg/kg, should be given.

c. Typically, the infant's tone and respiratory effort improve dramatically.

d. Caution must be maintained when delivering an infant of a mother who is addicted to drugs as acute drug withdrawal may be precipitated.

III. DISORDERS OF PREMATURE INFANTS. Birth at less than 37 weeks gestation occurs in about 10% of all pregnancies. The infant must adapt to extrauterine life with organs that are not fully mature. Despite this disadvantage, premature infants often do remarkably well with good medical care and support. This section deals with various problems of the preterm infant.

A. Respiratory distress syndrome is the most common and most serious problem of the preterm neonate. The more premature the infant, the more likely it is to occur. It is responsible for 50%–70% of deaths in preterm infants.

1. Clinical manifestations

a. Progressive respiratory insufficiency

b. Increased oxygen requirements

c. Grunting

d. Nasal flaring

e. Tachypnea

f. Intercostal retractions, indicating extrainspiratory effort

g. Cyanosis

2. Etiology. The cause of the respiratory distress syndrome is pulmonary immaturity. The lung is noncompliant and lacks normal elasticity as a result of a deficiency of surfactant, which is composed of phospholipids that increase in concentration as fetal maturity progresses. Surfactant acts as a detergent, decreasing the surface tension of the alveoli and allowing them to remain expanded. Hypoxia leads to acidosis, which further inhibits surfactant production and causes capillary endothelial damage. Fibrin leakage occurs, and hyaline membranes are formed in the lungs. Without surfactant, there is:

a. Alveolar collapse

b. Hypoventilation

c. Atelectasis

d. Poor gas exchange

3. Differential diagnosis

a. Transient tachypnea of the newborn

b. Pneumonia

c. Patent ductus arteriosus

d. Diaphragmatic hernia

4. Findings on chest x-ray

a. A "ground-glass" appearance

      b. Air bronchograms
      c. Atelectasis
  5. Treatment. The goal of treatment is to increase or initiate the production of surfactant by:
      a. Ventilatory support with a respirator capable of providing:
        (1) Positive end expiratory pressure (PEEP)
        (2) Continuous positive airway pressure (CPAP)
        (3) Intermittent mandatory ventilation (IMV)
      b. Monitoring of umbilical artery blood gases to maintain blood oxygen levels at 50–80 mm Hg and prevent hypoxemia
      c. Antibiotics
      d. Intravenous fluids
      e. Hyperalimentation
      f. General medical support with attention to body temperature and hematocrit
      g. Surfactant administration (experimental)

  6. Bronchopulmonary dysplasia is a chronic lung disease sometimes found in infants on respirators for more than 1 week. It results from high concentrations of oxygen or from barotrauma from positive pressure ventilation.
      a. Clinical manifestations
        (1) Chronic tachypnea
        (2) Persistent retractions
        (3) Oxygen requirements
        (4) Bronchiolar hypertrophy
        (5) Interstitial lung fibrosis
        (6) Emphysema
      b. Treatment to which most infants respond involves removal of the ventilatory source of lung injury by:
        (1) Reducing the respirator setting to an absolute minimum
        (2) Providing maximal nutritional support
        (3) Allowing the lung its great potential for postnatal growth

B. Necrotizing enterocolitis is a disease of preterm infants involving an acute inflammation of the bowel. The incidence in intensive care nurseries is approximately 2%, although 70% of cases are infants weighing less than 1500 g. It can be fatal.

  1. Clinical manifestations
      a. Presents within the first month of life, most often within the first week of feeding
      b. Gradual onset or acute onset with perforation
      c. Feeding intolerance with bilious vomiting
      d. Abdominal distension
      e. Bloody stools
      f. Evidence of sepsis with lethargy
      g. Apnea
      h. Bradycardia
      i. Temperature instability

  2. Predisposing factors
      a. Ischemia
      b. Shock
      c. Patent ductus ateriosus
      d. Umbilical artery or vein catheterization
      e. Infection
      f. Hypothermia
      g. Crowded nurseries

  3. Etiology. The cause of necrotizing enterocolitis is not fully understood, but it does appear to be an infectious process. Pathogenic bacteria combined with poor bowel perfusion in a stressed premature neonate can result in bowel ischemia, damage, and infection. This injury leads to reduced intestinal motility, bacterial proliferation, and endotoxin production. Septic shock and death may result.

  4. X-ray findings
      a. Abdominal x-rays show:
        (1) Intestinal ileus
        (2) Air–fluid levels
        (3) Interstitial intestinal gas

    b. Barium x-rays help to identify intestinal strictures, a major complication that involves the large intestine.

5. Pathology shows:
    a. Bowel ischemia
    b. Mucosal necrosis
    c. Infarction
    d. Intestinal gas (pneumotosis intestinalis), which results from:
        (1) Gas in the intestinal lining dissecting into the bowel wall
        (2) Gas-producing bacteria in the bowel

6. Treatment
    a. Intravenous fluids and hyperalimentation; nothing by mouth
    b. Antibiotics
    c. Decompression with nasogastric suction
    d. Plasma volume expanders, dopamine, and transfusion for infants with:
        (1) Hypotension
        (2) Poor perfusion
        (3) Shock
    e. Oxygen as needed
    f. Surgery in cases of intestinal perforations and obstruction

7. Summary
    a. Oral feedings are begun slowly after clinical improvement no earlier than 14 days after treatment.
    b. Clinical parameters for infection, including abdominal birth measurements and stool samples, are closely monitored.
    c. Prevention involves:
        (1) Slow and careful feedings to preterm compromised neonates
        (2) Good perinatal care
        (3) A high quality, clean nursery

C. Hyperbilirubinemia

    1. Elevated bilirubin in preterm infants is very common due to:
        a. Liver immaturity with little development of the enzyme conjugating system
        b. Reduced intestinal motility, resulting in increased reuptake of intestinal bilirubin
        c. Decreased red cell survival
        d. Delayed oral feedings, which further reduces the excretion of bilirubin

    2. Kernicterus, a destructive deposition of bilirubin in the brain and nervous system, is more likely to occur in preterm than in term infants.
        a. The blood–brain barrier, the capillary endothelial block to the passage of many substances, including bilirubin, into the brain is less developed. Bilirubin may, therefore, pass into the brain at lower blood concentrations in preterm infants.
        b. Hypoxia, sepsis, and hypoalbuminemia are also more likely in the preterm infant and can further damage the barrier and encourage bilirubin passage.
        c. To prevent kernicterus in the preterm infant, **phototherapy** is initiated early and **exchange transfusion** is used liberally.

D. Apnea is the interruption of spontaneous respiration for over 15 seconds.

    1. Incidence. The incidence of apnea is inversely proportional to gestational age. It occurs in approximately 84% of infants weighing less than 1000 g and 25% of infants weighing less than 2500 g. A "sleep study" is often done in infants with apneic episodes in which the heart rate and respiratory rate are monitored over periods up to 24 hours; if found to be abnormal, apnea monitors are used in the nursery and at home as such infants are at risk for the sudden infant death syndrome.

    2. Etiology. The cause of apnea is not fully known, but it may indicate immaturity of the respiratory drive centers. Nerve conduction in the brain stem is slower in the preterm infant than in the term infant. Other factors include:
        a. Decreased efficiency in the synapses
        b. Decreased response to carbon dioxide
        c. Increased periods of REM sleep

    3. Precipitating factors
        a. Fluctuating environmental temperature
        b. Patent ductus arteriosus

   c. Gastric dilation
   d. Rectal stimulation
   e. Nasal suctioning
   f. Pulmonary insufficiency
   g. Airway obstruction
   h. Central nervous system disease
   i. Metabolic abnormalities

  4. Treatment involves the elimination of any associated factors listed above. If no etiology is
     readily apparent, the following measures may help:
     a. Physical stimulation and the prone position to relieve occasional, mild episodes
     b. Nasal CPAP or ventilator support for frequent, severe episodes
     c. Theophylline, which acts by increasing the sensitivity of the respiratory center to carbon
          dioxide
     d. Small increases in ambient oxygen

 E. Intraventricular hemorrhage is a major cause of mortality and neurologic sequelae in the
    preterm infant.

  1. The incidence is inversely proportional to gestational age. It occurs in up to 50% of infants
     weighing less than 1500 g. All infants born before 34 weeks are at risk.

  2. Clinical manifestations, which may or may not be present, include:
     a. Acute hypotension
     b. Flaccidity
     c. A falling hematocrit without a clear etiology
     d. Cardiorespiratory arrest
     e. A bulging fontanelle
     f. Bloody cerebrospinal fluid
     g. Seizures (in serious cases)

  3. The diagnosis is made by real-time ultrasonography, which can be performed without dis-
     rupting a sick neonate. Serial scans can be performed with little risk to the neonate. Ultra-
     sonography has demonstrated intraventricular hemorrhage within minutes after birth. Four
     grades of severity have been demonstrated:
     a. Grade I: subependymal hemorrhage
     b. Grade II: no ventricular dilation
     c. Grade III: ventricular dilation
     d. Grade IV: parenchymal hemorrhage

  4. Pathology relates to prematurity of the nervous system and the following factors:
     a. Fragile ependymal blood vessels with poor connective tissue support
     b. Hypoxia leading to capillary damage and rupture

  5. Treatment has had mixed results. The goal is prevention of pressure damage to brain matter.
     Serial lumbar punctures and diuretics have been used. Prevention is the key to reducing mor-
     bidity.
     a. Posthemorrhagic hydrocephalus is a frequent sequela.
        (1) Death may occur from early aqueductal or intraventricular block in the acute phase.
        (2) A slowly evolving hydrocephalus due to obliterative arachnoiditis and meningeal
             thickening may appear.
     b. The prognosis is inversely proportional to the severity of intraventricular hemorrhage.
          Overall mortality is estimated at 30%.

IV. DISORDERS OF TERM INFANTS

 A. Infants of diabetic mothers

  1. Pathophysiology
     a. In utero, infants of diabetic mothers are exposed to varying degrees of glucose elevation
          due to an insulin resistant state in the mother secondary to pregnancy hormones.
     b. Glucose crosses the placenta via facilitated diffusion and travels to the fetus.
        (1) Elevated fetal glucose in the first trimester is associated with a greater incidence of fetal
             anomalies, particularly those of the skeletal and cardiac structures, such as spinal
             agenesis, ventricular septal defect, and transposition of the great vessels. The mecha-
             nism for this is unknown.
        (2) Glucose elevation in the second and third trimesters leads to fetal hyperinsulinemia
             and the development of four high-risk factors:

       (a) Fetal macrosomia
       (b) An enlarged placenta with a reduced functional capacity for oxygen transport, further increasing the likelihood of asphyxia and respiratory distress syndrome
       (c) Neonatal hypoglycemia from enlarged, overstimulated pancreatic islet cells that continue to produce increased amounts of insulin after birth, driving fetal glucose levels downward
       (d) Respiratory distress syndrome secondary to insulin interfering with surfactant production.

2. Treatment
    a. Infants of diabetic mothers are at risk for birth trauma if they are macrosomic. Shoulder dystocia and cesarean section are more common than in normal pregnancies. Good obstetric management is important.
    b. A pediatrician should be in attendance at birth in the event that unexpected anomalies are present.
    c. Neonatal hypoglycemia is managed with Dextrostix or Chemstrip glucose monitoring. If the glucose level is less than 25 mg/dl, a laboratory glucose determination is made, and oral glucose is administered. Blood glucose should be maintained at 40 mg/dl. In severe cases, intravenous glucose administration is necessary to prevent profound hypoglycemia and possible neurologic damage.
    d. Hyperbilirubinemia secondary to increased erythropoietin concentration and increased placental transfusion is treated with:
       (1) Phototherapy
       (2) Possibly exchange transfusion
    e. Less common complications include renal vascular thrombosis, hyperviscosity syndrome, and polycythemia. Management of these complications is controversial but includes:
       (1) Exchange transfusions
       (2) Fluid administration
       (3) Supportive care
    f. Hypocalcemia and hypomagnesemia are treated with intravenous supplementation.

3. Prevention. Good obstetric care is the key to a healthy infant of a diabetic mother. Rigid glucose control prior to conception and during the first trimester can help prevent fetal anomalies, which are certainly the most serious complications of these infants. Close monitoring of maternal glucose levels throughout pregnancy and good perinatal care at the time of delivery can optimize neonatal outcome.

B. Neonatal infection

1. Incidence. Serious neonatal infection occurs in approximately 0.2% of all live births. It should be suspected in the following clinical situations:
    a. Premature rupture of membranes over 24 hours *from*
    b. Maternal temperature or documented chorioamnionitis
    c. Unexplained birth asphyxia
    d. Fetal tachycardia in labor
    e. Foul-smelling amniotic fluid or neonate

2. Pathophysiology
    a. The three ways in which the infant can become infected are:
       (1) Transplacental passage
       (2) Rupture of membranes
       (3) Direct contact with the infectious agent on the genitalia of the mother at the time of vaginal delivery
    b. The most virulent organisms include:
       (1) Group B *Streptococcus*
       (2) *Escherichia coli*
       (3) *Chlamydia trachomatis*
       (4) *Neisseria gonorrhoeae*
       (5) *Listeria monocytogenes*
       (6) *Herpesvirus hominis*
    c. Neonatal sepsis is characterized by:
       (1) Cyanosis
       (2) Shock
       (3) Temperature instability
       (4) Acidosis
       (5) Tachycardia
       (6) Jaundice

d. The infant's immune system is fragile and can be easily overwhelmed by invasive organisms. Life-threatening infection can easily establish a foothold. The strength of the immune system is directly related to the infant's gestational age at birth.

3. Diagnosis
   a. Historical data are gathered from the prenatal, labor, and delivery records.
   b. Physical examination is performed with attention paid to:
      (1) Bulging fontanelle
      (2) Abdominal guarding
      (3) Pain in the joints and extremities
      (4) The state of the tympanic membranes
   c. Laboratory data include:
      (1) Complete blood count and platelet count. (Extremes of the neutrophil count and thrombocytopenia suggest sepsis.)
      (2) Cultures of urine, blood, and cerebrospinal fluid
      (3) Placental pathology
      (4) Chest x-ray
      (5) Arterial blood gases

4. Treatment
   a. Antibiotic therapy and supportive treatment are the keys to treatment. Broad-spectrum antibiotic combinations are generally used initially until culture results are available. Usually a combination of a penicillin derivative and aminoglycoside is chosen.
   b. Often sepsis is suspected in the neonate, but cultures prove negative. Antibiotics are either continued or withdrawn, depending on the clinical judgment of the neonatologist.

C. Intrauterine growth retardation

1. The incidence of intrauterine growth retardation is approximately 4% of all pregnancies where birthweight is less than the tenth percentile for the gestational age.

2. Categories of intrauterine growth retardation include the following:
   a. Symmetric intrauterine growth retardation occurs when the birthweight, length, and head circumference are all less than the tenth percentile for the gestational age.
   b. Asymmetric intrauterine growth retardation occurs when only the birthweight is less than the tenth percentile for the gestational age.

3. Etiology
   a. Symmetric intrauterine growth retardation indicates a long period of placental insufficiency secondary to a chromosomal anomaly or congenital viral infection (e.g., rubella and cytomegalovirus).
   b. Asymmetric intrauterine growth retardation indicates later placental insufficiency with brain-sparing phenomenon secondary to:
      (1) Hypertension
      (2) Insulin-dependent diabetes with vascular involvement
      (3) Multiple gestation
      (4) Preeclampsia
      (5) Collagen vascular diseases (e.g., systemic lupus erythematosus)
      (6) Poor nutrition

4. Management
   a. The intrauterine growth-retarded infant may sustain severe asphyxia or even intrauterine demise associated with anomalies or placental insufficiency. Anomalies may require surgical evaluation and treatment antepartum if detected by ultrasound or shortly after delivery. Asphyxia necessitates neonatal resuscitation and removal of meconium from the upper airway. Additionally, heat loss must be minimized with quick drying and radiant heat.
   b. Common problems of the intrauterine growth-retarded neonate include:
      (1) Congenital anomalies; thus, physical examination in the delivery room is especially important.
      (2) Hypoglycemia secondary to decreased glycogen reserve and decreased gluconeogenesis. Oral feeding should be instituted early and possibly with intravenous glucose.
      (3) Metabolic acidosis secondary to chronic hypoxia
      (4) Respiratory distress secondary to meconium aspiration, hyaline membrane disease, or cold stress
      (5) Persistent fetal circulation characterized by pulmonary hypertension, right-to-left shunting, and hypoxia. This is managed with assisted ventilation, pulmonary vasculature vasodilators (tolazoline), and possibly extracorporeal membrane oxygenation.
      (6) Infection

5. Long-term sequelae. Gestational age at onset of the growth retardation correlates with the severity of long-term sequelae.

  a. Onset prior to 26 weeks is generally severe and results in either death or a poor neurologic outcome.

  b. Little data are available for the 26–34-week age range.

  c. After 34 weeks, onset of intrauterine growth retardation generally causes no long-term damage unless associated with severe infection or anomalies. Growth in the postpartum period is rapid, and these infants usually reach normal physical growth patterns by 6 months of age and normal size and mental development by age 4.

  d. Treatment of these infants centers around:

   (1) Correction of anomalies

   (2) Testing for various causes of the intrauterine growth retardation

   (3) Nutritional support

   (4) Maintenance of a warm environment

D. Hyperbilirubinemia

  1. Incidence. Many newborn infants develop mild to moderate jaundice after birth. The incidence of visual jaundice during the first week of life is 60% of the term infants and 80% of preterm infants. The skin color results from the accumulation of lipid soluble bilirubin pigment formed as a product of hemoglobin molecular decomposition. This unconjugated material, at high concentrations, is neurotoxic.

  2. Etiology. Jaundice results from any disruption of the transition of bilirubin metabolism from the fetal stage where the placenta is the primary mode of bilirubin excretion to the adult stage where the liver conjugates bilirubin and excretes it into the bile and eventually the intestine. Disruptions include:

  a. Factors that increase the level of bilirubin to the liver, such as:

   (1) Rh disease and erythroblastosis

   (2) Other hemolytic anemias

   (3) Transfusions

   (4) Infections

   (5) Infant hematomas

  b. Factors that reduce the activity of the liver conjugating enzyme, such as:

   (1) Anoxia

   (2) Infection

   (3) Hypothermia

  c. Factors that compete for or block the enzyme, such as drugs

  d. Factors that lead to a decreased amount of the enzyme, such as:

   (1) Genetics

   (2) Prematurity

  e. Factors that reduce bilirubin retention in the blood and therefore increase the risk of toxic effects of bilirubin, such as:

   (1) Hypoproteinemia

   (2) Drugs that competitively bind with bilirubin to albumin

  f. Factors that increase the permeability of bilirubin to nerve cell membranes and therefore increase the toxic effects of bilirubin.

  3. Clinical manifestations

  a. It is characterized by yellow skin color.

  b. It may appear at any time during the neonatal period.

  c. The intensity of the color does not necessarily relate to the level of circulatory hyperbilirubinemia.

  d. The infant may be lethargic, feed poorly, and become dehydrated.

  4. Pathophysiology

  a. Normally infant bilirubin levels are 1–3 mg/dl at birth and peak at less than 10 mg/dl on the third to fourth day postpartum. The level decreases to below 2 mg/dl after 7 days. This "physiologic" jaundice results from the normal breakdown of red cells and transient limitation of conjugation and excretion by the liver.

  b. A search for other "pathologic" causes of the elevated bilirubin is initiated if:

   (1) Clinical jaundice is evident during the first 24 hours postpartum.

   (2) Serum bilirubin rises faster than 5 mg/dl/day.

   (3) Serum bilirubin is greater than 12 mg/dl in the full-term infant.

   (4) Jaundice persists after 7 days postpartum.

   (5) Serum conjugated bilirubin is greater than 1.0 mg/dl at any time.

    c. Kernicterus, neurologic damage caused by deposition of bilirubin into nerve cells, can occur if levels of bilirubin exceed 18–20 mg/dl.

5. Treatment

    a. The goal of therapy is the prevention of kernicterus.

    b. Phototherapy is the mainstay of treatment of hyperbilirubinemia.

        (1) It involves the use of high intensity fluorescent light, which is applied to the infant's skin.

        (2) The mechanism of action is not totally understood, but it involves the alteration of the bilirubin molecule in vivo, making biliary excretion more possible. *H₂O-soluble lumirub*

        (3) It should be used only after the cause of pathologic jaundice has been investigated and at least tenatively identified.

        (4) It is generally initiated if serum bilirubin levels are 10–15 mg/dl between 1 and 7 days postpartum.

        (5) It is discontinued when levels drop below 10 mg/dl.

    c. Exchange transfusion

        (1) It is used as frequently as is necessary to keep bilirubin levels under 20 mg/dl in the term infant.

        (2) The most common condition in which it is needed is Rh hemolytic disease of the newborn.

        (3) Exchange is initiated if bilirubin levels are over 15 mg/dl in the first 48 hours postpartum and any time over 20 mg/dl.

STUDY QUESTIONS

Directions: Each question below contains five suggested answers. Choose the **one best** response to each question.

1. All the following statements concerning the Apgar score are true EXCEPT

(A) it is formulated by assessing heart rate, respiratory effort, skin color, muscle tone, and reflex response
(B) it is used to determine the necessity and degree of resuscitative efforts
(C) it predicts the likelihood of the infant developing mental retardation
(D) severely depressed infants have Apgar scores of 3 or less
(E) resuscitative efforts should not be delayed to formulate the Apgar score

2. Mechanisms of heat loss in the newborn include all of the following EXCEPT

(A) evaporation
(B) convection
(C) condensation
(D) radiation
(E) conduction

3. All the following statements regarding a drug-depressed infant are true EXCEPT

(A) acute withdrawal symptoms can be precipitated with naloxone treatment in the infant of a mother addicted to narcotics
(B) immediate treatment with naloxone should be administered in the delivery room
(C) drug depression should be suspected in any newborn with poor respiratory effort at delivery
(D) drug depression does not occur with chronic maternal narcotic use irrespective of the time of last usage
(E) narcotic depression can occur if a narcotic analgesic has been given to the mother within several hours of delivery

4. A neonate's susceptibility to necrotizing enterocolitis is increased by all of the following factors EXCEPT

(A) excessive feeding
(B) crowded nurseries
(C) perinatal asphyxia
(D) phototherapy
(E) umbilical catheterization

5. A 30-year-old woman delivered a full-term infant weighing 7 lbs after prolonged rupture of membranes and prolonged induction of labor. Although the infant had initial Apgar scores of 7 at 1 minute and 8 at 5 minutes, it later had difficulty with temperature stability, cyanosis, and tachycardia. In addition, the mother developed a temperature of 102°F 2 hours after delivery. The most probable etiology for this set of clinical events is

(A) erythroblastosis fetalis
(B) hypoglycemia
(C) kernicterus
(D) respiratory distress syndrome
(E) neonatal sepsis

6. All of the following problems are associated with the intrauterine growth-retarded infant EXCEPT

(A) congenital anomalies
(B) shoulder dystocia
(C) metabolic acidosis
(D) persistent fetal circulation
(E) hypoglycemia

Directions: Each question below contains four suggested answers of which **one or more** is correct. Choose the answer

A   if **1, 2, and 3** are correct
B   if **1 and 3** are correct
C   if **2 and 4** are correct
D   if **4** is correct
E   if **1, 2, 3, and 4** are correct

7. Events at the time of delivery that initiate the conversion from fetal circulation to adult circulation include

(1) chest compression as the neonatal body is delivered
(2) ventilation of the lung
(3) cooling of the skin by evaporation
(4) clamping of the umbilical cord

8. True statements regarding congenital diaphragmatic hernia include which of the following?

(1) It results from a defect in fetal development in the eighth to ninth week of gestation
(2) The left side is more commonly affected than the right
(3) Pulmonary hypoplasia is associated with this condition
(4) Death occurs in 50% of cases

Directions: The group of questions below consists of lettered choices followed by several numbered items. For each numbered item select the **one** lettered choice with which it is **most** closely associated. Each lettered choice may be used once, more than once, or not at all.

Questions 9 and 10

For each clinical situation listed below, select the diagnosis that is most appropriate.

(A) Preeclampsia
(B) *Herpesvirus hominis*
(C) Gestational diabetes
(D) Narcotics addiction
(E) *Neisseria gonorrhoeae*

9. A 32-year-old woman who was pregnant for the first time had a routine prenatal course except that her infant seemed a bit larger than average. She went into labor at 41 weeks gestation and had a prolonged latent phase of labor. She also had a protracted active phase but progressed to complete dilation. She delivered a 10 lb 14 oz male infant by forceps; mild shoulder dystocia was encountered. The infant sustained no injuries. The second day after birth, a harsh, holosystolic murmer was heard across the precordium. Cardiac evaluation revealed a ventricular septal defect.

10. An 18-year-old woman who was pregnant for the first time had a normal prenatal course until 38 weeks gestation. In labor, however, her blood pressure rose from 140/90 to 156/95. Late decelerations developed, and she was delivered by cesarean section. The 4 lb 12 oz male infant had a 5 minute Apgar score of 7. He became jittery and developed hypoglycemia and hypocalcemia after birth. He subsequently did well after treatment.

ANSWERS AND EXPLANATIONS

1. The answer is C. (*II C, D 3*) The Apgar score assesses five characteristics of the newborn—heart rate, respiratory effort, skin color, muscle tone, and reflex response. This score is a useful measure of the need for resuscitative efforts. It does not predict ultimate outcome, although infants with a severely depressed Apgar score at 20 minutes are at high risk for developing cerebral palsy. Mental retardation is predicted on a multifactorial basis. Despite the usefulness of the Apgar score, resuscitation should not be delayed in order to compute the different parameters. This can be done after the infant is stabilized.

2. The answer is C. (*II D 1 a–d*) Newborns must be kept warm as they can lose heat rapidly by evaporation, convection, conduction, and radiation and become cold stressed. Evaporation occurs as amniotic fluid changes from a liquid to a gas, decreasing the newborn's skin temperature. Convection involves the cooling of the infant by room air currents. Conduction is the direct transfer of heat from the infant to a cooler object. Radiation of heat occurs from the surface of the infant out into the room. Condensation involves a cold object exposed to a warm, moist environment, which is the opposite of evaporation.

3. The answer is D. (*II E 3*) The neonatal effects of any drug taken by the mother may vary depending on the time of the last dose or the combined effects of several drugs. Naloxone should be given to any infant suspected of having narcotic depression at delivery. Naloxone (0.01 mg/kg) may be given intravenously or intramuscularly and may be repeated. Narcotics addiction should be considered in any woman who has had no prenatal care, who has signs of drug use or addiction, or who requires large or frequent doses of narcotics in the hospital.

4. The answer is D. (*III B 2 a–g, 3*) Although the cause of necrotizing enterocolitis is not fully understood, it relates to an inflammatory condition of the bowel in preterm infants where the intestine is compromised by hypoxia, asphyxia, or other perinatal events. Pathogenic bacteria seem to be related; thus, crowded nurseries may make it more likely for any infectious agent to be acquired. Excessive feeding may place a greater insult on an already stressed premature bowel. Phototherapy has no direct correlation with development of necrotizing enterocolitis. Umbilical catheterization has been shown to be related to necrotizing enterocolitis through mechanisms that are not fully understood.

5. The answer is E. (*IV B*) Although all of the conditions mentioned in the question are serious neonatal conditions, neonatal sepsis secondary to an infection in utero is the most likely diagnosis for the infant described in the question. This condition is often seen after prolonged rupture of membranes and prolonged labor. Additionally, given the maternal temperature elevation, the likelihood of neonatal infection is good.

6. The answer is B. (*IV C 3, 4 b*) The intrauterine growth-retarded infant is susceptible to many of the problems associated with poor nutrition and hypoxia, such as hypoglycemia, which is secondary to decreased glycogen reserve, and metabolic acidosis, which is secondary to chronic hypoxia. In addition, the symmetrically growth-retarded infant is more likely to have congenital anomalies or structural evidence of a viral infection. The persistent fetal circulation seen in growth-retarded infants is characterized by pulmonary hypertension, right-to-left shunting, and hypoxia. Shoulder dystocia is a problem encountered with the macrosomic infant of a diabetic mother.

7. The answer is C (2, 4). (*II B 1 a, b, 2 a–h*) Chest compression of the neonatal body is useful in clearing secretions from the neonatal lung to allow gas exchange, but it does not affect the transition from fetal to adult circulation. Cooling of the skin by evaporation can result in excess temperature loss and cold stress to the fetus, but it, too, has little to do with circulatory conversion. Ventilation of the lung decreases pulmonary vascular resistance, allowing greater pulmonary blood flow and less blood flow through the ductus arteriosus. Clamping of the umbilical cord increases aortic pressure, thereby further reducing flow through the ductus arteriosus and helping close the foramen ovale.

8. The answer is E (all). [*II E 2 a (1)–(9)*] Congenital diaphragmatic hernia results from the failure of the posterolateral pleuroperitoneal folds to close in the eighth to ninth week of gestation. The left side is affected 85% of the time, and thus more often than the right. Normal lung development is interrupted, which results in pulmonary hypoplasia and hypoxia, resulting in death in over 50% of cases.

9 and 10. The answers are: 9-C, 10-A. (*IV A 1 b, 2 a, C 3 b*) Gestational diabetes can result in fetal macrosomia from elevated maternal glucose levels throughout gestation. Shoulder dystocia is a potential complication of macrosomia. Fetal cardiac defects, such as ventricular septal defect, have a greater incidence in pregnancies associated with diabetes. Exposure in the first trimester to elevated glucose levels is important in the development of cardiac defects through unknown mechanisms.

Preeclampsia, a complication of pregnancy characterized by hypertension, proteinuria, and edema, can decrease uterine perfusion and is strongly associated with intrauterine growth retardation, placental insufficiency, hypocalcemia, and hypoglycemia. These clinical features do not characterize the other conditions listed in the question.

17
Operative Obstetrics
PonJola Coney

I. CESAREAN BIRTH. Cesarean (derived from the Latin *caedere* meaning to cut) section dates back to 700 BC in Rome when it was employed to remove infants from women who died late in pregnancy. In 1610, the first cesarean section was performed on a living patient. It is the most important surgical procedure in obstetrics. The maternal mortality rate was high up to the nineteenth century, most often due to hemorrhage and infection. However, advances in surgical and anesthetic techniques, safe blood transfusions, and the discovery of effective antibiotics have led to a dramatic decline in the mortality rate.

A. The incidence of cesarean sections has increased from 5%–22% of all births in most tertiary care centers, with an average of 15%. Cesarean section rates are lower in European countries (0.9%–12.7%) than in the United States.

    1. Perinatal mortality. Countries with the highest cesarean section rates have the lowest perinatal mortality rates, especially in the low-birth-weight groups (700–1500 g); however, factors other than cesarean sections have contributed to the decline in perinatal mortality, including:
        a. Fetal monitoring
        b. Steroids and tocolytic agents
        c. Sonography
        d. Up-to-date facilities
        e. Well-trained staff

    2. Indications. Cesarean section, however, is still accompanied by significant maternal risks and a morbidity greater than that with vaginal delivery; therefore, one or more of the following indications for cesarean section should exist before performing this procedure:
        a. Cephalopelvic disproportion
        b. Fetal and maternal anomalies
        c. Fetal malposition or posture
        d. Previous vaginal surgery (colporrhapy)
        e. History of uterine inversion
        f. Previous cesarean section
        g. Antepartum/intrapartum hemorrhage
        h. Medical or surgical disease of fetus or mother
        i. Failed trial or induction of labor
        j. Failed forceps or vacuum extractor delivery
        k. Cord prolapse
        l. Fetal distress

B. Complications. Less than 5% of cesarean sections are accompanied by complications, most of which are endometritis or wound infection.

    1. Endometritis/salpingitis

    2. Wound infection

    3. Hemorrhage

    4. Aspiration

    5. Atelectasis

    6. Urinary tract infection

    7. Deep venous thrombosis

8. Pulmonary embolus

9. Anesthetic complications

C. Types. There are two types of cesarean section that differ in the approach to the uterine wall.

1. Extraperitoneal cesarean section was devised for cases of amnionitis to avoid seeding the abdominal cavity. It has been virtually abandoned since the advent of effective antibiotics and because of the increased incidence of bladder and ureter injury incurred during the procedure.

2. Transperitoneal cesarean section is the approach almost exclusively used today.

D. Techniques

1. Patient preparation. The patient should be well hydrated and have a hematocrit of at least 30%. Blood should be readily available. The bladder should be empty. Prophylactic antibiotics are often given. Bacterial contamination is correlated with labor (duration, repeated vaginal examination, and status of membranes) before surgery. Antacids are also given. Informed consent should always be obtained.

2. Anesthesia can be **inhalational** (general) or **regional** (spinal, epidural). General anesthesia often results in depression of the infant immediately after delivery, the degree of depression increasing with delivery time. For this reason, patient preparation prior to the procedure (i.e., shaving, scrubbing, and draping) should be done before the induction of general anesthesia.

3. The abdominal incision can be **midline**, **paramedian**, or **Pfannenstiel**. The Pfannenstiel incision provides the most desired cosmetic effect but requires more time to perform. The infraumbilical vertical midline incision is less time consuming and less bloody.

4. Surgical techniques

   a. The pregnant uterus is palpated and inspected for rotation.

   b. The abdominal incision is made with the patient on the operating table with a lateral tilt of the body to the left to relieve any uteroplacental insufficiency that may result from compression of the inferior vena cava by the uterus when the patient is supine. The reflection of bladder peritoneum is incised and pushed down exposing the myometrium, the thickness of which varies according to the stage of labor. Incision of the myometrium is made as indicated or desired by the operating surgeon as follows:

   (1) Kerr (low transverse) is the incision most frequently employed today. It is made in the noncontractile portion of the uterus, minimizing chance of rupture or separation in subsequent pregnancies. The incision runs parallel with the muscle fibers of the cervix. It is essentially behind the peritoneal bladder reflection. The disadvantage of this incision is potential extension into the uterine vessels laterally.

   (2) Sellheim (low vertical) incision begins in the noncontractile portion of the uterus but almost always extends into the contractile portion (corpus).

   (3) Sanger (classical) is a longitudinal incision in the anterior fundus. It is infrequently used today but is indicated in cases of carcinoma of the cervix, lesions occupying the low segment of the uterus (myomas), and in the majority of cases of transverse lie. It is the simplest and quickest incision to perform. It carries a greater incidence of:

   (a) Postoperative adhesions

   (b) Hemorrhage from the incision site

   (c) Healing discomfort

   (d) Dehiscence during subsequent pregnancy and labor

   c. The infant is delivered with the **hand, forceps, vacuum extraction,** or **breech extraction**.

   d. The uterus is often exteriorized to massage the fundus, to inspect the adnexa, and for visualization of the wound for repair. Wound closure is as follows:

   (1) The uterus is closed in two layers. The first layer closes the main myometrial mass with interrupted or continuous heavy absorbable sutures. The first layer is then imbricated with adjacent myometrium to cover the suture line with the same type suture. This type of closure is peculiar to uterine myometrium for two reasons: coaptation and hemostasis. This is important in insuring the future integrity of the uterine scar.

   (2) The peritoneum of the bladder reflection is reattached with fine absorbable sutures, and the abdominal incision is closed in the usual manner.

5. Maternal morbidity and mortality are influenced by the indications for the surgery rather than by the procedure itself. The maternal mortality rate is 2/1000 (0.2%).

   a. Uterine rupture. The uterine scar from cesarean section has always been a major concern for subsequent pregnancies and labor.

(1) In 1957, Pedowitz and Schwartz reported the following incidences of uterine rupture, supporting the dictum, "Once a section, always a section":
    (a) Low transverse incision: 8.3%
    (b) Low vertical incision: 12.9%
    (c) Classical incision: 18.2%
(2) Today the incidence of uterine rupture is as follows:
    (a) Classical scar: 2%
    (b) Low segment incisions: 1%

   b. Vaginal delivery. Thus, because of the increased safety of cesarean section and the use of fetal monitoring, if scrupulous attention is given to surgical technique and if patients are carefully selected, a large number of patients with previous cesarean sections can achieve vaginal delivery.

II. EPISIOTOMY is an incision of the perineum at the end of the second stage of labor. It provides additional room for the fetal head during delivery, particularly with forceps and vacuum extractor deliveries, and prevents major perineal lacerations. Episiotomy is not practiced as routinely today as in the past; however, practice of routine episiotomy results in a decrease in the incidence of pelvic relaxation (i.e., cystocele and rectocele) and stress urinary incontinence in later years.

A. Median episiotomy results in less blood loss, is easier to repair, and is more comfortable during healing. The disadvantage is inadvertent cutting or extension into the anal sphincter and rectum. It is important to recognize and repair this complication during repair of the episiotomy because rectovaginal fistula may result from an unrecognized extension or inadequate repair.

B. Mediolateral episiotomy is incision of the perineum extended laterally to the anus onto the inner thigh, allowing more room than a median incision. This type of incision is more difficult to repair, results in more blood loss, and causes the patient more discomfort during healing. However, it is recommended in forceps deliveries and in deliveries where shoulder dystocia is expected (i.e., when more room is needed).

III. FORCEPS AND VACUUM EXTRACTOR OPERATIONS. Forceps and the vacuum extractor are used in obstetric operations to facilitate delivery in cases of failure of the second stage of labor secondary to malposition of the vertex, maternal fatigue, uterine inertia, and to avoid the voluntary forcing of the fetal head over the perineum. When using forceps or the vacuum extractor, if the head cannot be advanced with ordinary traction, the attempt should be abandoned. The success and results of both procedures depend upon the skill and judgment of the obstetrician.

A. Forceps. The forceps are two matched blades, which articulate and lock. The design of the blades provides standard **cephalic** (conforms to the shape of the fetal head) and **pelvic** (conforms to the axis of the vagina) curves.

  1. Application of the forceps is either **pelvic** or **cephalic.** Positions amenable to forceps application are occiput anterior (most customary), transverse, face (chin anterior), occiput posterior, and the aftercoming head in breech presentation.
    a. In pelvic application, the forceps are applied and locked with no reference to position of the head; however, this should never be done.
    b. In cephalic application, the forceps are applied to the occipitomental diameter of the head.

  2. Forceps operations
    a. High forceps. The forceps are applied before the head is engaged.
    b. Midforceps. The forceps are applied when the head is at or below the level of the ischial spines. Because of the safety of cesarean section and the potential damage to the infant and the birth canal, high and midforceps are almost anachronistic today.
    c. Low forceps. The forceps are applied when the head is visible at the introitus without separating the labia; that is, the skull is at the pelvic floor. This is the most popular use of forceps today. Forceps provide the final force (traction or rotation) required to deliver the head and, therefore, are considered "prophylactic." The head is lifted over the perineum, preventing damage to both the fetal head and the perineum. Forceps should never be applied to the breech, only the aftercoming head. Prerequisites for forceps delivery include:
      (1) The cervix must be completely dilated.
      (2) The correct position (vertex) must be known.
      (3) The membranes must be ruptured.
      (4) The bladder must be empty.

  3. Types of forceps commonly used include:

a. **Simpson's:** for traction in the occiput anterior position
b. **Tucker-McLean:** to rotate or deliver from the occiput posterior to occiput anterior position
c. **Kielland and Barton:** to rotate the occiput transverse to occiput anterior position
d. **Piper:** to deliver the aftercoming head of the breech

B. **Vacuum extractor.** There are two types of vacuum extractors; each type has some sort of cup, a rubber hose, and a vacuum pump.

1. **The Malmstrom vacuum extractor** consists of a metal cup (3–6 inches in diameter), which is applied to the fetal scalp and creates a vacuum, not exceeding 0.7–0.8 kg/cm². Traction is then applied to bring the infant's head through the introitus.

2. **The plastic cup extractor** consists of a flexible cup that is applied to the fetal scalp more easily and with less trauma than the Malmstrom extractor. The vacuum pressures attained are about the same but can be reached more quickly and with less trauma to the fetal scalp. This extractor is the more widely used of the two in the United States.

3. **Complications.** The major concern of the vacuum extractor is trauma to the scalp and brain. A caput succedaneum is always produced, which clears over a period of hours to days. The vacuum extractor is a definite improvement over the high and midforceps deliveries. Incidences of complications are:
   a. Scalp abrasion or laceration: 12.6%
   b. Cephalohematoma: 6%
   c. Intracranial hemorrhage 0.35% (little different from spontaneous vaginal deliveries)

IV. CERVICAL CERCLAGE

A. **Cervical incompetence** is characterized by painless dilation of the cervix, usually leading to second-trimester spontaneous abortion. This occurs secondary to insufficiency of the internal cervical os.

1. **The etiology** of cervical incompetence may be **acquired** or **congenital**. Acquired causes are primarily obstetric and surgical (e.g., rapid delivery, forceps, trauma, surgical dilation, conization, breech extraction, and induced labor).

2. **The diagnosis** is almost always from a clinical history of repeated late spontaneous abortions.
   a. Other etiologies for spontaneous abortion must be excluded (e.g., uterine anomalies, infection, hormonal dysfunction, and chromosomal aberrations).
   b. A cervix that allows insertion of a no. 8 Hegar dilator past the internal os may be regarded as incompetent.
   c. The widened os may also be demonstrated by hysterosalpingography.

B. **Cerclage of the cervix** involves the placement of an encircling suture about the cervical os, using a heavy, nonabsorbable suture or mercilene tape. The suturing prevents protrusion of the amniotic sac and consequent rupture by correcting the abnormal dilation of the cervical os. The following are two techniques used today for cervical cerclage:

1. **Shirodkar** is the most complicated procedure, whereby the suture is almost completely buried beneath the cervical mucosa. It can be left in place for subsequent pregnancies if a cesarean is performed.

2. **McDonald** is the simplest procedure incurring less trauma to the cervix and less blood loss than the Shirodkar procedure. It is a simple purse-string suture of the cervix.

C. **The success rate** of cerclage is 85%–95% of cases. It is usually performed between the fourteenth and sixteenth weeks of gestation but can be performed as late as the twenty-fourth week. The suture is removed at 38 weeks or earlier if labor begins. Labor is often rapid. Infection is infrequent but can occur. When the cervix is dilated and completely effaced, this operation is impractical. Fetal viability and the absence of anomalies should be documented before performing the procedure.

V. ABORTION is the termination of pregnancy before viability (i.e., capability of the fetus surviving extrauterine).

A. **Spontaneous abortion** is the expulsion of products of conception without medical or mechanical intervention. Five types of spontaneous abortion are as follows:

1. **Threatened abortion** occurs when bleeding and uterine cramping appear without cervical dilation. Therapy is often bed rest and observation.

2. **Inevitable abortion** occurs with profuse hemorrhaging, rupture of the membranes, and cramping with a dilated cervical os. Therapy is evacuation of the uterus via sharp or suction curettage.

3. **Incomplete abortion** occurs when some products of conception are expelled but some tissue remains in the uterine cavity. Therapy is evacuation of remaining tissue by curettage.

4. **Missed abortion** is death of the fetus or embryo without the onset of labor or the passage of tissue. Management is the same as in inevitable abortion.

5. **Habitual abortion** is three consecutive spontaneous abortions. This requires evaluation for etiologies, including:
   a. Cervical incompetence
   b. Uterine anomalies
   c. Infection
   d. Hormonal dysfunction
   e. Chromosomal aberrations

B. **Induced abortion.** Abortion first became legal in 1973 and can be induced up to 20 weeks gestation. Therapeutic abortions are those induced for the purpose of safeguarding the health of the mother and in cases of genetic disease and anomalies in the fetus.

1. **Medical means of inducing abortion** include extrauterine and intrauterine administration of abortifacients, such as prostaglandins, urea, hypertonic saline, and oxytocin.

2. **Mechanical means of inducing abortion** are far safer than medical induction and, therefore, more prevalent. *Laminaria* (seaweed) is used to gently and slowly dilate the cervix, incurring minimal if any cervical trauma before evacuation.
   a. Dilatation of the cervix and evacuation of the products of conception (D and E) by vacuum suction are used for both first- and second-trimester gestations.
   b. Other mechanical methods, which are now obsolete, include:
      (1) Sharp curettage
      (2) Hysterotomy
      (3) Hysterectomy

3. **Anesthesia** for induced abortion can be general or local. General anesthesia is accompanied by higher incidences of hemorrhage, cervical injury, and perforation than local anesthesia.

4. **Complications**
   a. Hemorrhage
   b. Cervical injury
   c. Coagulation defects
   d. Retained products of conception
   e. Infection
   f. Perforation
   g. Infertility
   h. Rh sensitization
   i. Embolism
   j. Live-born fetus
   k. Uterine rupture

5. **Mortality.** The overall mortality for abortion (induced) is approximately 30/100,000.

BIBLIOGRAPHY

Bergsjo P, et al: Differences in the reported frequencies of some obstetrical interventions. *Br J Obstet Gynecol* 90:628, 1983

Danforth D: *Obstetrics and Gynecology,* 3rd ed. New York, Harper & Row, pp 597, 630, 693-694, 1977

Pedowitz P, Schwartz RM: The true incidence of silent rupture of C-section scars. *Am J Obstet Gynecol* 74:1071, 1957

Plauche WC: Fetal cranial injuries related to delivery with the Malmstrom vacuum extractor. *Obstet Gynecol* 53:750, 1979

STUDY QUESTIONS

Directions: Each question below contains five suggested answers. Choose the **one best** response to each question.

1. The most important result of the increased number of cesarean sections being performed today is

(A) decreased maternal morbidity
(B) decreased maternal mortality
(C) decreased perinatal mortality
(D) increased maternal mortality
(E) increased use of fetal monitoring

2. Indications for a cesarean section include all of the following EXCEPT

(A) previous cesarean section
(B) failed forceps delivery
(C) fetal distress
(D) cervical cerclage
(E) cord prolapse

3. Habitual abortion can result from all of the following causes EXCEPT

(A) cervical incompetence
(B) hormonal dysfunction
(C) chromosomal abnormalities
(D) bicornuate uterus
(E) subserous myomas

4. Which of the following methods for induced abortion are no longer routinely practiced?

(A) Dilatation and evacuation after 12 weeks gestation
(B) Extrauterine administration of abortifacients
(C) Hysterotomy
(D) Intrauterine administration of abortifacients
(E) *Laminaria* for cervical dilation

Directions: Each question below contains four suggested answers of which **one or more** is correct. Choose the answer

> A if **1, 2, and 3** are correct
> B if **1 and 3** are correct
> C if **2 and 4** are correct
> D if **4** is correct
> E if **1, 2, 3, and 4** are correct

5. Which of the following complications could accompany an extraperitoneal cesarean section?

(1) Wound infection
(2) Pyelonephritis
(3) Endometritis
(4) Peritonitis

6. The advantages of an episiotomy include

(1) minimal trauma to the perineum
(2) few long-term incidences of pelvic relaxation and stress urinary incontinence
(3) additional room for the fetal head to deliver
(4) elimination of the need for forceps or vacuum extractor deliveries

7. Absolute prerequisites for the use of forceps or the vacuum extractor include

(1) a breech presentation
(2) uterine inertia
(3) fetal distress
(4) ruptured membranes

8. Which of the following types of abortion require surgical intervention?

(1) Incomplete
(2) Threatened
(3) Missed
(4) Habitual

ANSWERS AND EXPLANATIONS

1. The answer is C. (*I A 1*) The dramatic increase in cesarean section rates over the past 10 years has resulted in a decline in perinatal mortality, especially in the low-birth-weight groups (700–1500 g). Other factors, such as fetal monitoring, sonography, well-trained staff, and up-to-date facilities, have also had a major impact on decreasing perinatal mortality. Maternal morbidity is still significant but less so than before the advances in antimicrobial therapy and anesthetic techniques.

2. The answer is D. (*I A 2 a–l; IV B, C*) All of the possibilities listed in the question—previous cesarean section, failed forceps delivery, fetal distress, and cord prolapse—are accepted reasons for performing a cesarean section except for the cervical cerclage. However, a previous cesarean section is not as important an indication as previously because of the low incidence of uterine rupture with labor and because of the desire of many women to have a vaginal birth. Most cervical cerclages for incompetence today are of the McDonald type, which are used only for the pregnancy involved. The stitch is cut prior to or during labor, and cesarean section is not performed unless some other obstetric indication arises.

3. The answer is E. (*V A 5*) All of the possibilities listed in the question are associated with habitual abortion except subserous myomas. The myomas on the surface of the uterus (subserous) do not cause abortions; however, the myomas within the cavity of the uterus (submucous) can cause abortions. Cervical incompetence, luteal phase (progesterone) deficiencies, balanced chromosomal translocations, and abnormal uterine configurations can lead to repeated abortions.

4. The answer is C. (*V B 2 b*) With the legalization of abortion, many medical and mechanical means are now available to safely terminate pregnancy. Hysterotomy, popular many years ago, is no longer used in induced abortion. Procedures now widely practiced are safer than those used previously (e.g., sharp curettage, hysterotomy, and hysterectomy), particularly dilatation and evacuation via suction curettage.

5. The answer is A (1, 2, 3). (*I B 1–9, C 1*) Although it is not performed today, the extraperitoneal cesarean section had one advantage over the transperitoneal cesarean section: The potentially infected uterine contents with chorioamnionitis could not come in contact with or seed the peritoneal cavity. Therefore, peritonitis would be unlikely with the extraperitoneal section. However, any of the other complications that can accompany a transperitoneal section can occur, such as, wound infection because of the incision, pyelonephritis because of the catheterized bladder, and endometritis because of the susceptible endometrium with ruptured membranes and labor.

6. The answer is A (1, 2, 3). (*II*) With increasing demands from patient advocate groups for fewer traditional practices in obstetrics (e.g., shaving, enemas, or episiotomies), the episiotomy is not practiced as routinely today as in the past. However, it is well documented that in populations in which routine episiotomy is practiced, there are fewer cases of cystocele and rectocele. Protection is provided to the perineum from extensive lacerations, and additional room is provided for delivery, especially in forceps and vacuum extractor deliveries, minimizing damage to the birth canal and the fetal head.

7. The answer is D (4). [*III A 2 c (2), (3)*] The vacuum extractor and forceps must never be used with a breech presentation. The correct (cephalic) presentation must be known, and even then, care must be taken to secure delivery with minimal trauma to the fetus and the birth canal. It may be impossible to determine the correct presentation in the presence of bulging and intact membranes, which can obscure the head, making the correct application of instruments to the fetal head impossible. Uterine inertia and fetal distress often occur in the terminal stages of the second stage of labor and may or may not be managed with forceps or a vacuum extractor.

8. The answer is B (1, 3). (*V A 1–5*) Both the incomplete and the missed abortions imply an abnormal pregnancy, which requires the emptying of the uterus via suction curettage. The spontaneous process is incomplete in one and has not yet occurred in the other. The threatened abortion is manifested by no more than bleeding and, thus, needs no intervention yet. The habitual abortion describes three or more spontaneous abortions in one individual.

18

Obstetric Analgesia and Anesthesia
William W. Beck, Jr.

I. PHYSIOLOGIC FACTORS. The safety of the mother and the fetus must be a constant concern when considering analgesia and anesthesia for labor and delivery. Virtually all drugs administered during labor pass through the placenta; thus, a balance must be sought between pain relief for the mother and safety for the fetus.

A. Mother

1. **Cardiovascular and pulmonary function changes**
   a. There is a 33% *increase* in cardiac output during pregnancy between the twenty-fifth and thirty-sixth weeks.
   b. There is a 42% *increase* in pulmonary ventilation at term.
   c. Pregnancy requires a 10%–15% *increase* in oxygen consumption due to basic metabolic changes in the pregnant female and the fetus.
   d. There is an 18% *reduction* in the functional residual capacity of the lungs at the end of expiration; however, an *increase* in both the inspiratory capacity of the lungs and in the rate of respiration compensates for this reduction.
   e. The heavy uterus may cause a *reduction* in cardiac return, which, in turn, may reduce blood pressure and placental perfusion.

2. **Hazards of anesthesia**
   a. The onset of labor with its associated fear and pain may cause cessation of digestion; the stomach may contain food that was eaten 12–18 hours previously. Stomach contents must always be considered before anesthesia is administered.
   b. When inhalation anesthesia is used for delivery, there is an increased risk of aspirating the stomach contents.
   c. Since inhalation anesthesia may cause a reduction in uterine tone, it is important to monitor the depth of anesthesia closely so that it does not result in uterine atony.

B. Fetus

1. The maternal cardiovascular and pulmonary systems must work efficiently to provide oxygenated blood under sufficient pressure to perfuse the placenta. In addition, normal maternal acid–base balance must be maintained to prevent fetal acidosis. A reduced uterine blood flow may result from:
   a. Low maternal blood pressure
   b. Decreased maternal cardiac return
   c. A reduction in maternal pulmonary ventilation
   d. Vascular alterations due to anesthesia

2. Because there is greater resistance in the placental membranes than in the pulmonary alveoli (of the mother), the transfer of gases across the placenta is less efficient than across the alveoli.

3. Oxygen and carbon dioxide traverse the placenta by simple diffusion.
   a. The oxygen pressure gradient across the placenta is 20–25 mm Hg, and the carbon dioxide gradient is 4–5 mm Hg.
   b. The umbilical artery pH and the umbilical vein pH are essentially the same or only slightly less (0.02 units) than the maternal pH.

4. Fetal hemoglobin, which is more efficient than adult hemoglobin, is characterized by a shift to the left of the oxygen dissociation curve. Characteristics of fetal hemoglobin include the following:

a. It allows the efficient removal of oxygen from the placenta.

b. It allows a complete and an efficient unloading of oxygen in the fetal tissues.

c. It facilitates the transfer of carbon dioxide from fetal tissues to fetal blood and then to the maternal circulation.

C. Placental transfer. The placenta is not equipped with any natural barriers to anesthetic or analgesic agents. The respiratory center of the fetus is vulnerable to sedative and anesthetic drugs, leading to respiratory depression at birth.

1. The transfer of analgesic and anesthetic agents from the maternal circulation to the fetal circulation occurs by simple diffusion, which depends on:

a. The concentration gradient between maternal and fetal blood

b. The surface area and thickness of the placenta

c. The diffusion constant of a particular drug

2. Lipid substances, which are nonionized, diffuse into the placenta quite readily; therefore, anesthetic and analgesic agents that are lipid soluble and of low molecular weight enter the fetal circulation within 60 seconds. Muscle relaxants, on the other hand, are highly ionized, of low-lipid solubility, and diffuse poorly through the placenta and into the fetal circulation.

3. If only a single dose of an analgesic or anesthetic is administered, the mother absorbs most of it in her tissues, thus protecting the infant from the narcotizing effect of the drug.

4. If repeated doses of a drug are administered, the maternal tissues absorb relatively less medication.

a. Each succeeding dose increases the gradient between the fetal and maternal circulations.

b. The increased gradient allows the drug to accumulate in the fetal tissues and brain, producing a greater effect upon the respiratory center of the newborn.

II. ANALGESIA AND SEDATION DURING LABOR.
Uterine contractions and cervical dilation cause pain during labor. Medication for pain relief is often indicated to allow the mother to rest between contractions and to experience only moderate discomfort at the peak of the uterine contraction.

A. Meperidine and promethazine. A combination of a narcotic analgesic drug, such as meperidine, and a tranquilizer drug, such as promethazine, will effectively relieve pain during labor.

1. Meperidine (50–100 mg) with promethazine (25 mg) can be administered intramuscularly every 3–4 hours as needed. An intramuscular administration has a maximal analgesic effect in about 45 minutes.

2. When meperidine is administered intravenously, the dose is usually no more than 50 mg because analgesia occurs more rapidly by this route (about 5 minutes), and the depressant effect on the fetus is more predictable (about 90 minutes).

3. There is little evidence to suggest that meperidine affects the progress of labor, but it can cause a decrease in the beat-to-beat variability on the fetal monitor.

B. Butorphanol and nalbuphine are synthetic narcotic agonist–antagonist analgesics given intravenously, which cause less neonatal depression than meperidine.

C. Morphine. This powerful narcotic is not often used for analgesia in active labor. In doses of 10–15 mg intramuscularly, it is a particularly valuable analgesic for patients who are having the frequent painful contractions that are characteristic of a nonprogressive labor (i.e., hypertonic dysfunctional labor).

D. Narcotic antagonists. When narcotic agents are given close to delivery, the infant may be significantly depressed at birth. Naloxone is a narcotic antagonist that is capable of reversing the respiratory depression by displacing the narcotic from specific receptors in the central nervous system.

III. CONDUCTION ANESTHESIA

A. Neuropathways of obstetric pain. The complete relief of pain in obstetrics can be accomplished by blocking the sympathetic pathways of the eleventh and twelfth thoracic nerves and the parasympathetic and sensory fibers of the sacral nerves.

1. **Uterine contractions.** The pain of uterine contractions is transmitted from the uterus to the sympathetic nerves of the hypogastric plexus. The impulses are then transmitted by the paravertebral sympathetic chain and enter the grey rami of the eleventh and twelfth thoracic nerves.

2. **Cervical dilation.** The pain sensations of a dilating cervix are transmitted through the eleventh and twelfth thoracic nerves with overlap through the tenth thoracic and first lumbar nerves.

3. **Parturition.** The pain stimuli of parturition are transmitted to the cord by the pudendal nerve through the sensory fibers of the second, third, fourth, and fifth sacral nerves.

B. **Paracervical block** is effective for the relief of pain from uterine contractions but not for delivery.

1. **Route of administration.** By injecting local anesthetic—that is, lidocaine (Xylocaine)—paracervically at 3 and 9 o'clock or uterosacrally at 4 and 8 o'clock, the visceral afferent pain fibers are blocked. Pain relief for 1–2 hours is provided by 5–10 ml of 1% lidocaine injected on each side of the cervix.

2. **Complications.** Fetal bradycardia, a complication 10%–25% of the time, is not a sign of fetal asphyxia but is secondary to the transplacental transfer of the anesthetic agent or its metabolite, which has a depressant effect on the fetal heart. The bradycardia usually lasts from 6–10 minutes.

C. **Pudendal block**, which is basic to obstetric anesthesia, provides perineal anesthesia by anesthetizing the pudendal nerve. It works well for spontaneous delivery and episiotomy repair, but it is not likely to provide adequate anesthesia for a forceps delivery.

1. **Route of administration.** The main trunk of the pudendal nerve lies on the posterior surface of the sacrospinous ligament just medial to the ischial spine. A 1% lidocaine solution (10 ml) is injected on each side transvaginally around the tip of the ischial spine and through the sacrospinous ligament.

2. **Complications.** The intravascular injection of the local anesthetic can cause systemic toxicity characterized by stimulation of the cerebral cortex, leading to convulsions, and depression of the medulla, leading to respiratory depression.

D. **Spinal anesthesia** is a satisfactory method of alleviating the discomfort of uterine contractions and delivery since the level of anesthesia to the tenth thoracic nerve anesthetizes the sympathetic fibers of the eleventh and twelfth thoracic nerves and the parasympathetic and sensory fibers of the sacral plexus. Spinal anesthesia is satisfactory for both vaginal and cesarean deliveries, but is contraindicated in the presence of hemorrhage or overt pregnancy-induced hypertension.

1. **Route of administration.** Spinal anesthesia is administered by injecting a local anesthetic into the subarachnoid space. Pregnant patients need smaller amounts of anesthetic agents than nonpregnant patients because the subarachnoid space is smaller in a pregnant patient as a result of the engorgement of the internal vertebral venous plexus—a consequence of compression by the pregnant uterus on the inferior vena cava. Thus, a normal dose of an anesthetic agent could produce a much higher spinal blockade in a pregnant patient than in a nonpregnant patient. The level of the anesthesia is influenced by:
   a. The specific gravity of the agent
   b. The site of the injection
   c. The position of the patient
   d. The concentration of the anesthetic solution

2. **Complications of spinal anesthesia** include:
   a. **Hypotension**, which is the most common complication. It is due to the vasodilation from the sympathetic blockade compounded by obstructed venous return because of compression by the uterus on the inferior vena cava. It is treated by:
      (1) Uterine displacement to the left
      (2) Acute hydration with a saline solution
      (3) Intravenous ephedrine (10–15 mg)
   b. **High spinal blockade with respiratory paralysis.** This is a very dangerous complication as hypotension and apnea quickly develop and may progress to cardiac arrest. Ventilation with an endotracheal tube is indicated until the anesthesia wears off.
   c. **Spinal headache**, which is caused by leakage of cerebrospinal fluid from the puncture site.

The headache may persist for 3–5 days.

    (1) When the woman stands, the diminished volume of cerebrospinal fluid allows traction on pain-sensitive central nervous system structures, such as the pia–arachnoid.

    (2) Bed rest, analgesics, hydration, and the use of an abdominal binder are helpful.

  d. Meningitis. Because of sterile techniques and disposable equipment, contamination and infection of the meninges are now rare.

E. Epidural anesthesia. Caudal anesthesia and lumbar epidural anesthesia are accomplished by injecting suitable local anesthetic agents into the epidural or peridural space—a potential space that immediately surrounds the dura and extends from the foramen magnum to the sacral hiatus.

  1. Route of administration

    a. Caudal anesthesia is produced by injecting a local anesthetic, such as bupivacaine (0.25% or 0.5%), through the sacral hiatus into the caudal space.

      (1) The sacral hiatus is a foramen at the lower end of the sacrum, which results from the nonclosure of the last sacral vertebra.

      (2) This foramen leads to the caudal space—the lowest extent of the peridural space.

      (3) A rich network of sacral nerves runs through the caudal space; an anesthetic agent injected into this space abolishes the sensation of pain carried by the sacral nerves, producing anesthesia suitable for delivery.

    b. Lumbar epidural anesthesia is injected into the same anatomic space as caudal anesthesia, but the anesthetic agent is injected into the lumbar area of the space rather than through the sacral hiatus.

      (1) Anesthesia for the pain of labor and vaginal delivery depends on a block from the tenth thoracic nerve to the fifth sacral nerve; the block for an abdominal delivery must extend from the eighth thoracic nerve to the first sacral nerve.

      (2) The spread of lumbar anesthesia depends on:

        (a) The location of the catheter tip in the peridural space

        (b) The dose of the anesthetic agent

        (c) The head-down, horizontal, or head-up position of the patient

      (3) If the meninges are perforated with the needle and the usual amount of anesthetic agent is injected, the anesthesia will be subarachnoid and may rapidly produce a total spinal blockade.

  2. Complications of epidural anesthesia

    a. Inadvertent spinal anesthesia may occur with puncture of the dura and injection of the anesthetic agent. The complications of a high spinal block may follow (see section III D 2 b).

    b. Intravenous injection of the anesthetic agent can result in central nervous system toxicity with slurred speech, tinnitus, convulsions, or even cardiac arrest.

    c. Ineffective anesthesia may occur in a rapidly progressive labor because of the time it takes for peridural anesthesia to become effective. Perineal anesthesia for delivery may be difficult to obtain with the lumbar epidural anesthesia because the block does not include the sacral nerves.

    d. Hypotension and decreased placental perfusion occur because of the blockade of the sympathetic tracts and pooling of blood below the pregnant uterus.

    e. An epidural block induced prior to well-established labor may be followed by desultory labor. In addition, the patient's expulsive efforts may be hampered, leading to an increased incidence of forceps or vacuum extractor deliveries.

IV. GENERAL ANESTHESIA. Since the placenta is not a barrier to general anesthesia, all anesthetic agents that depress the central nervous system of the mother cross the placenta and depress the central nervous system of the fetus. General anesthesia is used in obstetric emergencies when the fetus must be delivered quickly or if conduction anesthesia (epidural or spinal) is containdicated because of back problems.

A. Gas anesthetics

  1. Nitrous oxide is used to provide pain relief during labor and delivery.

    a. Nitrous oxide does not prolong labor or interfere with uterine contractions.

    b. Satisfactory analgesia can be obtained with a concentration of 50% nitrous oxide and 50% oxygen with the patient breathing the mixture intermittently while pushing during the second stage of labor.

  2. Cyclopropane is infrequently used today for either vaginal or abdominal delivery because it is explosive and must be administered in a closed system.

    a. It is not a good myometrial relaxant that permits intrauterine manipulation of the fetus.

b. Because of the depressant effect of this gas, the infant often requires resuscitation at birth unless the time during which the anesthesia is administered prior to delivery is very short.

B. Volatile anesthetics

1. **Halothane** produces significant uterine relaxation and should be restricted to situations that require a relaxed uterus, such as internal podalic version, breech extraction, and replacement of the acutely inverted uterus. Prompt discontinuation of the anesthetic is necessary to prevent hemorrhage from an atonic uterus.

2. **Methoxyflurane** may be self-administered by a hand-held mask in low concentrations to provide analgesia during the first and second stages of labor as well as during delivery. It may depress myometrial contractility, leading to uterine inertia during labor and increased blood loss after delivery because of uterine atony.

3. **Enflurane**, like halothane, may cause myometrial depression and increased blood loss. It should not be used in a patient with impaired renal function.

C. Aspiration during general anesthesia. Pneumonitis from inhalation of gastric contents is the most common cause of anesthetic death in obstetrics.

1. **Prophylaxis.** Important factors in preventing aspiration include the following:
   a. The patient should fast for as long as possible prior to the induction of general anesthesia.
   b. After labor has begun, only clear liquids should be permitted.
   c. Before the induction of anesthesia, gastric acidity should be neutralized with antacids, such as sodium citrate.
   d. With intubation, cricoid pressure is administered to compress the esophagus just as the patient is being induced with sodium pentathol.

2. **Pathology.** When the pH of aspirated gastric fluid is below 2.5, a severe chemical pneumonitis develops.
   a. Aspiration of particles without acidic fluid leads to:
      (1) Patchy atelectasis
      (2) Bronchopneumonia
   b. Aspiration of acidic fluid leads to:
      (1) Tachypnea
      (2) Bronchospasm
      (3) Rhonchi
      (4) Rales
      (5) Atelectasis
      (6) Cyanosis
      (7) Hypotension
   c. Exudate into the lung interstitium and alveoli causes:
      (1) Decreased pulmonary compliance
      (2) Shunting of blood
      (3) Severe hypoxemia

3. **Treatment**
   a. Suction. As much inhaled material as possible must be removed immediately from the mouth, pharynx, and trachea.
   b. Bronchoscopy. This procedure is indicated if large particulate matter is causing airway obstruction.
   c. Corticosteroids. Large doses of intravenous corticosteroids should be administered every 8 hours for 24 hours in an attempt to maintain cell integrity in the presence of strong acid.
   d. Oxygen and ventilation. Endotracheal intubation with intermittent positive pressure may be necessary to maintain the arterial P_{O_2} at 60 mm Hg. Frequent suction is necessary to remove secretions and edema fluid.
   e. Antibiotics. Infection after aspiration is most frequently caused by anaerobes. Therefore, coverage with clindamycin or metronidazole is indicated.

STUDY QUESTIONS

Directions: Each question below contains five suggested answers. Choose the **one best** response to each question.

1. All of the following statements concerning maternal physiology during pregnancy are correct EXCEPT

(A) cardiac output is increased
(B) pulmonary ventilation is increased
(C) oxygen consumption is increased
(D) functional residual capacity of the lungs is increased
(E) inspiratory capacity of the lungs is increased

2. Epidural anesthesia in a pregnant woman may result in all of the following conditions EXCEPT

(A) hypotension
(B) decreased placental perfusion
(C) decreased venous return
(D) increased venous pooling
(E) increased cardiac output

Directions: Each question below contains four suggested answers of which **one or more** is correct. Choose the answer

A if **1, 2, and 3** are correct
B if **1 and 3** are correct
C if **2 and 4** are correct
D if **4** is correct
E if **1, 2, 3, and 4** are correct

3. Correct statements concerning placental transfer of analgesic agents include which of the following?

(1) It occurs by simple diffusion
(2) It depends on the concentration gradient between maternal and fetal blood
(3) It is a function of placental surface area and thickness
(4) It is rapid with ionized substances

4. Perineal anesthesia is provided by anesthetizing the

(1) pudendal nerve
(2) parasympathetic fibers of the second through fourth sacral nerves
(3) sensory fibers of the second through fourth sacral nerves
(4) hypogastric plexus

5. A spinal headache after spinal anesthesia for labor and delivery is caused by

(1) leakage at the puncture site
(2) traction on the pia–arachnoid
(3) diminished cerebrospinal fluid volume
(4) hypotension

6. Anesthetic agents associated with increased postpartum blood loss include which of the following?

(1) Methoxyflurane
(2) Halothane
(3) Enflurane
(4) Cyclopropane

7. Standard treatment of aspiration pneumonitis includes

(1) antibiotics
(2) corticosteroids
(3) ventilation
(4) antacids

Directions: The group of questions below consists of lettered choices followed by several numbered items. For each numbered item select the **one** lettered choice with which it is **most** closely associated. Each lettered choice may be used once, more than once, or not at all.

Questions 8 and 9

For each clinical presentation listed below, select the type of anesthesia that is most likely to have been administered.

(A) General anesthesia
(B) Paracervical block
(C) Spinal anesthesia
(D) Lumbar epidural anesthesia
(E) Meperidine

8. A woman is in labor, and her cervix is 2 cm dilated. She is having regular contractions, which occur every 3 minutes. She requests pain relief but is allergic to meperidine. Within 10 minutes of receiving the anesthetic agent, the fetal heart tones drop to 60 beats/min.

9. A woman is in active labor, and her cervix is 5 cm dilated. She requests something for pain relief. Within 5 minutes of receiving the anesthesia, she is in respiratory arrest.

ANSWERS AND EXPLANATIONS

1. The answer is D. *(I A 1 a–d)* Due to an increased fluid volume and changes in the basic metabolic rate in pregnant women, cardiac output, pulmonary ventilation, oxygen consumption, and the inspiratory capacity of the lungs are increased. However, because of the enlarging uterus, which pushes the intra-abdominal contents under the diaphragm, there is an actual decrease in the functional residual capacity of the lungs at the end of expiration.

2. The answer is E. *(I A 1 a, e; III D 2, E 2)* Because of the blockade of the sympathetic tracts with epidural anesthesia in a pregnant woman, there is pooling of blood in the lower extremities below the large uterus with a decreased venous return. This can result in hypotension and decreased placental perfusion, which in turn can cause fetal distress. There would not be an increased cardiac output because the anesthesia would cause a decrease in the venous return to the heart, resulting in a decreased maternal cardiac output.

3. The answer is A (1, 2, 3). *(I C 1 a–c, 2)* The placental transfer of analgesic agents occurs by simple diffusion, which, in turn, is influenced by concentration gradients and surface area. Most anesthetic agents are lipid soluble, of low molecular weight, and nonionized, which allow for rapid transfer across the placenta. Ionized agents traverse the placenta slowly.

4. The answer is B (1, 3). *(III A 3, C)* Pain from the perineum travels to the spinal cord through the pudendal nerve, which involves the sensory fibers, not the parasympathetic fibers, of the second through fourth sacral nerves. The hypogastric plexus is not involved.

5. The answer is A (1, 2, 3). *(III D 2 a, c)* Spinal headaches are caused by leakage of cerebrospinal fluid from the puncture site through the dura. As a result of diminished cerebrospinal fluid volume, there is traction on the pain-sensitive structures of the central nervous system, such as the pia–arachnoid, with a resultant headache. Hypotension is not a factor in the usual spinal headache.

6. The answer is A (1, 2, 3). *(IV A 2, B 1–3)* Halothane, methoxyflurane, and enflurane can cause depressed myometrial contractility and significant uterine relaxation. This, in turn, may be related to increased blood loss after delivery of the placenta due to uterine atony. Cyclopropane is not a good uterine relaxant and is not associated with an atonic postpartum uterus.

7. The answer is A (1, 2, 3). *(IV C 1, 2, 3 a–e)* Once gastric contents have been aspirated and pneumonitis is a fact, prophylaxis, such as antacids, is no longer effective. The problem, mostly a chemical pneumonitis, ultimately involves exudate into the lung interstitium. Bronchoscopy, oxygen, ventilation, and corticosteroids are used to combat the aspiration and the chemical pneumonitis. Antibiotics are used to treat the infection following aspiration; this infection is frequently caused by anaerobes.

8 and 9. The answers are: 8-B, 9-D. *(III B 1, 2, D 2 a–c, E 1 b, 2 a–e)* For women in early labor (2 cm dilated in this case), spinal anesthesia is out of the question because delivery is hours away. Epidural anesthesia is not advisable either this early in labor as it is usually given when the cervix is 4–5 cm dilated. The woman described in the question is allergic to meperidine, the commonly used intravenous narcotic for pain relief in early labor. Paracervical block is perfect for such cases to help with the pain of uterine contractions. However, one of the complications of paracervical block is a transient fetal bradycardia.

The woman in active labor who is 5 cm dilated is a perfect candidate for epidural anesthesia. Spinal anesthesia is not an option at this point because delivery is not in the immediate future. Paracervical block would be possible, but it would not last until delivery. The woman received lumbar epidural anesthesia, which became a spinal when the dura was inadvertently punctured. The larger dose of anesthetic agent used in epidural anesthesia (as opposed to spinal anesthesia) was injected and caused the equivalent of a high spinal block with respiratory paralysis.

19
Gestational Trophoblastic Disease
William W. Beck, Jr.

I. INTRODUCTION. Gestational trophoblastic disease (GTD) is the general term for a spectrum of proliferative abnormalities of the trophoblast associated with pregnancy.

A. Clinical classification

1. **Hydatidiform mole** is characterized by proliferation of the trophoblast, which may fill the uterine cavity, suggesting an advanced normal pregnancy. Hydatidiform moles may be complete or partial.

2. **Gestational trophoblastic neoplasia (GTN)** is malignant trophoblastic disease, which arises from the trophoblastic elements of the developing blastocyst, retains the invasive tendencies of the normal placenta, and retains the ability to secrete the polypeptide hormone, human chorionic gonadotropin (HCG). GTN can be either metastatic or nonmetastatic.

B. Incidence

1. **Benign GTD** (hydatidiform mole) occurs in 1 out of 1200 pregnancies in the United States and 1 out of 120 pregnancies in other parts of the world (e.g., the Far East).
   a. There is an increased incidence among women with low socioeconomic status and women in underdeveloped areas, such as Southeast Asia.
   b. Moles tend to occur in older women.
   c. Spontaneous remission is common in 80%–85% of patients after dilatation and evacuation.
   d. Malignant GTD (GTN or choriocarcinoma) develops in 3%–5% of moles.

2. **Malignant GTD** occurs in 1 out of 20,000 pregnancies in the United States and may follow:
   a. Hydatidiform mole (50%)
   b. Normal pregnancy (25%)
   c. Abortion and ectopic pregnancy (25%)

II. HYDATIDIFORM MOLE

A. Characteristics (microscopic features)

1. **Complete mole**
   a. Marked edema and enlargement of the villi
   b. Disappearance of the villous blood vessels
   c. Proliferation of the lining trophoblast of the villi
   d. Absence of fetus, cord, or amniotic membrane
   e. A normal karyotype (usually XX, rarely XY)

2. **Partial mole**
   a. Marked swelling of the villi with atrophic trophoblastic cells
   b. Presence of normal villi
   c. Presence of a fetus, cord, and amniotic membrane
   d. An abnormal karyotype, usually triploidy or trisomy

B. Symptoms

1. Bleeding usually occurs in the first trimester.

2. The uterus is often larger than expected with respect to the last menstrual period.

3. Nausea and vomiting occur in about one-third of patients.

4. Preeclampsia in the first trimester is almost pathognomonic of a molar pregnancy.

5. There is an occasional occurrence of clinical hyperthyroidism, hypothesized to be caused by binding of the HCG molecule (with elevated levels of HCG) by the thyroid-stimulating hormone (TSH) receptor site and hyperfunction of the gland.

6. Abdominal pain secondary to theca lutean cysts is found in 15% of patients due to the excessive HCG produced by the molar pregnancy.

C. Diagnosis

1. The first evidence of a molar pregnancy may be the passage of vesicular tissue.

2. A quantitative HCG of greater than 100,000 mIU/ml with an enlarged uterus and bleeding is suggestive of a mole.

3. Amniography can make the definitive diagnosis by demonstrating the characteristic honeycomb appearance on x-ray.

4. A flat plate of the abdomen after 15 weeks fails to show any fetal skeleton.

5. Ultrasonography can be very specific by demonstrating multiple echoes without the normal gestational sac or fetus.

D. Management

1. Suction curettage is the primary tool for evacuation of a mole even when the uterus is larger than 20 weeks.
   a. Suction curettage has almost eliminated the need for hysterotomy, which was commonly used before suction was available when the uterus was larger than 12–14 weeks.
   b. Suction curettage is used in conjunction with intravenous oxytocin, which is begun after a moderate amount of tissue has been removed.

2. Primary hysterectomy may be selected as the method of evacuation if the patient does not desire future pregnancies.
   a. If theca lutean cysts are encountered, the ovaries are left untouched as the cysts will regress as the HCG level falls to normal.
   b. Despite the hysterectomy, the follow-up is no different from the suction evacuation of the molar pregnancy.

3. Prophylactic chemotherapy. Since 80% of patients with molar pregnancies have spontaneous remission and do not require any therapy and since serial HCG determinations can identify the 20% who will develop malignancies, it is not appropriate to treat all patients. The toxicity from prophylactic chemotherapy can be severe, and deaths have occurred.

E. Follow-up. The average time to expect complete elimination of HCG is 73 days; however, this time period depends on the initial level of HCG, the amount of viable trophoblastic tissue remaining after evacuation, and the serum half-life of HCG. Follow-up of a molar pregnancy should include:

1. HCG determinations every 1–2 weeks until they are negative twice, then monthly for 1 year. Patients must be advised to use contraception for 1 year.

2. Physical examination, including a pelvic examination every 2 weeks until remission, then every 3 months for 1 year.

3. Chest film initially and then a repeat film if the HCG titer plateaus or rises to rule out pulmonary metastases.

4. Chemotherapy should be started immediately if the HCG titer rises or plateaus during follow-up or if metastases are detected at any time.

III. GESTATIONAL TROPHOBLASTIC NEOPLASIA (GTN)

A. Characteristics

1. Abnormal uterine bleeding due to GTN may appear within a relatively short time or years after a pregnancy.

2. Bleeding from lesions in the lower genital tract can occur at any time.

3. Metastatic disease can be found in the gastrointestinal tract, the genitourinary system, the liver, the lung, and the brain, often associated with hemorrhage because of the propensity of trophoblastic tissue to invade vessels.

B. Diagnosis

1. With a high index of suspicion, a quantitative HCG is diagnostic.

2. Workup of the patient with GTN should include the following:
   a. Chest film and intravenous pyelogram
   b. Liver and CT scans
   c. Hematologic survey and serum chemistries
   d. Pretreatment HCG titer
   e. Ultrasound of the pelvis

C. Nonmetastatic GTN. This is the most common form of the disease and is confined to the uterus.

1. **Treatment.** Treatment of nonmetastatic GTN has been almost 100% successful.
   a. Patients with nonmetastatic disease can be treated with single-agent chemotherapy (e.g., methotrexate, actinomycin D, and high-dose methotrexate with folic acid rescue) at 7-day intervals until negative HCG titers are obtained for 3 consecutive weeks or unless one of the following toxic reactions occurs:
      (1) Thrombocytopenia
      (2) Leukopenia
      (3) Oral or gastrointestinal ulceration
      (4) Febrile course
      (5) Abnormal BUN, SGPT, and SGOT
   b. In patients who failed chemotherapy, secondary hysterectomy can be performed followed by remission.
   c. In patients who no longer desire fertility, primary hysterectomy is recommended during the first course of chemotherapy.
   d. Almost 50% of those desiring pregnancy following treatment for nonmetastatic GTN have been successful with normal infants in 80%–85% of cases being reported.

2. **Follow-up**
   a. Three consecutive normal weekly HCG assays
   b. HCG titers every 2 weeks for 3 months, then monthly for 3 months, then every 2 months for 6 months, then every 6 months
   c. Frequent pelvic examinations
   d. Chest x-ray every 3 months for a year
   e. Contraception for 1 year

D. Metastatic GTN is disease outside the uterus. Patients have various symptoms, such as hemoptysis (pulmonary metastases) or neurologic signs (brain metastases).

1. **Good prognosis metastatic GTN**
   a. The following factors are associated with a good prognosis:
      (1) Short duration (last pregnancy less than 4 months previously)
      (2) Low pretreatment HCG titer (HCG titer less than 40,000 mIU/ml)
      (3) No metastatic spread to the brain or liver
      (4) No significant prior chemotherapy
   b. **Treatment** is the same as the treatment for nonmetastatic GTN with similar results (see section III C 1); however, when compared with nonmetastatic GTN, more courses of chemotherapy are required in patients being treated for good prognosis metastatic GTN.
      (1) Once negative titers have been achieved, one additional course of chemotherapy is routinely given.
      (2) If resistance to methotrexate occurs (rising or plateauing HCG titers) or if negative titers are not achieved by the fifth course, patients are switched to actinomycin D.
      (3) If there is resistance to both drugs, patients are started on a multiple-agent protocol of methotrexate, actinomycin D, and chlorambucil.
      (4) Primary and secondary hysterectomy are used in a similar manner as in treatment for nonmetastatic GTN.
   c. **Follow-up** is the same as with nonmetastic GTN (see section III C 2).

2. **Poor prognosis metastatic GTN**
   a. The following factors are associated with a poor prognosis:
      (1) Long duration (last pregnancy more than 4 months previously)
      (2) High pretreatment HCG titer (titer greater than 40,000 mIU/ml)
      (3) Liver and brain metastases
      (4) Failure of prior chemotherapy

    b. Treatment. There is a significant problem in treating patients with a poor prognosis because many have been treated previously with chemotherapy and are thus resistant to therapy; these patients are also likely to experience considerable toxicity and to deplete bone marrow reserves.

      (1) These patients should be treated with multiple-agent chemotherapy, and a multiple modality approach is necessary.

      (2) Patients should be treated in centers that have special interest and expertise in this disease, especially when the life-threatening toxicity from therapy is a factor.

      (3) The remission rate for these patients is about 66% with patients treated with chemotherapy and concurrent radiation therapy having the best prognosis. If primary or secondary hysterectomy is necessary, the prognosis worsens.

    c. Follow-up

      (1) Three consecutive normal weekly HCG assays

      (2 HCG titers every 2 weeks for 3 months then monthly for a year, then every 6 months for 4–5 years

      (3) Chest x-ray every 3 months

      (4) Contraception until 1 year of negative titers have been achieved

E. Recurrence rates

    1. Nonmetastatic GTN (2%)

    2. Good prognosis metastatic GTN (5%)

    3. Poor prognosis metastatic GTN (21%)

STUDY QUESTIONS

Directions: Each question below contains five suggested answers. Choose the **one best** response to each question.

1. Signs and symptoms associated with a hydatidiform mole include all of the following EXCEPT

(A) first-trimester bleeding
(B) a uterus larger than the expected gestational age
(C) hypothyroidism
(D) preeclampsia at 14 weeks gestation
(E) nausea and vomiting

2. Follow-up of the management of a hydatidiform mole should routinely include all of the following EXCEPT

(A) human chorionic gonadotropin level determinations
(B) pelvic examinations
(C) contraception
(D) chest films
(E) chemotherapy

Directions: Each question below contains four suggested answers of which **one or more** is correct. Choose the answer

A   if **1, 2, and 3** are correct
B   if **1 and 3** are correct
C   if **2 and 4** are correct
D   if **4** is correct
E   if **1, 2, 3, and 4** are correct

3. Usual treatment of a hydatidiform mole includes

(1) suction dilatation and evacuation
(2) hysterotomy
(3) hysterectomy
(4) resection of the accompanying ovarian cysts

4. Treatment modalities for nonmetastatic gestational trophoblastic neoplasia are characterized by

(1) a success rate of approximately 80%
(2) treatment with single-agent chemotherapy
(3) treatment with hysterectomy without chemotherapy
(4) treatment with chemotherapy until negative human chorionic gonadotropin titers are obtained for 3 consecutive weeks

5. Characteristics of poor prognosis metastatic gestational trophoblastic neoplasia include

(1) pretreatment human chorionic gonadotropin values of more than 40,000 mIU/ml
(2) recurrence rate of 5%
(3) brain metastases
(4) no prior chemotherapy

Directions: The group of questions below consists of lettered choices followed by several numbered items. For each numbered item select the **one** lettered choice with which it is **most** closely associated. Each lettered choice may be used once, more than once, or not at all.

Questions 6–8

For each clinical presentation that follows, select the therapeutic modality that is most appropriately indicated.

(A) Chemotherapy
(B) Chemotherapy and hysterectomy
(C) Hysterectomy
(D) Suction dilatation and evacuation
(E) No treatment is indicated

6. A 23-year-old nullipara presents with irregular vaginal bleeding. Her first pregnancy ended in a spontaneous abortion 3 months previously. Her human chorionic gonadotropin (HCG) titer is 35,000 mIU/ml. Chest x-ray is negative. Liver and brain scans are negative. Pelvic examination reveals a normal uterus. Dilatation and curettage (D and C) reveals gestational trophoblastic neoplasia (GTN).

7. A 35-year-old multigravida had a therapeutic abortion and tubal ligation 3 months previously. She presents with uterine bleeding and an HCG titer of 30,000 mIU/ml. The uterus is a normal size. Chest x-ray is negative, and an ultrasound of the pelvis reveals no masses or abnormalities. D and C reveals GTN.

8. A 40-year-old grand multipara presents 12 weeks after her last menstrual period. She had had a postpartum tubal ligation that obviously failed. She complains of vaginal bleeding and has a uterus enlarged to the level of the umbilicus and an HCG titer of 100,000 mIU/ml. Flat plate of the abdomen reveals no fetal skeleton. Ultrasound reveals no gestational sac or fetus.

ANSWERS AND EXPLANATIONS

1. The answer is C. (*II B 1–6*) Bleeding from a uterus that is larger than the expected gestational age is suggestive of a hydatidiform mole. Nausea and vomiting are also frequent findings and may take the form of hyperemesis gravidarum. Preeclampsia, except with a molar pregnancy, is uncommon before the third trimester. Occasionally, hyperthyroidism is seen in a molar pregnancy, but not hypothyroidism, as a result of binding of the human chorionic gonadotropin molecule by the thyroid-stimulating hormone receptor sites and hyperfunction of the gland.

2. The answer is E. (*II E 1–4*) Follow-up of the management of a hydatidiform mole should routinely include human chorionic gonadotropin (HCG) level determinations every 1–2 weeks until two consecutive negative titers are obtained and pelvic examinations every 2 weeks until remission. A chest film should be obtained initially and repeated if the HCG level plateaus or rises to rule out pulmonary metastases. Contraception is important so that the pregnancy HCG does not obscure the plateauing or rising of the molar HCG levels. Chemotherapy is not used routinely but only if the HCG level plateaus or rises.

3. The answer is B (1, 3). (*II D 1, 2*). Suction dilatation and evacuation (D and E) is the primary approach in the treatment of a mole. In conjunction with intravenous oxytocin, the suction D and E has practically eliminated the use of hysterotomy in the treatment of a molar pregnancy. Hysterectomy is appropriate therapy if there is no desire for future pregnancies, but the theca lutean cysts should be left untouched because they will resolve once the mole is evacuated and the human chorionic gonadotropin level drops.

4. The answer is C (2, 4). (*III C 1 a–d*) The usual treatment of nonmetastatic gestational trophoblastic neoplasia (GTN) is single-agent chemotherapy. If the patient does not desire future pregnancies, a primary hysterectomy can be performed in conjunction with single-agent chemotherapy. Therapy is continued until negative human chorionic gonadotropin titers are obtained for 3 consecutive weeks. Treatment for nonmetastatic GTN has been almost 100% successful.

5. The answer is B (1, 3). (*III D 2 a, E 3*) High pretreatment human chorionic gonadotropin values, a long duration between the last pregnancy and the gestational trophoblastic neoplasia (GTN), liver and brain metastases, and failed prior chemotherapy comprise the criteria for poor prognosis metastatic GTN. After treatment, poor prognosis metastatic GTN has a recurrence rate of 21% not 5%.

6–8. The answers are: 6-A, 7-B, 8-C. (*II D 2; III C 1 a, c*) The 23-year-old nullipara has a nonmetastatic gestational trophoblastic neoplasia (GTN). She is young and probably desires future pregnancies; thus the treatment should be single-agent chemotherapy.

The 35-year-old multigravida has nonmetastatic GTN. She is an older woman who has had a tubal ligation and thus obviously desires no future pregnancy. In patients who no longer desire fertility, primary hysterectomy is recommended during the first course of chemotherapy.

The 40-year-old grand multipara has a molar pregnancy that needs to be treated. She does not desire future pregnancies as indicated by her previous (failed) tubal ligation; therefore, a primary hysterectomy would be the indicated therapy.

Part II
Gynecology

20
Pediatric and Adolescent Gynecology
PonJola Coney

I. INTRODUCTION. An awareness of the problems that are unique to pediatric and adolescent gynecology is required for proper management of the young patient. Particular care is essential in performing a pelvic examination because both physical and emotional trauma may be inadvertently inflicted. Often a complete physical examination, in addition to a pelvic examination, can help to establish rapport and reassurance in a patient unaccustomed to examination of sexual areas. The adolescent patient should have a pelvic examination at menarche or at least by high school age and then regularly after becoming sexually active, or whenever she feels the need.

A. Pelvic examination of a pediatric patient may reveal the following:

1. A mucoid vaginal discharge and even vaginal bleeding for up to 2 weeks after birth as a result of maternal estrogens

2. An introitus that is located more anteriorly and a clitoris that is more prominent than normal (1–2 cm)

3. A redundant hymen that may protrude on straining and that remains essentially the same size until age 10, allowing the passage of instruments

4. A vaginal epithelium that is uncornified and erythematous with an alkaline pH

5. A small uterus (2.5–3 cm) with the cervix comprising two-thirds of the organ—the reverse of adult proportions

6. A cervical os that normally appears as an ectropion

B. Visualization of the vagina. Instruments for visualizing the vagina include the vaginoscope, the urethroscope, and the pediatric speculum. Stirrups are usually not necessary for the preadolescent; a simple "frog-leg" position is usually sufficient. Anesthesia or a "pediatric cocktail"* may be necessary, particularly in cases of rape.

C. Rectal examination is often more informative because the short posterior vaginal fornix cannot be distended and a cul-de-sac does not exist.

II. VULVOVAGINAL LESIONS

A. Lichen sclerosus et atrophicus

1. **Clinical picture.** A white, papular lesion resembling leukoplakia may cover the vulva and perianal regions.

2. **Etiology.** The etiology is unknown.

3. **Diagnosis.** Biopsy, which shows superficial hyperkeratosis with basal atrophic and sclerotic changes, should be performed to clarify the diagnosis.

4. **Therapy.** This condition is benign and self-limiting, rarely requiring therapy; however, cortisone may be used temporarily for itching.

B. Trauma

1. **Clinical picture**
   a. Tears, abrasions, ecchymoses, and hematomas are common in preadolescent girls.

---

*A pediatric cocktail is a combination of meperidine (Demerol), promethazine (Phenergan), and chlorpromazine (Thorazine) for analgesia and amnesia.

b. Rape trauma necessitates immediate medical attention, including a complete physical examination, cervical and rectal smears, serologic tests, and psychological evaluation and follow-up.

2. Therapy
a. Conservative therapy for most trauma consists of rest, heat, and analgesics.
b. With rape, penicillin therapy is advised as prophylaxis for venereal infection.

C. Labial agglutination

1. Clinical picture. Adhesion of the labia minora in the midline, usually the result of irritation or skin disease (epidermolysis bullosa) is the usual presentation. A line extends vertically downward and distinguishes labial agglutination from imperforate hymen or vaginal atresia. The agglutination encourages retention of urine and infection.

2. Therapy
a. Topical estrogen* twice daily is used to induce cornification of the epithelium and to promote spontaneous separation.
b. Surgical separation is sometimes necessary.

D. Imperforate hymen

1. Clinical picture. The usual presentation is a bulging introitus, which is usually an isolated anomaly.

2. Therapy
a. Surgical correction prior to puberty is imperative.
b. Cruciate incisions into the membrane maintains patency.

E. Prolapsed uretha

1. Clinical picture. A red mass at the vaginal orifice occludes the vagina and usually causes dysuria. This lesion must be differentiated from ureterocele. If it is not reduced promptly, the urethra may become gangrenous.

2. Therapy
a. Reduction is rarely possible without surgical excision of the redundant tissue.
b. Attempts should be made to catheterize the center of the mass or perform retrograde cystourethrography.

F. Vaginal discharge

1. Clinical picture
a. A mucoid discharge is common in infants for up to 2 weeks after birth as a result of maternal estrogen. It is also a common finding in pre- and postpubertal girls, perhaps as a result of increased estrogen production by maturing ovaries.
b. Discharge may result from any of the following conditions:
(1) Infections with organisms, such as *Escherichia coli*, *Proteus*, *Pseudomonas*, yeast, *Gardnerella*, *Neisseria gonorrhoeae*, and *Trichomonas*
(2) Hemolytic streptococcal vaginitis, which results in a bloody or serosanguineous discharge, generally following a streptococcal infection elsewhere (e.g., skin or throat)
(3) Monilial vaginitis, which is common in diabetic children or following antibiotic therapy
(4) A foreign body, which can cause persistent vaginal discharge, sometimes with pain and bleeding
(5) Nonspecific vaginitis from local irritation, scratching, or manipulation

2. Therapy. Conservative management is advisable, consisting of the following:
a. A culture to identify causative organisms and saline/potassium hydroxide preparations to treat appropriately
b. An urinalysis to rule out cystitis
c. Questioning for unhygienic practices, such as use of irritating soaps and powders or tight underclothing
d. A perianal examination with Scotch tape to test for pinworms
e. Administration of estrogen,* which decreases the vaginal pH and cornifies the epithelium, to alleviate symptoms resistant to other therapy

---

*The use of estrogen in the prepubertal female may cause breast stimulation.

III. CONGENITAL ANOMALIES

A. Vaginal atresia

1. Clinical picture. Vaginal atresia represents a failure of caudal müllerian duct or sinovaginal bulb development of the urogenital sinus. Ovarian development is normal, but there is less than a 10% chance that the uterus is functional.

2. Therapy. Surgical correction should be deferred until the structures are well developed unless a functional uterus is present.

B. Ectopic ureter with vaginal terminus

1. Clinical picture
   a. Ectopic ureter, the most common cause of vaginal cysts in infants, presents as a ureterocele, which appears as a cystic mass protruding from the vagina. If the ureter is patent, constant irritation and vaginitis may be presenting signs.
   b. The ectopic ureter is usually one of a pair to a single kidney, and it almost always drains the rudimentary upper renal pole of the kidney.
   c. Hydroureter and hydronephrosis may also develop.

2. Diagnosis is made with an intravenous pyelogram to outline the tract and allow visualization of the entire urinary tract.

3. Therapy. Resection of the lowest portion of the ureter and implantation into the bladder is preferable to removal of the ureter and the associated portion of the kidney.

C. Vaginal ectopic anus

1. Clinical picture. Vaginal ectopic anus is an imperforate anus associated with rectovaginal communication. Only a skin dimple is found at the normal anal site.

2. Therapy. Surgical correction is indicated.

IV. NEOPLASMS

A. Tumors of the vagina, while uncommon, are most often malignant when they do occur.

1. Vaginal adenosis
   a. Clinical picture. Vaginal adenosis is a benign condition that presents as strawberry red areas in the vagina.
   b. Diagnosis
      (1) There is a history of maternal ingestion of diethylstilbestrol (DES).
      (2) Diagnosis is by cytologic studies, colposcopy, and biopsy.

2. Clear cell adenocarcinoma
   a. Clinical picture. Vaginal bleeding, discharge, and pain are common presenting symptoms, but many patients are asymptomatic.
   b. Diagnosis. Clear cell adenocarcinoma, which is found at or after puberty, is a malignancy associated with maternal ingestion of DES.

3. Sarcoma botryoides
   a. Clinical picture
      (1) Sarcoma botryoides is a tumor that arises from mesenchymal tissue of the cervix or vagina, usually on the anterior wall of the upper vagina.
      (2) It grows rapidly, fills the vagina, and then protrudes through the introitus.
      (3) It appears as an edematous, grape-like mass that bleeds readily on touch.
      (4) It is usually multicentric, and extension is usually local with rare instances of distant metastases.
   b. Therapy. It is curable only by radical surgery.

B. Ovarian tumors

1. Clinical picture. Though uncommon in children, ovarian tumors present as torsion (twisting). Forty percent of ovarian neoplasms are of non–germ-cell origin (coelomic epithelium), and sixty percent are of the germ-cell origin.
   a. Non–germ-cell origin
      (1) Lipoid cell tumors (feminizing)
      (2) Granulosa–theca cell tumors (feminizing), of which approximately 20% are malignant

b. Germ-cell origin
   (1) Benign cystic teratomas
   (2) Benign cysts
   (3) Arrhenoblastomas (virilizing)
   (4) Germinomas and gonadoblastomas (tumors of dysgenetic gonads)
   (5) Endodermal sinus tumors
   (6) Embryonal carcinomas (gonadotropin-secreting)
   (7) Immature teratomas, which account for 20% of malignant germ-cell tumors

2. Therapy is surgical, alone or in combination with radiation and chemotherapy, depending on the tumor.

V. DEVELOPMENTAL DEFECTS OF THE GENITALIA. Early diagnosis is important so that proper assignment of sex can be made during the neonatal period in order to establish a management plan that will minimize psychological problems and facilitate establishment of the gender role.

A. Congenital adrenal hyperplasia results when enzymatic regulation of the biosynthesis of cortisol and aldosterone is impaired at various steps in the pathway. The increase in the precursors immediately preceding the impaired step and by-products have biologic activity that can lead to the clinical and biochemical features observed. The sites on the steroid nucleus that can be affected are carbons 21, 20, 17, 18, 11, and 3. The most common sites are 21, 11, and 3. The 21-hydroxylase defect is the most common cause of distinct virilization of the female newborn. Its incidence is 1/5,000 births, and it accounts for 95% of all cases of congenital adrenal hyperplasia, which is inherited as an autosomal recessive trait.

   1. Clinical picture. The chromosomes, gonads, and internal genitalia are female, and the degree of closure of the urogenital orifice varies. Clitoral enlargement and accentuation of labial folds are characteristic. The disorder is progressive if untreated.

   2. Diagnosis. Urinary pregnanetriol, urinary 17-ketosteroids, and plasma 17-hydroxyprogesterone are elevated.

   3. Therapy. Hydrocortisone is administered indefinitely to all patients.

B. Adrenal tumors, which may cause virilization of the external genitalia after infancy should be suspected in children with very high levels of urinary 17-ketosteroid excretion.

C. Maternal ingestion of synthetic progestins can result in masculinization of the female fetus.
   1. Clinical picture. Masculinization is limited to the external genitalia. The clitoris is enlarged, and the labia are fused, but the vagina, tubes, and uterus are normal. Growth and development are normal, and progressive virilization does not occur.

   2. Diagnosis can be made from a positive history and by exclusion.

   3. Therapy. Clitoral reduction and surgical correction of fused labia may be necessary.

D. Androgen ingestion by children is usually through preparations with androgenic activity (e.g., hair and scalp ointments and medications).

E. Androgen insensitivity syndrome (testicular feminization)
   1. Clinical picture. Androgen insensitivity is characterized by a 46,XY genotype and a female phenotype. The vagina ends as a blind pouch, and testicles can be found in the labia. These patients who are often raised as females, have a deficiency of the androgen receptors. The external genitalia can appear virilized in the incomplete form (Rifenstein syndrome).

   2. Therapy. The testicles should be removed after puberty and maturation because of an increased risk of malignancy (3%–4% before age 25).

F. True hermaphroditism
   1. Clinical picture. The genotype of most true hermaphrodites is most commonly 46,XX. The external genitalia may appear male, female, or ambiguous. Both male and female internal genitalia may be present. Sex assignment and rearing should be consistent with the dominant appearance of the external genitalia and with surgical correctability.

   2. Therapy. The genitalia inconsistent with sex assignment should be surgically removed or modified.

G. Maternal virilizing tumor during pregnancy (luteoma of pregnancy) can result in masculinization of the female fetus. The clinical picture and the therapy are similar to the maternal ingestion of synthetic progestins (see section V C).

VI. SPECIAL PROBLEMS OF THE ADOLESCENT

A. Dysmenorrhea

  1. Clinical picture
  a. Dysmenorrhea may be secondary to obstructive and other anatomic causes.
  b. Nausea, vomiting, and diarrhea are common accompaniments.

  2. Etiology. Frequently, no organic etiology is found.

  3. Therapy
  a. Antiemetics
  b. Prostaglandin inhibitors

B. Dysfunctional uterine bleeding (DUB). Most adolescent girls have anovulatory menstrual periods for the first 2–3 years after menarche; approximately 2% of adolescents ovulate in the first 6 months, and 18% by the end of the first year after menarche. This bleeding is not considered pathologic unless the menses last more than 7 days and anemia is present, in which case the condition is known as DUB.

  1. Etiology. The usual etiology of DUB is an immature hypothalamic–pituitary axis. Other causes include psychogenic factors, juvenile hypothyroidism, and coagulation disorders (von Willebrand's disease).

  2. Clinical picture
  a. Menometrorrhagia is the most characteristic symptom.
  b. The condition is usually self-limited, but if symptoms persist for more than 4 years, there is a 50% chance of future DUB.

  3. Therapy is cyclic hormonal manipulation with estrogens and progestins.

C. Amenorrhea. Primary amenorrhea categorizes menarche that has not yet occurred, and secondary amenorrhea categorizes menstruation that ceases for more than 6 months. Late menarche or oligomenorrhea are common before age 16. Evaluation is indicated if menarche is delayed beyond age 16. Chromosomal abnormalities account for approximately 30%–40% of all cases of primary amenorrhea. Other etiologies for amenorrhea include malnutrition; delayed puberty; systemic illness; central nervous system lesions; tumors; and psychogenic (anorexia nervosa), anatomic, hypothalamic, and metabolic disorders.

  1. Müllerian anomalies and **vaginal atresia** represent 20% of cases. Forty-five percent of these patients have associated urinary tract abnormalities. **Anatomic causes** include imperforate hymen and hematometra.

  2. Hypogonadotropic hypogonadism, which is characterized by a deficiency of pituitary or hypothalamic hormone secretion (particularly gonadotropin), accounts for 40%–50% of all cases of amenorrhea. **Kallmann's syndrome** is an autosomal dominant disorder in which there is a deficiency of gonadotropin-releasing hormone (GnRH). Hypopituitarism with obesity (adiposogenital dystrophy) manifests as adiposity of breasts, mons pubis, pelvic girdle, and atrophy of the genitalia. The etiology is unknown.

  3. Systemic illnesses, including infections; hepatic, thyroid, and adrenal diseases; diabetes mellitus; cystic fibrosis; and hemoglobinopathies (e.g., sickle cell anemia and thalassemia) may be responsible for amenorrhea.

  4. Central nervous system lesions, including space-occupying lesions (e.g., craniopharyngioma, pinealomas, adenomas), trauma, and vascular lesions may play a role in amenorrhea and delayed adolescent development.

  5. Anorexia nervosa, characterized by extreme weight loss with no known organic etiology, can affect adolescent development and cause amenorrhea. Psychiatric symptoms can be present, and occasionally the outcome is fatal.

  6. Gonadal dysgenesis (hypergonadotropic hypogonadism) is characterized by absence of secondary sex characteristics, infantile but normal genitalia, and streak-like gonads that are devoid of germ cells and appear as fibrous white streaks. The presence of a Y chromosome dictates early removal of the gonads because of their propensity to malignancy (25% of cases by age 15). The different forms of gonadal dysgenesis are listed below:

a. **Turner's syndrome** (45,X) is characterized at birth by low birth weight, short stature, edema of the hands and feet, and loose skin folds on the neck. Adolescent patients present with short stature, lack of sexual maturation, low posterior hairline, prominent ears, broad chest, and epicanthal folds.

b. **Swyer's syndrome** (46,XY) is characterized by a female phenotype with a lack of secondary sex characteristics and amenorrhea. Growth is usually normal and some virilization may occur after puberty, especially when gonadal tumors are present. This clinical picture without virilization and tumor propensity can also occur in 46,XX individuals, whose condition is termed "**pure gonadal dysgenesis**." Swyer's syndrome is inherited as an X-linked recessive trait. Pure gonadal dysgenesis is compatible with autosomal recessive inheritance.

c. **Mixed gonadal dysgenesis** (45,X/46,XY mosaicism) is characterized by sexual ambiguity in the newborn. Internal structures include müllerian and wolffian derivatives. There is asymmetrical development of the gonads expressed as a testis or gonadal tumor on one side with a rudimentary gonad, a streak, or no gonad on the other side.

d. **Abnormalities of the X-chromosome** (mosaicism, isochromosome, long arm, short arm X deletion, long arm X deletion, and translocation) result in amenorrhea and varying degrees of Turner's syndrome features.

D. **Delayed puberty** Although most adolescents with delayed puberty prove to have no underlying physiologic or anatomic abnormality (constitutional), evaluation is indicated if there are no secondary sex characteristics by age 13.

1. **Etiology.** The causes of amenorrhea mentioned previously apply to delayed puberty as well. Disorders that are only associated with delayed puberty include Hand-Schüller-Christian disease, developmental defects of the midbrain, dwarfism, Prader-Willi syndrome, and Laurence-Moon-Biedl syndrome).

2. **Diagnosis** is based on neurologic, physical, and pelvic examinations; measurement of gonadotropin levels; karyotype; and endocrine profiles.

3. **Therapy** is simply gonadal steroid replacement (estrogen/progesterone).

E. **Precocious puberty** is characterized by early sexual maturation with menarche before the age of 9.

1. **Types of precocious puberty**
   a. **Heterosexual precocious puberty** is the development of secondary sex characteristics that are inconsistent with genetic sex. The etiology may include tumors (arrhenoblastomas), congenital adrenal hyperplasia, and chronic ingestion of androgenic preparations.
   b. **Isosexual precocious puberty** is the development of secondary sex characteristics consistent with genetic sex. Precocious puberty can be divided into true sexual precocity in which the homones are secreted by maturing gonads and precocious pseudopuberty in which maturing normal gonads are not the source of the sex steroids.
      (1) **Clinical picture.** It has been found that 80%–90% of cases of isosexual precocious puberty have no obvious underlying etiology (idiopathic). A family history can sometimes be elicited. The clinical course is usually benign. Patients are larger than normal for chronologic age (height, weight, and bone age). Somatic and genital development are consistent with bone age. There is early closure of the epiphyses, so that final height is less than normal. Intellectual capacity is not accelerated or abnormal, although electroencephalographic abnormalities have been noted in most of these patients. Psychological development and mental capacity are consistent with chronologic age. Heterosexual activity is usually not premature. Reproductive potential is not adversely affected, and the patient can become pregnant.
      (2) **Therapy.** Progestational agents and GnRH analogues are effective and represent the most significant advance in the management of precocious puberty. The agents are potent and long-acting. They can be given intranasally and subcutaneously. Within 1 week of therapy, gonadotropin secretion is decreased.

2. **Causes of precocious puberty**
   a. **Central nervous system disorders**
      (1) Trauma to the hypothalamus
      (2) Postinflammatory reactions (e.g., toxoplasmosis, congenital syphilis, tuberculosis, encephalitis, or meningitis)
   b. **Congenital anomalies**
      (1) McCune-Albright syndrome, a polyostotic fibrous dysplasia characterized by café au

lait spots distributed unilaterally over the osseous lesions with fractures and deformities of the long bones

(2) Hemartoma of the hypothalamus

(3) Tuberous sclerosis

(4) Hydrocephalus

(5) Neurofibromatosis

(6) Intracranial neoplasms that occupy the floor of the third ventricle

c. **Chronic ingestion of estrogens,** usually oral contraceptives or tonics, lotions, or creams containing estrogen

d. **Adrenal estrogen-secreting tumor** (rare)

e. **Estrogen-producing ovarian neoplasm or cyst**, such as granulosa–theca cell tumor

3. **Diagnosis** of precocious puberty is based on physical, ophthalmologic, and radiologic signs; endocrine profile; and possibly laparoscopy or laparotomy to diagnose occult tumors.

4. **Therapy** is aimed at slowing down the accelerated growth, reducing pituitary, ovarian, or adrenal function, and inducing regression of secondary sex characteristics. In cases of known or organic etiology, therapy is with surgery, chemotherapy, or radiation as indicated.

F. **Contraception.** Most sexually active adolescents do not use contraception, especially at the time of the first sexual act. In addition, the young patient will not mention contraception; therefore, a discussion of contraception should follow a physical examination whether or not the patient is sexually active.

BIBLIOGRAPHY

Carrington ER: Gynecologic problems in infants and prepubertal girls. *Surg Clin N Am* 34:1615, 1954

Huffman JW: Gynecologic endocrine disorders in childhood and adolescence. *Clin Obstet Gynecol* 16:51, 1973

Robboy SJ, et al: *Gynecologic and Obstetric Pathology.* Cambridge, Massachusetts, Harvard Medical School, 1980

Smith DR: *General Urology,* 8th ed. Los Altos, California, Lange Medical, 1975

Southam AL, Richart RM: Prognosis for adolescents with menstrual abnormalities. *Am J Obstet Gynecol* 94:637, 1966

Styne D, et al: Treatment of true precocious puberty with a potent luteinizing hormone–releasing factor agonist: effect on growth, sexual maturation, pelvic sonography and the use of hypothalamic–pituitary gonadal axis. *J Clin Endocrinol Metab* 61:142, 1985

Wilson JR, et al: *Obstetrics and Gynecology,* 5th ed. St Louis, CV Mosby, 1975

STUDY QUESTIONS

Directions: Each question below contains five suggested answers. Choose the **one best** response to each question.

1. All of the following statements concerning congenital adrenal hyperplasia are true EXCEPT that

(A) the incidence is 1/5,000 births
(B) it is self-limiting and rarely requires therapy
(C) the internal genitalia are normal
(D) it is the most common cause of virilization in the newborn female
(E) the most common defect is of 21-hydroxylase

2. Sexual ambiguity may be seen in which of the following conditions?

(A) Androgen insensitivity syndrome
(B) Pure gonadal dysgenesis
(C) Swyer's syndrome
(D) Mixed gonadal dysgenesis
(E) Structural abnormalities of the X chromosome

3. In idiopathic precocious puberty, the parents should be warned that

(A) final height will be less than that of peers
(B) premature heterosexual activity is common
(C) future reproductive potential is adversely affected
(D) mental capacity is also advanced
(E) there is no satisfactory therapy

Directions: Each question below contains four suggested answers of which **one or more** is correct. Choose the answer

A if **1, 2, and 3** are correct
B if **1 and 3** are correct
C if **2 and 4** are correct
D if **4** is correct
E if **1, 2, 3, and 4** are correct

4. A newborn female could naturally have which of the following conditions?

(1) A mucoid vaginal discharge
(2) An enlarged clitoris
(3) Labial fusion
(4) A prolapsed urethra

5. Potential etiologic agents of a prepubertal vaginal discharge include

(1) foreign body
(2) hemolytic *Streptococcus*
(3) *Escherichia coli*
(4) *Candida*

6. Neoplasms associated with the maternal ingestion of diethylstilbestrol include which of the following?

(1) Vaginal adenosis
(2) Sarcoma botryoides
(3) Clear cell adenocarcinoma
(4) Granulosa–theca cell tumor

7. Characteristics of ovarian neoplasms in pediatric and adolescent patients include which of the following?

(1) They are predominantly of coelomic epithelial origin
(2) They commonly present with torsion
(3) The majority are of non–germ-cell origin
(4) The majority of granulosa–theca cell tumors are benign

8. Dysfunctional uterine bleeding is characterized by

(1) prolonged, heavy, and irregular menses
(2) a lesion in the hypothalamic–pituitary region
(3) menses that last longer than 7 days accompanied by anemia
(4) permanence in more than 60% of cases

Directions: The group of questions below consists of lettered choices followed by several numbered items. For each numbered item select the **one** lettered choice with which it is **most** closely associated. Each lettered choice may be used once, more than once, or not at all.

Questions 9–12

For each clinical presentation that follows, select the therapy that would be most appropriate.

(A) Estrogens and progestins
(B) Hydrocortisone
(C) Progestational agents
(D) Prostaglandin inhibitors
(E) None of the above

9. Congenital adrenal hyperplasia

10. Isosexual precocious puberty

11. Dysfunctional uterine bleeding

12. Dysmenorrhea

ANSWERS AND EXPLANATIONS

1. The answer is B. (*V A 1–3*) Elevation of androgenic steroids preceding the block in the biosynthetic pathway lead to persistent virilization of the external genitalia and heterosexual precocity if therapy is not instituted. The steroids secreted do not affect the negative feedback upon adrenocorticotropic hormone production, which is also increased. Hydrocortisone is administered indefinitely to all patients.

2. The answer is D. (*V E; VI C 6 b–d*) Most patients with mixed gonadal dysgenesis have the genotype XO/XY or some form of mosaicism. The Y chromosome results in a unilateral testis and, therefore, ambiguous genitalia. Patients with testicular feminization and other types of gonadal dysgenesis have female external genitalia. Androgen insensitivity is characterized by a 46,XY genotype and a female phenotype.

3. The answer is A. [*VI E 1 b (1)*] In idiopathic precocious puberty, early tall stature is the rule followed by short adult height secondary to early closure of the epiphyses. This may cause emotional problems, but these children do not exhibit accelerated intellectual and psychological development. Ongoing studies have shown that gonadotropin-releasing hormone analogues are the most effective therapy.

4. The answer is A (1, 2, 3). (*II C, E, F 1 a; V C 1*) Because of increased secretion of maternal estrogen during pregnancy, a female newborn may have both a mucoid discharge and nipple enlargement for up to 2 weeks after birth. Maternal ingestion of progestins during pregnancy can result in masculinization of the female fetus with enlargement of the clitoris and fusion of the labia. A prolapsed urethra is not found in the newborn.

5. The answer is E (all). (*II F 1 b*) Organisms from the gastrointestinal tract (*Escherichia coli*) or from the skin or throat (*Streptococcus*) have been associated with vaginal discharge in the prepubertal female. A foreign body can be an irritant, which may also cause a discharge. *Candida* causes a monilial vaginitis, possible due to lack of resistance secondary to decreased estrogen levels in the prepubertal female.

6. The answer is B (1, 3). (*IV A 1–3, B 1 a*) Vaginal adenosis is a benign condition that has been associated with the maternal ingestion of diethylstilbestrol (DES). Clear cell adenocarcinoma of the vagina, found at or after puberty, is also associated with maternal DES ingestion. Neither sarcoma botryoides nor granulosa–theca cell tumor is associated with maternal ingestion of any substance.

7. The answer is C (2, 4). (*IV B 1*) Most ovarian neoplasms in adolescents are endocrine secreting whether of germ-cell origin or non–germ-cell origin. The germ-cell variety are the most common. The minority are of the non–germ cell or coelomic epithelium origin. Torsion, as the presenting symptom, correlates with the size (rapid growth) of the tumor. Eighty percent of granulosa–theca cell tumors are benign.

8. The answer is B (1, 3). (*VI B*) Anovulatory cycles tend to be heavy and irregular; thus, cycles that tend to be prolonged with anemia constitute dysfunctional uterine bleeding. The pathophysiology is unknown but requires the exclusion of any detectable organic etiology.

9–12. The answers are: 9-B, 10-C, 11-A, 12-D. [*V A 3; VI A 3 b, B 3, E 1 b (1)–(2)*] Congenital adrenal hyperplasia results when the enzymatic regulation of the biosynthesis of cortisol and aldosterone is impaired. A 21-hydroxylase defect is the most common cause of distinct virilization of the female newborn (95% of all cases of congenital adrenal hyperplasia). Hydrocortisone is administered indefinitely to all patients.

Isosexual precocious puberty is the early development of secondary sex characteristics (before 9 years of age) consistent with genetic sex. Although 80%–90% of all cases of isosexual precocious puberty have no obvious underlying etiology, progestational agents and gonadotropin-releasing hormone analogues have been found to be effective in suppressing the socially unacceptable (because of the child's age) uterine bleeding.

Dysfunctional uterine bleeding (bleeding unaccompanied by ovulation) in adolescent girls is usually self-limited; however, if symptoms persist, cyclic hormonal manipulation with combination estrogens and progestins is recommended.

Although dysmenorrhea may be secondary to obstructive or anatomic causes, frequently no organic etiology is found. Prostaglandins are present during the menses and are known to cause painful uterine contractions. Therapy includes antiemetics for the nausea and vomiting and prostaglandin inhibitors for the pain.

21

The Menstrual Cycle
William W. Beck, Jr.

I. INTRODUCTION. The menstrual cycle is characterized by the regular occurrence of ovulation throughout the reproductive life of a woman. The cycle is divided into two phases: the follicular (or proliferative) phase and the luteal (or secretory) phase.

A. Length of the cycle

    1. The mean duration of the cycle is 28 days plus or minus 7 days.

        a. Menstrual cycles that occur at frequent intervals (less than 21 days) are called **polymenor-rhea**.

        b. Menstrual cycles that occur at long intervals (more than 35 days) are called **oligomenor-rhea**.

    2. Menstrual cycles are the most irregular during the 2 years after menarche (i.e., the first menses) and the 3 years before menopause during which times anovulation (i.e., absent ovulation) is most common.

B. Follicular or proliferative phase. This phase lasts from the first day of menses until ovulation during which time the endometrial glands proliferate under the influence of estrogen, primarily estradiol. It is characterized by:

    1. A variable length

    2. A low basal body temperature

    3. Development of ovarian follicles

    4. Vascular growth of the endometrium

    5. Secretion of estrogen from the ovary

C. Luteal or secretory phase. The second part of the cycle extends from ovulation until the onset of menses. Under the influence of progesterone, the endometrial glands develop the secretory status necessary for implantation of the embryo. It is characterized by:

    1. A fairly constant duration of 12–16 days

    2. An elevated basal body temperature (over 98°F)

    3. The formation of the corpus luteum in the ovary with the secretion of progesterone and estrogen

    4. An endometrium that reveals gland tortuosity and secretion, stromal edema, and a decidual reaction

D. Cycle integration. The integration of the menstrual cycle involves the interaction among gonadotropin-releasing hormone (GnRH), the gonadotropins [i.e., follicle-stimulating hormone (FSH) and luteinizing hormone (LH)], and the sex steroids (i.e., androstenedione, estradiol, estrone, and progesterone).

II. GnRH is the hypothalamic hormone that controls gonadotropin release.

A. Characteristics

    1. GnRH is a decapeptide with 10 amino acids.

2. It is produced by hypothalamic neurons and is transported along axons that terminate in the median eminence around capillaries of the primary portal plexus.

3. It is secreted into the portal circulation, which carries it to the anterior lobe of the pituitary gland.

B. Secretion

1. GnRH is secreted in a pulsatile manner; the amplitude and frequency of the secretions vary throughout the cycle.
   a. One pulse every hour is typical of the follicular phase.
   b. One pulse every 2–3 hours is typical of the luteal phase.

2. The amplitude and frequency are regulated by:
   a. Feedback of estrogen and progesterone
   b. Neurotransmitters within the brain, mainly the catecholamines, dopamine and norepinephrine

C. Action

1. GnRH stimulates the synthesis and release of both FSH and LH from the same cell.

2. When GnRH binds to specific receptors on the surface membrane of target cells, it:
   a. Activates or inhibits a second messenger, adenyl cyclase
   b. Changes the concentration of cyclic adenosine monophosphate (cAMP)

3. With GnRH stimulation, there is a rapid (30 minute) increase in serum FSH and LH with a later (90 minute) release of LH.
   a. The stored pool is released first.
   b. The synthesized pool is released second.

III. GONADOTROPINS: FSH AND LH

A. FSH receptors exist primarily on the granulosa cell membrane.

1. FSH acts primarily on the granulosa cells to stimulate follicular growth.

2. It stimulates formation of LH receptors.

3. It activates the aromatase and 3-hydroxysteroid dehydrogenase enzymes.

4. It stimulates follicular growth by increasing both FSH and LH receptor content in granulosa cells; this action is enhanced by the estradiol being produced by the granulosa cells.

B. LH receptors exist on theca cells at all stages of the cycle and on granulosa cells after the follicle matures under the influence of FSH and estradiol.

1. LH stimulates androgen synthesis by the theca cells.

2. With a sufficient number of LH receptors on the granulosa cells, LH acts directly on the granulosa cells to cause luteinization (i.e., the formation of the corpus luteum) and the production of progesterone.

C. Two-cell hypothesis of estrogen production

1. LH acts on the theca cells to produce androgens, that is, androstenedione and testosterone.

2. Androgens are transported from the theca cells to the granulosa cells.

3. Androgens are aromatized to estrogens (i.e., estradiol and estrone) by the action of FSH on the enzyme aromatase in the granulosa cells.

IV. OOGENESIS

A. Primordial follicle

1. The primordial follicle is covered by a single layer of granulosa cells.

2. Even without gonadotropin stimulation, some primordial follicles develop into preantral follicles.
   a. This process occurs during times of anovulation (i.e., childhood, pregnancy, and with use of oral contraceptives) as well as during ovulatory cycles.
   b. Nearly all of the preantral follicles become atretic.

B. Preantral follicle

1. Under the influence of FSH, the number of granulosa cells in the primordial follicle increases.

2. There is a parallel increase in estradiol secretion. Estradiol, in turn:
   a. Stimulates preantral follicle growth
   b. Reduces follicle atresia
   c. Increases FSH action on the granulosa cells.

C. Antral follicle

1. The follicle destined to become dominant secretes the greatest amount of estradiol, which, in turn, increases the density of the FSH receptors on the granulosa cell membrane.

2. Rising estradiol levels result in negative feedback on FSH secretion levels; this halts the development of other follicles, which then become atretic.

3. The follicular rise of estradiol exerts a positive feedback on LH secretion.
   a. LH levels rise steadily during the late follicular phase.
   b. LH stimulates androgen production in the theca.
   c. The dominant follicle uses the androgen as substrate and further accelerates estrogen output.

4. FSH induces the appearance of LH receptors on granulosa cells.

D. Preovulatory follicle

1. Estrogens rise rapidly, reaching a peak approximately 24–36 hours before ovulation.

2. LH increases steadily until midcycle when there is a surge, which is accompanied by a lesser surge of FSH.

3. LH initiates luteinization and progesterone production in the granulosa layer.

4. The preovulatory rise in progesterone facilitates the positive feedback action of estrogen and is required to induce the midcycle FSH peak.

E. Ovulation   *peak ~~(estrat)~~ LH surg = best predictor of ovulation 10-12°*

1. Ovulation occurs approximately 10–12 hours after the LH peak and 24–36 hours after the estradiol peak; the *onset* of the LH surge, which occurs 28–32 hours prior to ovulation is the most reliable indicator of the timing of ovulation.

Onset of LH surg

2. The LH surges stimulates the following:
   a. Completion of reduction division in the oocyte
   b. Luteinization of the granulosa cells
   c. Synthesis of progesterone and prostaglandins within the follicle

3. Prostaglandins and proteolytic enzymes are responsible for the digestion and rupture of the follicle wall.

4. The progesterone-dependent midcycle rise in FSH serves to free the oocyte from follicular attachments and to ensure sufficient LH receptors for an adequate luteal phase.

F. Corpus luteum

1. Peak levels of progesterone are attained 8–9 days after ovulation, which approximates the time of implantation of the embryo.

2. Normal luteal function requires optimal preovulatory follicular development.
   a. Suppression of FSH during the follicular phase is associated with:
      (1) Low preovulatory estradiol levels
      (2) Depressed midluteal progesterone production
      (3) A small luteal cell mass
   b. The accumulation of LH receptors during the luteal phase sets the stage for the extent of luteinization and the functional capacity of the corpus luteum.
   c. A defective luteal phase can contribute to both infertility and early pregnancy wastage.

3. In early pregnancy, HCG maintains luteal function until placental steroidogenesis (with the production of progesterone) is established.

V. MENSTRUATION

A. In the absence of a pregnancy, decreasing steroid levels lead to increased coiling and constriction of the spiral arteries, which supply the upper two-thirds of the functional endometrium.

1. The decreased blood flow to the functional portion of the endometrium causes ischemia and degradation of endometrial tissue.

2. The bleeding, or menses, is the result of the degraded endometrial tissue, which is desquamated or shed into the uterine cavity.

B. Within 2 days of the onset of menses, regeneration of the surface epithelium begins under the influence of estrogen and continues to occur at the same time that the endometrium is shedding.

VI. CLINICAL PROBLEMS ASSOCIATED WITH THE MENSTRUAL CYCLE

A. Dysmenorrhea. Painful menses usually begin with ovulatory menstrual periods and are the most common medical problem in young women.

1. Clinical aspects
   a. Dysmenorrhea begins just before or with the onset of menses and lasts 24–48 hours.
   b. The pain is suprapubic, sharp, and colicky.
   c. Nausea, diarrhea, and headache may accompany the pain.
   d. Dysmenorrhea does not occur in anovulatory cycles.

2. Physiology
   a. Menstrual cramps are the result of uterine contractions.
   b. Prostaglandins are potent stimulators of uterine contractions.
   c. Endometrial prostaglandins are produced during the luteal phase. If ovulation does not occur, there is no luteal increase in prostaglandins.
   d. In the first day menstrual endometrium, the prostaglandin level is increased several times over the concentrations in the luteal phase.

3. Management
   a. Prostaglandin synthetase inhibitors (e.g., nonsteroidal anti-inflammatory drugs) have the following properties:
      (1) They decrease levels of endometrial prostaglandin.
      (2) They lessen uterine contractions.
      (3) They relieve dysmenorrhea.
   b. Combination (estrogen/progestin) oral contraceptive agents eliminate ovulation.
      (1) Estrogen followed by progesterone (ovulatory cycles) is necessary to produce high menstrual levels of prostaglandin in the endometrium.
      (2) Combination oral contraceptives prevent dysmenorrhea by eliminating the natural estrogen/progesterone progression found only in the ovulatory cycle.
      (3) In the absence of ovulation, there is little or no dysmenorrhea.

B. Premenstrual syndrome (PMS). This syndrome is a set of symptoms or molimina that occur with the approach of the menses and usually end abruptly with the onset of bleeding.

1. Clinical aspects
   a. Over 100 symptoms have been attributed to PMS. The most common symptoms are:
      (1) Abdominal bloating
      (2) Anxiety
      (3) Breast tenderness
      (4) Crying spells
      (5) Depression
      (6) Fatigue
      (7) Irritability
      (8) Weight gain
   b. Premenstrual symptoms can exist in women with stable or unstable personalities.

2. Etiology. The etiology of PMS is elusive and has been associated with excesses or deficiencies of progesterone, estrogen, prolactin, aldosterone, pyridoxine, opioids, unrecognized mineralocorticoids, and monoamine oxidase activity.

3. Management. Both the physiologic and the psychosocial aspects of PMS must be considered when designing a therapeutic program. Basic measures include:
   a. Regular exercise and a balanced diet
   b. Vitamin B_6 on a daily basis
   c. Luteal phase progesterone or estrogen, depending on perceived need
   d. Diuretics
   e. Oral contraceptives and elimination of the ovulatory sequence

STUDY QUESTIONS

Directions: Each question below contains five suggested answers. Choose the **one best** response to each question.

1. The average length of the menstrual cycle is

(A) 22 days
(B) 25 days
(C) 28 days
(D) 35 days
(E) 38 days

2. The establishment and maintenance of the menstrual cycle is dependent upon

(A) prolactin release by the anterior pituitary
(B) pulsatile secretion of gonadotropin-releasing hormone
(C) a follicular phase that has a variable length
(D) progesterone synthesis by the corpus luteum
(E) estrogen secretion by the ovary

3. Gonadotropin-releasing hormone controls the synthesis and secretion of which of the following substances?

(A) Follicle-stimulating hormone and luteinizing hormone
(B) Dopamine
(C) Prolactin
(D) Norepinephrine
(E) Thyrotropin-releasing hormone

4. The best predictor of ovulation is

(A) estrogen peak
(B) luteinizing hormone (LH) surge
(C) follicle-stimulating hormone surge
(D) onset of the LH surge
(E) preovulatory rise in progesterone

Directions: The question below contains four suggested answers of which **one or more** is correct. Choose the answer

A if **1, 2, and 3** are correct
B if **1 and 3** are correct
C if **2 and 4** are correct
D if **4** is correct
E if **1, 2, 3, and 4** are correct

5. Changes in the endometrium that occur during the menstrual cycle include

(1) proliferation of glandular cells
(2) vascular growth
(3) stromal edema
(4) decidual reaction

6. Correct statements concerning the two-cell hypothesis of estrogen production include which of the following?

(1) Theca cells produce androstenedione
(2) Luteinizing hormone stimulates the granulosa cells
(3) Aromatization of androgens takes place in the granulosa cells
(4) Estradiol is transported to the theca cells

Directions: The group of questions below consists of lettered choices followed by several numbered items. For each numbered item select the **one** lettered choice with which it is **most** closely associated. Each lettered choice may be used once, more than once, or not at all.

Questions 7–10

For each activity listed, select the hormone that is most likely to be responsible for it.

(A) Follicle-stimulating hormone
(B) Luteinizing hormone
(C) Both
(D) Neither

7. Stimulates androgen secretion

8. Stimulates aromatase activity

9. Stimulates prolactin release

10. Stimulates target cells in the ovary

ANSWERS AND EXPLANATIONS

1. The answer is C. (*I A 1, 2*) The length of the normal menstrual cycle varies between 21 and 35 days with the average being about 28–30 days. The preovulatory phase of a normal cycle is often variable in length, ranging from 8–21 days, while the length of the postovulatory phase (about 2 weeks) is usually fairly constant.

2. The answer is B. (*II B 1, 2, C 1*) It has been demonstrated that hourly pulses of gonadotropin-releasing hormone (GnRH) given intravenously lead to the onset and establishment of menses in prepubertal monkeys. Discontinuation of the GnRH infusion results in amenorrhea. Thus, this pulsatile activity is a prerequisite for the establishment and maintenance of the menstrual cycle; what follows this activity are the components of a normal menstrual cycle: estrogen secretion from the ovary, a follicular phase of variable length, ovulation, the establishment of the corpus luteum, and the secretion of progesterone from the corpus luteum.

3. The answer is A. (*II B 2, C 1*) Gonadotropin-releasing hormone (GnRH) controls the synthesis and secretion of the gonadotropins, follicle-stimulating hormone and luteinizing hormone. The catecholamines, dopamine and norepinephrine, are neurotransmitters that influence the release of GnRH. Thyrotropin-releasing hormone stimulates prolactin and thyroid-stimulating hormone secretion. Prolactin is not affected by GnRH.

4. The answer is D. (*IV D 1, 2, E 1*) The onset of the luteinizing hormone (LH) surge, which occurs 28–32 hours prior to ovulation is the most reliable indicator of the timing of ovulation. The estrogen peak occurs about 24–36 hours and the LH peak about 10–12 hours before ovulation, and a small FSH rise occurs along with the LH surge; however, none of these are as predictive of ovulation as the onset of the LH surge. The preovulatory rise in progesterone is important in stimulating the midcycle rise in FSH, but it is not a predictor of ovulation.

5. The answer is E (all). (*I B 4, C 4*) Under the influence of estrogen, the endometrium proliferates with replication of both glandular and stromal cells and vascular growth. During the postovulatory phase, under the influence of progesterone, there is an increase in the tortuosity and secretory activity of the glands with stromal edema and a decidual reaction present toward the end of the cycle.

6. The answer is B (1, 3). (*III C 1–3*) In the two-cell hypothesis of estrogen production, luteinizing hormone acts on the theca cells to stimulate the production of the androgens, androstenedione and testosterone, which are transported to the granulosa cells. The androgens are aromatized in the granulosa cells to form the estrogens, estradiol and estrone.

7–10. The answers are 7-B, 8-A, 9-D, 10-C. (*III A 1, 2, B 1, C 1–3*) Luteinizing hormone (LH) stimulates the theca cells to produce androgens, which are important precursors in the synthesis of estrogens. Follicle-stimulating hormone (FSH) stimulates the granulosa cells, follicular growth and maturation, and aromatase activity, which is necessary for the synthesis of estradiol. The two-cell hypothesis for estrogen production involves the aromatization of theca cell androgen to estradiol in the granulosa cells. Both FSH and LH stimulate target cells in the ovary, and neither is responsible for prolactin release.

22
Family Planning: Contraception and Complications
William W. Beck, Jr.

I. NATURAL FAMILY PLANNING entails planning or avoiding pregnancies by abstaining from sexual intercourse during the fertile phase of the menstrual cycle. Drugs, devices, and surgical procedures are not used. In western countries, there is a pregnancy rate of 10–15/100 woman years of exposure among women using natural family planning.

A. **Fertility cycle.** The fertile and infertile phases of the menstrual cycle are indicated by bodily signs and symptoms that result from the changing concentrations of estrogen and progesterone over the cycle. Estrogen and progesterone have their most marked effects on the cervical mucus and the basal body temperature. The fertility cycle can be divided into three phases.

1. **Phase 1, the relatively infertile phase**, covers the time from menstruation to the beginning of the development of the egg follicle.
   a. This phase of the menstrual cycle varies in length, depending on the rapidity of the follicular response to the pituitary hormones.
   b. This phase can be a problem in terms of fertility assessment because of the potential variation from cycle to cycle.

2. **Phase 2, the fertile phase**, extends from the beginning of follicular development until 48 hours after ovulation.
   a. The 48 hours allow 24 hours for the fertilizable life span of the ovum and 24 hours for the clinical imprecision of detecting ovulation.
   b. Spermatozoa retain the capacity to fertilize the ovum for up to 5 days in the cervical mucus, which is produced abundantly during this phase of the cycle.
   c. This combined fertile phase, therefore, averages approximately 6–8 days a cycle.

3. **Phase 3, the absolutely infertile phase**, extends from 48 hours after ovulation until the onset of menstruation. This phase lasts approximately 10–16 days and is much more consistent than phase 1.

B. **Cervix.** Changing concentrations of estrogen and progesterone affect the cervix, causing changes in the quantity and quality of mucus.

1. **Phase 1.** Just after menstruation, little, if any, mucus is produced.
   a. If mucus is found at the vulva, it will be thick, tacky, and opaque.
   b. When held between the thumb and forefinger and stretched, mucus of this type breaks quickly.
   c. When mucus is present, women have a feeling of stickiness at the entrance to the vagina.
   d. When mucus is not present, women have a sensation of dryness in the vulva.

2. **Phase 2.** As the follicles produce increasing amounts of estrogen, the cervix responds with increased mucus production.
   a. The mucus becomes more abundant, increasingly thin, stretchy, clear, and watery.
   b. If held between the thumb and forefinger, mucus of this type can be stretched for several inches before it breaks.
   c. Women have a sensation of wetness and slipperiness in the vulva at this time.
   d. Peak cervical mucus occurs at the height of estrogen secretion, preceding ovulation by not more than 3 days; peak cervical mucus can only be identified in retrospect—that is, after the mucus again changes characteristics and becomes thick, sticky, and opaque.
   e. If 24 hours is allowed for ovum fertilization, then the fourth day after the peak indicates the end of the fertile phase.

3. **Phase 3.** With ovulation and the production of progesterone, there is a rapid change in the amount and characteristics of the mucus.

   a. The quantity of mucus drops sharply and sometimes disappears altogether.

   b. Mucus, if present, becomes thick, sticky, and opaque as in the infertile-type mucus in the first stage of the cycle.

C. Basal body temperature is the temperature of the body at complete rest after a period of sleep and before normal activity, including eating, begins.

   1. There is an increase in the basal body temperature of 0.4°F–1.0°F during the postovulatory phase of the cycle due to the secretion of progesterone, which has a thermogenic effect.

   2. As an indicator of fertility, the basal body temperature can only detect the end of the fertile phase, which is identified by a sustained elevation of the temperature for 3 days after the shift.

   3. To avoid pregnancy using the basal body temperature method alone, sexual intercourse must be restricted to the period from the third day of temperature elevation until the end of the cycle.

II. BARRIER METHODS OF CONTRACEPTION

II. BARRIER METHODS OF CONTRACEPTION—diaphragms, condoms, sponges, and spermicides—protect users against sexually transmitted diseases and, thus, indirectly against carcinoma of the cervix; they are also thought to be relatively free from side effects.

A. Condoms are one of the oldest surviving forms of birth control. They are effective, safe, relatively inexpensive, and reversible. Although condoms are highly effective, couples must be encouraged to use them with *every* act of coitus.

   1. Pregnancy rates range from 5–10/100 woman years of use; effectiveness depends on the following features:
   a. Age of the couple
   b. Family income
   c. Desires to space or prevent further children
   d. Education level of the couple

   2. Sexually transmitted diseases. Because condoms are airtight, watertight, and impermeable to microorganisms, it is reasonable to expect them to prevent the spread of sexually transmitted diseases. Transmission of the following organisms is prevented by the use of condoms:
   a. Herpes simplex virus
   b. *Neisseria gonorrhoeae*
   c. *Chlamydia trachomatis*
   d. *Ureaplasma urealyticum*
   e. Human papillomavirus
   f. *Mycoplasma hominis*
   g. *Trichomonas vaginalis*
   h. *Treponema pallidum*
   i. Human immunodeficiency virus (HIV)

   3. Carcinoma of the cervix. Barrier contraception is thought to protect the cervix from sexually transmitted agents that promote cervical neoplasia, such as herpesvirus, papillomavirus, and *Chlamydia*. It has also been suggested that the use of condoms may help to reverse the progression of cervical dysplasias.

B. Spermicides—including creams, jellies, aerosol foam, nonfoaming and foaming suppositories—are commonly used with other forms of contraception, such as diaphragms, sponges, and condoms. Only about 3% of women use spermicides alone.

   1. Mode of action
   a. The barrier substances are important for the following reasons:
      (1) The speed with which they release the active ingredient
      (2) Their ability to spread over the cervix and vagina
      (3) Their ability to act as physical barriers at the cervix to prevent sperm penetration
   b. The active agents work by either killing the sperm, decreasing sperm motility, or inactivating the enzymes necessary for the sperm to penetrate the ova.
      (1) Surface-active agents (e.g., nonoxynol 9, octoxynol 9, and menfegol) are spermicidal agents that disrupt the outer lipoprotein surface layer of spermatozoa.
      (2) Enzyme inhibitors (e.g., gossypol) are spermostatic and either attack the enzymes necessary for sperm motility or the enzymes of the acrosome (e.g., hyaluronidase and proacrosin), which are necessary for the sperm to fertilize the egg.

   2. Pregnancy rates vary from 5–25/100 woman years of use and reflect a wide range of factors. Effectiveness depends on the motivation of the couple to use this form of contraceptive correctly for *every* act of coitus.

3. Safety. No serious side effects have been reported with the currently available spermicides. A report citing a higher spontaneous abortion rate and a higher incidence of congenital abnormalities among users of spermicides compared to nonusers is controversial. The study did not have adequate controls and did not control for other variables, such as drugs and cigarette smoking.

C. **Vaginal sponges.** The most widely used sponge is the Today Collatex sponge. It is made of polyurethane impregnated with 1 g of nonoxynol 9.

   1. Mode of action. Vaginal sponges release spermicide during coitus, absorb ejaculate, and block the entrance to the cervical canal. They may be used for 24 hours regardless of the frequency of coitus.

   2. Pregnancy rates have been reported to be 10–15/100 woman years of use.

   3. Safety. Toxic shock syndrome (TSS) has been reported among sponge users; however, TSS is no more frequent in women who use the sponge than in women who use no contraception. TSS is a serious illness characterized by a sudden onset of a high fever, vomiting, diarrhea, and body rash; it is caused by toxins produced by *Staphylococcus aureus*.

D. **Diaphragms.** All diaphragms are dome-shaped and made of latex rubber with diameters of 50–105 mm. The base of the dome is made of a metal spring, which is either a flat spring, a coil spring, or an arcing spring. Diaphragms rest between the posterior aspect of the symphysis pubis and the posterior fornix of the vagina, covering the anterior vaginal wall and the cervix.

   1. Mode of action. Diaphragms act as physical barriers to sperm and are effective vehicles by which to carry spermicidal creams or jellies. They prevent the cervical mucus from neutralizing the vaginal acidity so that the vagina remains hostile to sperm.

   2. Pregnancy rates have been reported to be 5–10/100 woman years of use. Effectiveness depends on leaving the diaphragm in place for 6 hours after intercourse and introducing more spermicide if intercourse occurs again.

   3. Safety. There are few side effects associated with use of the diaphragm. There has been a reported increase in the frequency of urinary tract infections due possibly to urethral compression. The diaphragm may protect against pelvic inflammatory disease.

III. INTRAUTERINE DEVICES (IUDs)

A. **Advantages** include:

   1. A high level of effectiveness

   2. A lack of associated systemic metabolic effects

   3. A single act of motivation (the IUD insertion) required for long-term use

B. **Mode of action**

   1. Contraception is due to the production of a local sterile inflammatory reaction caused by the presence of the foreign body in the uterus.

   2. Tissue breakdown products from the increased number of endometrial leukocytes are toxic to all cells, including sperm and the blastocyst.

   3. The addition of copper increases the inflammatory reaction.

   4. With removal of both copper-bearing and noncopper-bearing IUDs, the inflammatory reaction rapidly disappears and resumption of fertility is not delayed.

C. **Types.** There were four types of IUDs in general use, which are listed below. All IUDs except for the progesterone-releasing device (Progestasert) and the recently released copper-containing device (Paragard) are no longer being produced because of medicolegal costs.

   1. The barium-impregnated plastic device (Lippes loop and Saf-T-Coil). The pure plastic devices may be left in situ indefinitely.

   2. The copper-bearing Copper 7 and the Copper T. Because of the constant dissolution of copper, the copper IUDs have to be replaced every 3–4 years.

   3. The progesterone-releasing T-shaped device. The progesterone-releasing IUD must be replaced each year; the reservoir of progesterone becomes depleted after 18 months of use.

D. Adverse effects

1. **Uterine bleeding.** Heavy or prolonged menses and intermenstrual bleeding are the major reasons for discontinuing use of the IUD.
   a. Vascular erosions have been seen in areas of the endometrium in direct contact with the IUD, and evidence of increased vascular permeability has been seen in areas not in direct contact with the IUD.
   b. Excessive bleeding in the first few months after IUD insertion should be treated with reassurance and supplemental oral iron; the bleeding frequently diminishes with time as the uterus adjusts to the presence of the foreign body. If bleeding continues, the IUD should be removed.

2. **Perforation.** Perforation of the uterine fundus is one of the potentially serious complications associated with IUD use.
   a. Perforation initially occurs at insertion in about 1 in 1000 insertions.
   b. Perforation should be suspected if a patient reports she cannot feel the attached string and did not notice that the device was expelled. Rotation of the device can occur with the string being drawn into the cavity.
      (1) X-ray film or sonography can be used to locate the device.
      (2) Contrast media in the uterine cavity with an x-ray will help to locate the IUD within or outside the uterus.
   c. If an IUD is found outside the uterus, it should be removed because complications, such as adhesions and bowel obstruction, have been reported.

3. **Infection.** In the first 24 hours after insertion of an IUD, the normally sterile cavity is infected with bacteria; the natural defenses destroy these bacteria in most cases.
   a. Pelvic infection rates are highest in the first 2 weeks after insertion and then steadily diminish.
   b. The incidence of salpingitis is about three times greater in IUD users than in diaphragm or oral contraceptive users with the highest incidence in nulliparous women under 25 years of age.
   c. The risk of developing pelvic infection is greatest in women who have:
      (1) A prior history of pelvic infection
      (2) No children and who are under 25
      (3) Multiple sexual partners
   d. It is prudent not to insert the IUD in a nulliparous woman at the risk of impairing her future fertility.
   e. Treatment
      (1) Salpingitis can usually be treated effectively with removal of the IUD and antibiotics.
      (2) The unilateral tubo-ovarian abscess occasionally found in IUD users may be removed without a pelvic cleanout, which is unique among IUD users.

E. Complications related to pregnancy

1. **Congenital anomalies.** The IUD is always extra-amniotic in a pregnancy, and there is no evidence of an increased incidence of congenital anomalies in infants born to women with an IUD in utero.

2. **Spontaneous abortion.** The rate of spontaneous abortion is about 50% if an IUD is left in situ. If the IUD is removed in early pregnancy, the subsequent abortion rate is about 20%–30%. Because of the possibility of serious infection associated with an IUD pregnancy, there should be an attempt at IUD removal.

3. **Ectopic pregnancy.** If pregnancy occurs with an IUD in place, there is a greater chance that it will be an ectopic pregnancy than if no IUD were used, possibly as a result of the effectiveness of an IUD in preventing a uterine pregnancy; chances of having an ectopic pregnancy range from 3%–9%.

4. **Prematurity.** There is a 12%–15% chance of prematurity in pregnancies producing live-births with an IUD in situ. This may be due to an irritative influence by the IUD on the myometrium during the third trimester.

F. Pregnancy rates among IUD users are 2–3/100 woman years of use.

IV. ORAL CONTRACEPTIVES

A. Composition. The oral contraceptive agents contain either an estrogen/progestogen combination or a progestogen alone.

1. The combination pills contain various amounts of estrogen (ethinyl estradiol or mestranol) and one of a variety of progestogens. The current preparations contain low doses of estrogen, (20–50 mcg per pill is the usual dose). They are taken for 21 days with a week between pill packs.

2. The progestogen only pills are taken continuously without a break.

B. Mode of action

1. Suppression of ovulation is the primary mechanism of action. Either the estrogen or the progestogen is capable of suppressing gonadotropins and inhibiting ovulation.

2. The cervical mucus is changed into a thick, rather viscous material, which is hostile to sperm migration through the endocervix.

3. The endometrium, under the influence of the progestogens, becomes flat and inactive and, thus, unprepared for the implantation of the embryo.

C. Side effects.
The frequency of side effects appears to be related to estrogen dosage. These side effects include the following:

1. Serious thromboembolic complications

2. Troublesome breakthrough bleeding, which is often seen with very low-dose preparations

3. Nausea, headaches, weight gain, and breast tenderness, which usually disappear or lessen in severity after two or three cycles of pill use

D. Complications

1. **Thromboembolism.** Estrogen causes an increase in plasma levels of a number of clotting factors, especially factor VII, presumably by acting on the liver. Antithrombin III levels fall within 10 days of starting oral contraceptives.
   a. Both superficial and deep vein thromboses are increased in oral contraceptive users.
   b. The relative risk of dying from all vascular diseases for women currently taking oral contraceptives is increased fourfold.
      (1) Most deaths are due to myocardial infarction; there is no relationship between the incidence of death due to cardiovascular disease and the length of oral contraceptive use.
      (2) Cardiovascular disease morbidity and mortality, which are related to the estrogen content of the oral contraceptives, are significantly reduced in preparations containing 50 μg or less.
      (3) Age and cigarette smoking have been found to have an important influence on the risk of death from myocardial infarction among oral contraceptive users; women who smoke and are 35 years of age and older are at greatest risk.

2. **Hypertension**
   a. Renin substrate, plasma renin activity, and angiotensin are elevated in oral contraceptive users. There is an increase in aldosterone secretion and renal retention of sodium.
   b. The resulting hypertension in a small number of oral contraceptive users may represent the failed suppression of renin substrate and plasma renin activity with elevated levels of angiotensin.
   c. There seems to be an association between the length of oral contraceptive use and the development of hypertension; about 5% of users develop hypertension after 5 years of use.
   d. Almost all women who develop hypertension while taking oral contraceptives return to normotensive levels when the medication is discontinued.

3. **Postpill amenorrhea.** The occurrence of amenorrhea after cessation of oral contraceptive use is estimated to range between 0.2% and 3.1%.
   a. Studies indicate that preexisting menstrual irregularities were present in 35%–56% of women who developed amenorrhea after discontinuation of oral contraceptives.
   b. The possibility of a pituitary adenoma with any amenorrhea must be explored even when the amenorrhea seems to result from oral contraceptive use.

4. **Liver tumor.** An association between the use of the oral contraceptives and the subsequent development of a rare liver tumor, the hepatocellular adenoma, has been reported; the risk of developing this tumor increases with use of oral contraceptives for 5 years or more. It occurs at a rate of 3/100,000 woman years of use.

E. Continued use

  1. There is no scientific basis for the impression that the oral contraceptives should be discontinued every 2–3 years.
   a. There is no lowered incidence of complications with such a break.
   b. There is a high incidence of unwanted pregnancies during such "rest" periods.

  2. Oral contraceptives should be discontinued when elective surgery is scheduled. Any estrogen-containing formulation should be stopped 1 month prior to planned surgery to lessen the incidence of postoperative thrombophlebitis.

F. Neoplasia.
At the present time, there is no statistically valid data to support a cause and effect relationship between oral contraception and neoplasia in the breast, cervix, endometrium, or ovary.

  1. Breast
   a. Progestogens antagonize the stimulating effects of estrogen on breast tissue.
   b. There is a decreased incidence of benign breast disease in oral contraceptive users.
   c. The incidence of breast cancer has remained fairly constant during the past 15–20 years despite widespread use of the birth control pill.

  2. Cervix
   a. Cervical hypertrophy and eversion is seen in pill users.
   b. The pill does not induce carcinoma of the cervix, but it is not protective because its non-barrier mode of action does not prevent exposure to potential carcinogenic agents, such as the papillomavirus or herpesvirus.

  3. Endometrium
   a. Progestogens compete with estrogen for binding sites in the endometrial cells.
   b. Progestogens reduce the stimulating effect of estrogen and prevent the normal proliferative endometrium from progressing to hyperplasia.
   c. The regressive effect of the pill on the endometrium has led to its use as a therapeutic agent in treating adenomatous hyperplasia in some cases.

  4. Ovary
   a. Functional cysts are lower in oral contraceptive users than in nonusers.
   b. Oral contraceptive use suppresses ovarian activity and inhibits ovulation.
   c. An hypothesis suggests that the interruption of a significant number of ovulatory cycles in oral contraceptive users could actually lead to a decreased incidence of ovarian cancer.

G. Effectiveness.
The combination oral contraceptives are the most effective reversible method of birth control known to exist. When properly used, these preparations are virtually 100% effective.

V. OTHER HORMONAL CONTRACEPTION

A. Injectable contraception—medroxyprogesterone

  1. Medroxyprogesterone (Depo-Provera), a progestogen, acts on the hypothalamic–pituitary–ovarian axis to inhibit ovulation. As a consequence of this, it also has an effect on the endometrium and on the cervical mucus.

  2. The usual dose is 150 mg intramuscularly every 3 months. At this dosage schedule, the drug is a very effective contraceptive with reported failure rates of zero.

  3. The main reason for discontinuing this drug, or any other progestogen-only contraception, is menstrual disturbances, ranging from frequent, irregular, but sometimes heavy menses to amenorrhea.

  4. There is some initial delay in the return of fertility following medroxyprogesterone use because of the time it takes to eliminate the drug completely and to resume ovulation. The median time to conception is 9 months, which is double the median time for conception after stopping other forms of birth control.

B. Luteinizing hormone-releasing hormone (LH–RH) analogues

  1. Agonistic analogues of LH–RH were originally developed for facilitating treatment of hypogonadism. Paradoxically, chronic LH–RH agonist treatment resulted in desensitization or down-regulation, or both, of the pituitary processes responsible for gonadotropin synthesis and release.

2. The superagonist, buserelin, a LH–RH analogue, can be absorbed when given intranasally—a fact that has stimulated further clinical trials of this new approach to birth control.
   a. One study revealed that women given daily doses of 400 μg or 600 μg of buserelin intranasally over 3–6 months had safe and effective birth control by interfering with normal ovulation; no pregnancies occurred.
   b. The bleeding pattern during the chronic superagonist treatment varied from fairly regular menstrual-like bleeds to oligomenorrhea or amenorrhea; dysfunctional bleeding did not occur.
   c. No side effects, except bleeding disturbances caused by the induced anovulation, occurred.

3. The main mechanism of action of chronic LH–RH agonist treatment seems to be pituitary desensitization of the processes responsible for gonadotropin secretion. The reserve capacity for gonadotropin secretion is rapidly reduced during repeated administration of LH–RH agonists.

C. Postcoital contraception

1. This is sometimes called the "morning after pill" and can be used after unprotected coitus around the time of ovulation.
   a. It must be taken within 72 hours of coitus; however, use within 24 hours is preferable.
   b. The high doses of steroids just after ovulation may disrupt the endometrium enough so that implantation of the embryo does not take place.

2. The usual regimen is diethylstilbesterol (DES) 25 mg twice a day for 5 days. An antiemetic must be given to counteract the nausea and vomiting.

3. Four combination ethinyl estradiol and norgestrel (Ovral) tablets (two given twice over 12 hours) or ethinyl estradiol alone (5 mg/day for 5 days) are alternative forms of treatment.

4. Because of the potential teratogenic effects of the steroids, a therapeutic abortion must be recommended if the postcoital contraception fails and a pregnancy is established.

STUDY QUESTIONS

Directions: Each question below contains five suggested answers. Choose the **one best** response to each question.

1. Characteristics of the fertile phase of the menstrual cycle include all of the following EXCEPT

(A) peak levels of estrogen
(B) clear, abundant cervical mucus
(C) ovulation
(D) production of progesterone
(E) sensation of vulvar slipperiness

2. Negative side effects of the barrier methods of contraception include all of the following EXCEPT

(A) toxic shock syndrome
(B) urinary tract infection
(C) pregnancy rate between 5% and 15%
(D) congenital anomalies
(E) salpingitis

3. Spermicides effect their contraceptive action in all of the following ways EXCEPT by

(A) killing the sperm
(B) decreasing sperm motility
(C) inactivating acrosomal enzymes
(D) disrupting the outer lipoprotein surface layer
(E) neutralizing vaginal acidity

4. Physiologic changes effected by oral contraceptives include all of the following EXCEPT

(A) suppression of ovulation
(B) hostile cervical mucus
(C) a hypoestrogenic state
(D) inactive endometrium
(E) reduction of gonadotropins

Directions: Each question below contains four suggested answers of which **one or more** is correct. Choose the answer

A if **1, 2, and 3** are correct
B if **1 and 3** are correct
C if **2 and 4** are correct
D if **4** is correct
E if **1, 2, 3, and 4** are correct

5. Amenorrhea is associated with which of the following methods of contraception?

(1) Oral contraception
(2) Gonadotropin-releasing hormone agonists
(3) Medroxyprogesterone
(4) Progesterone-releasing intrauterine device

6. A woman presents with lower abdominal pain, a low-grade temperature, and a tender uterus. She is using an intrauterine device (IUD) for birth control. The plan of treatment should include

(1) x-ray of the pelvis to locate the IUD
(2) removal of the IUD
(3) ultrasound examination to determine the position of the IUD
(4) antibiotics

7. Increased thromboembolic activity with oral contraception may be the result of

(1) increased levels of factor VII
(2) increased plasma renin activity
(3) decreased levels of antithrombin II
(4) increased platelet counts

8. Which of the following conditions are associated with the prolonged use of birth control pills?

(1) Amenorrhea
(2) Hypertension
(3) Thromboembolism
(4) Liver tumor

9. Reasons for postpill amenorrhea include which of the following?

(1) Pituitary adenoma
(2) Previous oligomenorrhea
(3) Pregnancy
(4) Length of usage

ANSWERS AND EXPLANATIONS

1. The answer is D. (*I A 2, 3, B 2 a–d, 3*) The fertile phase of the menstrual cycle is characterized by ovulation. Estrogen levels rise to a peak just prior to ovulation; it is this peak that triggers ovulation. With the rise of estrogen, the cervix is stimulated to produce clear, abundant mucus, which gives the vulva a feeling of slipperiness. Progesterone production occurs after ovulation and characterizes the infertile phase of the menstrual cycle.

2. The answer is E. (*II A 1, B 2, 3, C 2, 3, D 2, 3*) Barrier methods of contraception (i.e., diaphragms, condoms, sponges, and spermicides) are thought to be relatively free from side effects; they also protect users against sexually transmitted diseases (and therefore salpingitis) and, thus, indirectly against carcinoma of the cervix. However, some negative side effects have been reported: (1) A few cases of toxic shock syndome have been reported among vaginal sponge users. (2) Recurrent urinary tract infections have been associated with the diaphragm because of its pressure on the urethra. (3) Pregnancy rates between 5% and 15% have been reported for all barrier methods of contraception. (4) The possibility that spontaneous abortion rates and incidences of congenital anomalies may be higher than normal with spermicide use has been reported; however, these findings are controversial.

3. The answer is E. (*II B 1 a, b*) Spermicides have two basic components: the active agent and the carrier substance. The active agent works by disrupting the outer lipoprotein surface layer of the spermatozoa, which kills it. In addition, the spermicides decrease sperm motility and inactivate the enzymes necessary for the sperm to penetrate the ovum. If the spermicides neutralized the vaginal acidity, they would decrease their effectiveness because sperm are naturally inactivated in an acidic vagina.

4. The answer is C. (*IV A 1, B 1–3*) The oral contraceptives are effective for several reasons. They cause a reduction of gonadotropins, which, in turn, inhibits ovulation. Because of the dominant progestogen effect, they also cause the cervical mucus to be scant and viscous and the endometrium to be inactive; both of these features contribute to contraception. Patients on oral contraceptives are not hypoestrogenic. Either mestranol or ethinyl estradiol are pill components, both of which maintain normal estrogen levels.

5. The answer is A (1, 2, 3). (*III C 3, D 1; IV D 3; V A 3, 4, B 2 b*) Any medication that suppresses hypothalamic–pituitary function and, consequently, suppresses ovarian activity can result in amenorrhea. When the ovary produces little or no estrogen, the endometrium is so minimally stimulated that there is no tissue to slough and, thus, no menses. Oral contraceptive agents, gonadotropin-releasing hormone agonists, and medroxyprogesterone all have the ability to shut down the hypothalamic–pituitary–ovarian axis. Women who use the progesterone-bearing intrauterine device continue to have menses, which may be scant because of the regressive action of the progesterone on the endometrium.

6. The answer is C (2, 4). (*III D 3 a–e*) With an intrauterine device (IUD) in situ, a low-grade temperature, and a tender uterus, one must suspect an IUD-related pelvic infection. Because the patient has not complained of abnormal bleeding or of not being able to feel the attached string, x-ray and ultrasound would not be indicated to help locate the IUD. The IUD should be removed, and the patient started on antibiotics to guard against an infection that could compromise future fertility.

7. The answer is B (1, 3). (*IV D 1–2*) Superficial and deep vein thromboses are increased in oral contraceptive users. This may be due to an increase in the number of clotting factors, such as factor VII, and a decrease in antithrombin III. Platelet counts do not increase in pill users. There is an increase in plasma renin activity in pill users, but this is associated with the pathophysiology of hypertension, not thromboembolic disease.

8. The answer is C (2, 4). (*IV D 1–4*) Hypertension and liver tumors are two complications associated with prolonged use (more than 5 years) of oral contraception. There is no relationship between the length of pill use and amenorrhea; thus, a "rest period" to prevent amenorrhea is unnecessary. Both superficial and deep vein thromboses are increased in *all* oral contraceptive users as antithrombin III levels fall within 10 days of starting oral contraceptives; thromboembolism is, therefore, not associated with prolonged use.

9. The answer is A (1, 2, 3). (*IV D 3 a–b*) The incidence of postpill amenorrhea is very small (0.2%–3.1%). Many of the women who experience postpill amenorrhea had preexisting menstrual abnormalities (35%–56%), such as oligomenorrhea. Any amenorrhea following cessation of contraceptive use should suggest pregnancy; it is the first cause to be ruled out. Since a pituitary adenoma occasionally develops in women who use oral contraceptives and since it is the most dangerous reason for the amenorrhea, it must be ruled out promptly with measurement of serum prolactin levels. Length of usage is not related to the occurrence of amenorrhea.

I. INTRODUCTION. The evaluation of pelvic pain and abdominal pain—the most frequent complaints in a gynecologic practice—is often difficult. Not only do innumerable pathologic entities and functional disorders cloud the diagnostic picture, but also individual responses to pain and pain thresholds make localization of pain a taxing diagnostic dilemma.

II. NEUROPHYSIOLOGY. Nerve endings extend into all internal pelvic organs. However, they are few in number, and because there is no great concentration of sensory nerve ganglia in the pelvis, it is difficult for the central nervous system to differentiate the pain that arises from the deep pelvic viscera. Moreover, pelvic pain is characterized as a second type of pain, that is, it is poorly localized, slowly conducted, and persists after a stimulus is removed.

A. Sources of pelvic pain. Pelvic pain is visceral and thus does not respond to thermal, chemical, or tactile sensations. Visceral pain is referred or splanchnic.

1. Referred pain occurs when autonomic impulses arise from a diseased organ and elicit an irritable focus within the spinal cord, exciting cells receiving somatic impulses. Pain is then sensed by the corresponding central nervous system site as originating in the superficial site.

2. Splanchnic pain occurs when an irritable stimulus is appreciated in the specific organ secondary to:
a. Tension
  (1) Distension and subsequent contraction of a hollow viscus
  (2) Traction as a result of fibrosis or a fibrotic process
  (3) Stretching of the capsule of a solid organ
b. Peritoneal irritation or inflammation
  (1) Inflammation from an adjacent viscus tends to be well localized and well defined.
  (2) Generalized peritonitis may result from spillage (i.e., pus, blood, or intestinal contents) of an irritant.
  (3) Chemical irritation
  (4) Tissue ischemia

B. The autonomic nervous system innervates the pelvic organs. Visceral abdominal pain tends to be poorly localized because sensory impulses from several viscera overlap within the same segment of the spinal cord. Sensations from the pelvic organs are transmitted by the following three pathways:

1. The parasympathetic nerves (S2, S3, and S4) transmit sensations to the spinal cord via the hypogastric plexus from the:
  a. Upper third of the vagina
  b. Cervix
  c. Lower uterine segment
  d. Posterior urethra
  e. Trigone of the bladder
  f. Lower ureters
  g. Uterosacral ligaments
  h. Cardinal ligaments
  i. Rectosigmoid
  j. Dorsal external genitalia

2. The thoracolumbar sympathetic nerves (T11, T12, and L1) transmit impulses to the spinal cord via the hypogastric and inferior mesenteric plexus from the:
  a. Uterine fundus

      b. Proximal third of the fallopian tube
      c. Broad ligaments
      d. Upper bladder
      e. Appendix
      f. Cecum
      g. Terminal large bowel

3. The superior mesenteric plexus (T5–T11) transmits impulses to the spinal cord from the:
      a. Ovaries
      b. Lateral two-thirds of the fallopian tubes
      c. Upper ureters

III. HISTORY. Since pelvic pain is often difficult to describe, it is imperative that a meticulous history be taken. It is important to consider the onset (acute or chronic), location, quality, duration (constant or cyclic), and severity of the pain episode as well as any associated complaints, such as fever, chills, anorexia, nausea, vomiting, or bleeding. It is also important to determine whether or not the pain is related to the menstrual cycle, is life-threatening, necessitates resuscitative efforts, or is related to reproductive processes.

A. Onset

1. Sudden onset suggests an acute intraperitoneal event, such as perforation, hemorrhage, rupture, or torsion. Acute colic of the urinary or gastrointestinal tract may present similarly.

2. Gradual onset suggests inflammation, obstruction, or a slowly evolving problem.

B. Location

1. Abdominal pain that is generalized suggests extensive peritoneal irritation.

2. Epigastric pain suggests problems in structures innervated by T6–T8.
      a. Stomach
      b. Duodenum
      c. Pancreas
      d. Liver
      e. Gallbadder

3. Periumbilical pain suggests problems in structures innervated by T9 and T10.
      a. Small intestine
      b. Appendix
      c. Upper ureters
      d. Ovaries

4. Hypogastric or suprapubic pain suggests problems in structures innervated by T11 and T12.
      a. Colon
      b. Bladder
      c. Lower ureters
      d. Uterus

5. Pelvic pain suggests problems in structures innervated by S2, S3, and S4 (e.g., cervix) or T10–T12 (e.g., ovaries and fallopian tubes).

6. Shoulder pain may indicate referred pain from diaphragmatic irritation.

C. Quality

1. Cramping, rhythmic pain suggests:
      a. Muscular contractions of a hollow viscus
      b. Intraluminal pressure in a hollow viscus

2. Constant pain suggests:
      a. An inflammatory process
      b. Overdistension of a solid organ
      c. Compromise of blood supply

3. Sharp pain suggests obstruction or an acute peritoneal event.

4. Dull pain suggests an inflammatory process.

D. Duration. Duration and recurrence of pain episodes help to establish whether the problem is acute or chronic. If the patient has had similar pain in the past or similar pain for a prolonged period, an acute problem is unlikely. Acute attacks of pain over long periods, which last less than 48 hours and are recurrent, may be secondary to a chronic problem (e.g., ovulatory pain).

E. Severity. The appearance of the patient must be evaluated for the presence or absence of pallor and diaphoresis.

F. Associated symptoms

1. **Vaginal bleeding** associated with pelvic pain generally indicates reproductive tract pathology.

2. **Fever and chills** often indicate a pelvic infection that has spread systemically.

3. **Anorexia, nausea, and vomiting**, while nonspecific, often indicate intestinal tract pathology.

4. **Syncope, vascular collapse, and shock** usually indicate intraperitoneal hemorrhage and instability secondary to hypovolemia.

5. **Frequency, dysuria, flank pain, or hematuria** generally indicate urinary tract pathology.

6. **Shoulder pain** indicates irritation of the undersurface of the diaphragm by blood or inflammatory fluid.

7. **Dyspareunia** must be investigated as it can have many etiologies.

8. **Other.** A history of ectopic pregnancy, pelvic inflammatory disease, appendectomy, tubal repair, and endometriosis should be invesigated.

IV. PHYSICAL SIGNS

A. General examination

1. **Vital signs**
   a. Blood pressure
   b. Pulse
   c. Respiration
   d. Temperature

2. **General appearance**

3. **Heart and lungs.** Abdominal pain may be referred from pulmonary and cardiac disease.

4. **Activity level**

B. Abdominal examination

1. **Inspect** to evaluate distension and contour and determine the location of the pain. Initially, the area of maximum pain should be avoided.

2. **Auscultate** gently to evaluate hypoactive or hyperactive bowel sounds, concomitantly evaluating for guarding, rebound tenderness, and abdominal rigidity.

3. **Percuss** to localize the area of tenderness and to evaluate ascites, distension, masses, or organ size.

4. **Palpate** gently to evaluate tenderness or masses.

C. Pelvic examination The identification of tenderness or masses needs further evaluation. Careful evaluation of the cervix, uterus, and adnexa is imperative.

1. Inspect external genitalia and cervix for evidence of trauma, infection, hemorrhage, or asymmetry.

2. Without placing the hand on the abdomen, palpate the vaginal wall for tenderness, and palpate the cervix for cervical motion tenderness, localizing the side of tenderness.

3. Palpate the adnexa, starting with the side of least tenderness as elicited by the cervical motion test.

4. Use the hand on the abdomen to evaluate masses or tenderness.

V. LABORATORY TESTS. The evaluation of pelvic pain presents the clinician with a diagnostic challenge. Valuable diagnostic information can be gleaned with:

A. **A complete blood count** with a differential smear. An increased white blood cell count, especially with a shift to the left, may indicate systemic infection. Decreased hemoglobin levels may indicate blood loss.

B. **An urinalysis** with microscopic examination and culture and sensitivity testing. The presence of bacteria, white blood cells, or red blood cells suggests that the urinary tract is the site of disease.

C. **Blood type and antibody screen.** If intra-abdominal bleeding is suspected or diagnosed, then blood should be sent to the blood bank for typing and crossmatched. In addition, if the patient has a miscarriage, then Rh status must be evaluated (see Chapter 11, Rh Isoimmunization).

D. **A pregnancy test** with serial human chorionic gonadotropin (HCG) β-subunit measurements if indicated. This is important in the evaluation of the patient who may be pregnant. A negative serum pregnancy test essentially excludes this possibility. A positive serum pregnancy test needs to be followed with serial β-subunit measurements if the exact location of the pregnancy is in doubt. Anything other than the 2–3 day doubling time needs to be viewed with suspicion and evaluated carefully. Until this value is obtained, however, a urine pregnancy test will be useful if positive.

E. **Cervical cultures** for gonorrhea and *Chlamydia* are indicated if a pelvic infection is suspected.

F. **Culdocentesis,** which may be helpful in evaluating the posterior cul-de-sac for intraperitoneal blood or free fluid.

G. **Erythrocyte sedimentation rate,** which may be elevated in cases of infection. It is an acute phase reactive protein that is nonspecific but that indicates an inflammatory reaction.

H. **X-rays.** Abdominal x-rays, including upright, supine, and lateral decubitus films, may reveal evidence of:

  1. Intestinal obstruction

  2. Free air under the diaphragm, suggesting perforation of an air-filled viscus

  3. Free fluid, suggesting bleeding or a ruptured cyst

  4. Calcifications, suggesting renal stones, gallstones, calcified myomas, and dermoid cysts

I. **Ultrasound**, which is particularly useful in evaluating the pelvis for the diagnosis of:

  1. An early intrauterine pregnancy or ectopic pregnancy

  2. An adnexal mass

J. **Laparoscopy** is quite useful in the assessment of pelvic pain since it is a well-controlled procedure, it allows visualization of the pelvic structures, it allows time for reflection upon optimal mode of management, and it is an opportunity to diagnose and treat a problem without extensive surgery. It is, however, contraindicated in patients with hypovolemic shock or gastrointestinal obstruction. Despite the usefulness of this procedure, approximately 30% of pelvic pain patients will have a normal pelvis.

VI. DIFFERENTIAL DIAGNOSIS

A. **Acute pelvic pain**

  1. **Pregnancy related**
    a. **Abortion** is characterized by vaginal bleeding and abdominal pain that is suprapubic, crampy, and of variable intensity. It is classified as:
      (1) **Spontaneous.** Four categories of spontaneous abortion include:
        (a) **Threatened abortion** in which blood exits from the cervical os even though it is closed
        (b) **Inevitable abortion**, which is manifested by prolonged, profuse bleeding with an open cervical os
        (c) **Incomplete abortion**, which is characterized by a partial passage of tissue through the cervical os
        (d) **Complete abortion**, which is characterized by a complete passage of tissue, resulting in resolution of symptoms

(2) **Induced.** Subsequent to an induced abortion, pelvic pain can occur secondary to:
  (a) **Incomplete evacuation**
  (b) **Septic abortion**, which is characterized by abortion symptoms along with fever and sepsis secondary to infection of the uterine contents. Treatment consists of:
      (i) Obtaining appropriate cultures
      (ii) Dilatation and evacuation
      (iii) Instituting intravenous broad-spectrum antibiotics

b. **Ectopic pregnancy**
  (1) Ninety-five percent of all ectopic pregnancies are found in the fallopian tubes. A pregnancy may exist in any portion of the tube, including the cornua, interstitium, isthmus, ampulla, or infundibulum, each of which are associated with particular complications and surgical considerations. Ectopic pregnancies may also be found in the abdomen, cervix, or ovary, although these are uncommon.
  (2) The mechanism of pain may involve distension of the tube due to the growing pregnancy. The presenting symptoms may be so vague that the physician must always suspect ectopic pregnancy when a patient presents with pelvic pain. The low abdominal pain is usually unilateral; however, it may be bilateral or generalized. The pain may be either crampy due to tubal distension by the enlarging pregnancy, sudden and sharp due to acute rupture with intra-abdominal bleeding, or dull and aching associated with a chronic ectopic and a surrounding organized hematoma. The pain may wax and wane over a few days, and it may be aggravated by motion.
  (3) A patient who has a history of an ectopic pregnancy or a pelvic infection or who uses an intrauterine device is at increased risk for a future ectopic pregnancy.
  (4) Associated symptoms include:
      (a) Vaginal bleeding or spotting
      (b) Delayed or missed menses
      (c) Syncope
      (d) Orthostatic changes
      (e) Rectal pressure and the urge to defecate as a result of blood in the posterior cul-de-sac
      (f) The nonspecific symptoms of pregnancy:
          (i) Nausea
          (ii) Vomiting
          (iii) Breast enlargement
  (5) Laboratory evaluations
      (a) HCG β-subunit radioimmunoassay is particularly useful since it is extremely sensitive and specific. In a normal pregnancy, the serum HCG β-subunit levels double every 1.4–2.2 days. Thus a fall, plateau, or prolonged doubling rate in serial values indicate a necessity for evaluation.
      (b) Ultrasound can localize an intrauterine pregnancy at HCG β-subunit levels of greater than 5800 mIU/ml, and with a vaginal probe, earlier gestations may be visualized. Additionally, it may localize fetal heart activity either in the adnexa or within the uterine cavity and the presence of free fluid within the cul-de-sac.
      (c) Culdocentesis yielding nonclotting blood is an indication for laparotomy.
      (d) Laparoscopy yields more information and allows for more conservative surgery.

2. **Unrelated to pregnancy**
  a. **Mittelschmerz** is pain in the lower abdomen occurring around ovulation and believed to be secondary to chemical irritation of the peritoneum from ovarian follicular cyst fluid. The pain generally lasts only a few hours but usually no longer than 2 days.
  b. **Ovarian accidents.** Bleeding, rupture, and torsion may be associated with inflammatory cysts, endometriomas, benign or malignant cysts or solid tumors, or variations in the normal ovarian cycle. The mechanisms of pain involve acute distension, peritoneal irritation by blood or cyst fluids, or ischemia.
  (1) Bleeding may cause pain by irritation of the peritoneal cavity by extruded blood or acute distension of the ovary.
  (2) Rupture of a cyst releases cyst fluid, which is quite irritating to the peritoneum.
  (3) Torsion (i.e., rotation of a tumor around its pedicle) leads to ischemia and tissue necrosis; the clinical presentation depends upon the extent of interference with the ovarian blood supply. Torsion can also involve the fallopian tube. The more complete the vascular occlusion, the more extensive the ischemia, and then the more severe the pain. The pain is usually paroxysmal and unilateral but becomes more constant if infarction occurs. In pregnancy, torsion is more likely to occur during the period of rapid uterine growth (8–16 weeks) or involution postpartum.

(a) Associated symptoms may include:

(i) Nausea

(ii) Vomiting

(iii) Syncope

(iv) Shock

(v) Shoulder pain

(b) Therapy involves laparotomy with isolation and clamping of the infundibulopelvic ligament prior to untwisting torsed adnexae with subsequent excision.

c. Ovarian hyperstimulation syndrome may occur in patients with a history of infertility who are currently being treated with fertility hormones (e.g., clomiphene or human menopausal gonadotropins). The ovaries are enlarged with multiple follicular cysts, a large cystic corpus luteum, and stromal edema. Associated symptoms include the following:

(1) Mild cases

(a) Weight gain

(b) Abdominal distension

(c) Abdominal pain

(2) Severe cases may also include:

(a) Ascites

(b) Pleural effusion

(c) Hypovolemia

(d) Oliguria

(e) Electrolyte disturbances

(f) Dyspnea

(3) Therapy involves:

(a) Hospitalization

(b) Observation

(c) Bedrest

(d) Fluid and electrolyte replacement

d. Pelvic inflammatory disease (PID) is an infection of the pelvic organs by pathogenic microorganisms, usually *Neisseria gonorrhoeae*, *Chlamydia trachomatis*, and *Mycoplasma hominis*.

(1) The infectious process. The route of bacterial infection is usually an ascending infection via the vagina and cervix; however, it may also involve infection via the veins and lymphatics of the broad ligaments. If not treated, the infectious process may spread, causing peritonitis or abscess formation. The course of the disease depends upon the virulence of the invading organism and the ability of the host to respond. Pelvic infection may be characterized by the following entities:

(a) Endometritis, inflammation of the endometrium, usually develops postpartum or postabortal, especially if there has been a preceding chorioamnionitis. This may progress to a parametritis, which is an inflammation of the connective tissue surrounding the uterus. The typical symptoms include:

(i) Chills, sweats, and fever

(ii) Lower abdominal pain

(iii) Vaginal bleeding

(iv) Mucopurulent vaginal discharge

(b) Salpingo-oophoritis, inflammation of the fallopian tubes and the ovary, presents as lower abdominal pain that is gradual in onset but increases in severity over a few hours to a few days. It usually becomes bilateral and develops during or shortly after the menses. The pain is aggravated by motion once the inflammatory process extends to peritoneum. Associated symptoms include:

(i) Vaginal bleeding

(ii) Vaginal discharge

(iii) Chills

(iv) Fever

(v) Anorexia

(vi) Nausea

(vii) Vomiting

(c) Tubo-ovarian abscess is the result of an infected tube that involves the ovary. Pus accumulates, resulting in the development of a tender, nonmobile, poorly defined, pelvic mass. Severe, constant, and diffuse abdominal pain is the most characteristic symptom when the abscess is forming; however, the pain later becomes localized to the abscess site. Rupture of the tubo-ovarian cyst should be suspected if the pain is sudden, severe, diffuse, abdominal pain that is associated with shock. Associated symptoms may include:

(i) Abnormal vaginal bleeding due to an associated endometritis
(ii) Fever
(iii) Chills
(iv) Anorexia
(v) Nausea
(vi) Vomiting
(vii) Gastrointestinal or genitourinary symptoms due to extrinsic pressure from the abscess

(2) Laboratory evaluation of PID includes:
(a) Cervical cultures for *Neisseria, Chlamydia,* and *Mycoplasma*
(b) Sedimentation rate and leukocyte count
(c) Consideration of laparoscopy if the diagnosis is in question

(3) Therapy
(a) If present, an intrautrine device (IUD) should be removed.
(b) Intravenous antibiotics should include one of the following three combinations:
(i) Doxycycline and cefoxitin
(ii) Gentamicin and clindamycin
(iii) Doxycycline and metronidazole
(c) Abscess rupture must be managed by laparotomy with excision of the infected tissue and subsequent drainage in addition to above measures.
(d) Colpotomy may be performed to drain a pelvic abscess provided the abscess is fluctuant, dissects the rectovaginal septum, and is in the midline.

e. Appendicitis. The pain is not well localized and is referred initially as a result of distension of the lumen of the appendix by inflammatory exudate. The pain is colicky with a gradual onset. It localizes to the right lower quandrant (i.e., to the site of the appendix) once the overlying parietal peritoneum becomes locally involved in the inflammatory process. In pregnancy the appendix is usually displaced upward by the enlarging uterus, and symptoms tend to localize at the site where the appendix might be for that stage of pregnancy. Associated symptoms include:
(1) Anorexia
(2) Nausea
(3) Vomiting

B. Chronic pelvic pain

1. Cyclic
a. Mittelschmerz. Pain is sudden, episodic, and usually unilateral in the lower abdomen. Therapy relies on reassurance and consideration of suppression of ovulation with oral contraceptives.
b. Dysmenorrhea is defined as pain accompanying menstruation. It is further categorized as:
(1) Primary dysmenorrhea, which is defined as painful menstruation in the absence of organic pelvic lesions. Primary dysmenorrhea generally accompanies ovulatory cycles. The pain is spasmodic and throbbing and located in the lower abdomen, often radiating to lower back and the front of the thighs. Its onset is concurrent with the menses and lasts for 1–3 days. Associated symptoms include backache, nausea, vomiting, diarrhea, headache, and fatigue.
(a) While there may be a psychological component to primary dysmenorrhea, it is generally thought that decreasing progesterone levels at the end of the menstrual cycle cause a release of phospholipase A_2 from the endometrial cells. This acts on the lipid cell membrane to produce arachidonic acid, and through the action of prostaglandin synthetase, prostaglandin E_2 (PGE_2) and F_{2a} (PGF_{2a}) are formed. These prostaglandins cause uterine contraction, resulting in areas of ischemia, which ultimately causes pain.
(b) Therapy entails the following:
(i) Discussions regarding the nature of the pain
(ii) Suppression of ovulatory cycles with oral contraceptives to decrease prostaglandin levels in menstrual fluid
(iii) Use of prostaglandin synthetase inhibitors, such as ibuprofen, naproxen, and mefenamic acid. These should be administered 48 hours prior to onset of menses and for 1–3 days of menstrual flow.
(iv) Laparoscopy if the above medications are not effective
(2) Secondary dysmenorrhea, which is defined as painful menstruation in the presence of organic disease, occurring more than 2 years after menarche. Numerous conditions may precipitate this complaint, including:

 (a) Endometriosis, which is characterized by the proliferation of foci of normal endometrium outside the uterine cavity. The usual affected areas include the ovaries, uterosacral ligaments, and posterior cul-de-sac; however, the intestinal tract and urinary tract may also be involved. Endometriosis can cause local destruction, distortion, obstruction, adhesions, and scar formation.

  (i) The pain is usually recurrent and aggravated by menstruation, maybe due to hemorrhagic distortion, peritoneal irritation, or escaped bloody fluid.

  (ii) Associated symptoms include dyspareunia, irregular vaginal bleeding, infertility, and intestinal or urinary symptoms, if these organ systems are involved.

  (iii) Therapy depends on the extent of the disease process as determined by laparoscopy. Medical treatment may involve continuous oral contraceptives, danazol, medroxyprogesterone, or gonadotropin-releasing hormone agonists. Severe disease may necessitate surgical excision and even removal of the uterus and adnexa (see Chapter 25).

 (b) Adhesive disease secondary to chronic PID, endometriosis, or postsurgical formation. Therapy is comprised of surgical lysis of adhesions.

 (c) Uterine pathology

  (i) Adenomyosis is a uterine pathology characterized by the presence of ectopic foci of endometrial glands and stroma in the myometrium. It is associated with heavy menstrual bleeding secondary to swelling of the ectopic endometrial islands in the myometrial wall. Antiprostaglandin medications may decrease both dysmenorrhea and heavy menstrual flow. Hysterectomy should be considered in refractory cases.

  (ii) Leiomyomas (i.e., fibroids or myomas) are benign uterine tumors composed of muscle and fibrous connective tissue in various locations: pedunculated, intramural, subserosal, or submucosal. Chronically, they may cause a crampy secondary dysmenorrhea associated with vaginal bleeding, which may progressively worsen. Therapy involves hysteroscopic resection of submucosal myomas, abdominal myomectomy, or hysterectomy (see Chapter 31).

 (d) Congenital anomalies may cause an obstruction to menstrual flow with resultant hematometra (i.e., accumulation of menstrual blood in the uterus secondary to cervical obstruction) or hematocolpos (i.e., accumulation of menstrual blood in the vagina secondary to introital obstruction). Imperforate hymen or noncommunicating horn of uterus are examples. These conditions must be repaired surgically.

 (e) Cervical stenosis secondary to previous surgery. Treatment involves dilation or laser-directed opening of the cervical os.

2. Acyclic pelvic pain is prolonged intractable pelvic pain that is unrelated to menstrual function. The goal in treating this type of pain is to localize the organic problem and separate this from any psychogenic influence.

 a. Organic etiologies

  (1) Endometriosis [see section VI B 1 b (2) (a) and Chapter 25]

  (2) Pelvic adhesions

  (3) Pelvic congestion syndrome. The existence of this syndrome as a true pathologic entity is controversial, although many claim that this is secondary to dilated pelvic varicosities.

  (4) Urinary tract. Although the kidney is located at a distance from the urinary tract, it can, along with the more distal ureters and the bladder, refer pain to the lower abdomen. As a result any pathology in the urinary tract may be responsible for chronic pelvic pain. These include:

  (a) Cystitis

  (b) Ureteral colic secondary to renal calculi

  (5) Intestinal tract. Gastrointestinal disease should be regarded as one possible explanation for the etiology of pelvic pain (lower abdominal pain) and should be appropriately evaluated. These include:

  (a) Diverticulitis

  (b) Colitis

  (6) Orthopedic conditions. There are a number of disease processes, congenital deformities, or inflammatory processes that may cause pain with an abdominal reference. These include:

  (a) Spina bifida

  (b) Scoliosis

  (c) Osteoarthritis

  (d) Fibromyositis

  (e) Herniated intervertebral disc

b. Psychogenic etiologies. When organic disease has been eliminated as the source of pelvic pain, patients should be evaluated for evidence of borderline personality, hypochondriasis, depression, and hysteria. Additionally, studies have shown that these patients may also have difficulty with interpersonal relationships and a history of sexual abuse as a child and instability during the growing years (adolescence). Results of the Minnesota Multiphasic Personality Index show that patients with chronic pelvic pain have a fourfold increase in the manifestation of somatization, depression, and borderline personality. Management should revolve around a team approach, including a social worker or psychiatrist, to evaluate psychosocial difficulties that may be responsible in part for the pain.

STUDY QUESTIONS

Directions: Each question below contains five suggested answers. Choose the **one best** response to each question.

1. The parasympathetic nerves innervate all of the following structures EXCEPT the

(A) cervix
(B) lower uterine segment
(C) uterine fundus
(D) uterosacral ligaments
(E) cardinal ligaments

2. All of the following statements concerning pain episodes are true EXCEPT

(A) the sudden onset of pain usually suggests an acute episode
(B) generalized abdominal pain suggests extensive peritoneal irritation
(C) crampy, rhythmic pain usually suggests muscular contractions or increased intraluminal pressure of a hollow viscus
(D) primary dysmenorrhea is usually unilateral and associated with a specific structural or organic abnormality
(E) vaginal bleeding in association with pelvic pain generally indicates reproductive tract pathology

3. In evaluating abdominal and pelvic pain, the correct order of examining the patient's abdomen is

(A) inspection, percussion, auscultation, palpation
(B) palpation, inspection, auscultation, percussion
(C) inspection, auscultation, percussion, palpation
(D) auscultation, inspection, palpation, percussion
(E) palpation, inspection, percussion, auscultation

4. A 19-year-old woman comes to a physician for evaluation of sharp pain that occurs in her lower abdomen for 2–3 days every month since her menses at 14 years of age. Approximately 2 weeks after she experiences this pain, she has her menses. The most probable etiology for her pain is

(A) endometriosis
(B) dysmenorrhea
(C) pelvic infection
(D) mittelschmerz
(E) ectopic pregnancy

5. A 29-year-old woman comes to see the physician with the complaint of chronic pelvic pain. The pain is dull and continuous. She has a history oligomenorrhea as well as several hospitalizations for suicidal ideation. She is taking numerous medications for arthritic complaints, asthma, peptic ulcer disease, and depression. The most likely etiology for her chronic pain is

(A) endometriosis
(B) uterine fibroids
(C) mittelschmerz
(D) pelvic adhesions
(E) psychogenic

Directions: Each question below contains four suggested answers of which **one or more** is correct. Choose the answer

    A if **1, 2, and 3** are correct
    B if **1 and 3** are correct
    C if **2 and 4** are correct
    D if **4** is correct
    E if **1, 2, 3, and 4** are correct

6. Which of the following symptoms are associated with an ectopic pregnancy in the fallopian tube?

(1) Unilateral lower abdominal pain
(2) Vaginal bleeding or spotting
(3) Missed menstrual period
(4) Rectal bleeding

ANSWERS AND EXPLANATIONS

1. The answer is C. (*II B 1 a–j, 2 a–g*) The parasympathetic nerves (S2, S3, and S4) transmit sensations to the spinal cord via the hypogastric plexus from the upper third of the vagina, cervix, the lower uterine segment, the uterosacral and cardinal ligaments, the posterior urethra, the trigone of the bladder, the lower ureters, and the rectosigmoid. The uterine fundus is innervated by the thoracolumbar sympathetic nerves (T11, T12, and L1).

2. The answer is D. [*III A 1, 2, B 1, 2, C 1, 2, F 1; VI B 1 b (1), (2)*] Sudden onset of pain usually suggests an acute episode, whereas a gradual onset suggests inflammation, obstruction, or a more slowly evolving entity. Extensive peritoneal irritation is usually associated with generalized abdominal pain, whereas peritoneal inflammation associated with specific structures is generally more localized. Crampy, rhythmic pain is usually associated with muscular contractions, while a steady persistent pain suggests an inflammatory process. Primary dysmenorrhea is generally symmetrical with no associated pelvic disease and often improves with pregnancy. On the other hand, secondary dysmenorrhea is usually associated with a structural or organic abnormality and more frequently is unilateral. Vaginal bleeding in association with pelvic pain generally indicates reproductive tract pathology.

3. The answer is C. (*IV B 1–4*) In evaluating the abdomen of a patient with pelvic pain, the physician must be careful not to elicit further pain, which may confuse the evaluation. To put the patient at ease, the abdomen should be inspected while conversing with the patient. Next, the patient should be asked to identify the area of maximum tenderness, and the area must be avoided until more information has been gathered. Auscultation follows; the physician may gently press down on the abdomen and then release pressure. True rebound tenderness will be elicited if peritoneal irritation exists. Percussion localizes the pain further and determines its severity. Palpation determines the presence of a mass.

4. The answer is D. (*VI A 2 a*) The presence of cyclic pain related to menses indicates a reproductive etiology for the pelvic pain of the young woman described in the question. Given that the pain is sharp and occurs 2 weeks prior to menses, it is most likely due to ovulation, namely mittelschmerz. Although dysmenorrhea is cyclic, by definition it occurs during the menses. Endometriosis may be chronic or cyclic, but it occurs at irregular intervals. Pelvic infection and ectopic pregnancy are not cyclic types of pain, although they present acutely.

5. The answer is E. (*VI B 2 b*) Although it is apparent that the etiology of the pelvic pain of the woman described in the question is psychogenic, this type of patient is one of the most difficult for a gynecologist to manage. Not only must the physician be alert to the real possibility of organic pain, but he or she must be aware of the numerous medical problems, real or imagined, that are possible. Given the history of somatization and depression, chronic pelvic pain is most apt to be another manifestation of deep-rooted psychological difficulties. A team approach, using a gynecologist, internist, psychiatrist, and social worker, would most benefit the patient described in the question.

6. The answer is A (1, 2, 3). [*VI A 1 b (1)–(5)*] The presenting symptoms of an ectopic pregnancy may be so vague that the physician should always consider the possibility of an ectopic pregnancy in the differential diagnosis of pelvic pain. The lower abdominal pain is usually unilateral; however, it may be bilateral or generalized. The patient may also present with vaginal bleeding or spotting and a delayed or missed menstrual period. Nonspecific symptoms of pregnancy may also exist. Rectal bleeding is not usually an associated symptom.

all can be involved in

endometritis
salpingitis
oophoritis
myometritis
peritonitis

12/26 – 12/28 / 98

24
Pelvic Inflammatory Disease
William W. Beck, Jr.

I. INTRODUCTION. Pelvic inflammatory disease (PID) is a term that describes an infection of the upper genital or reproductive tract. PID can involve infection of the endometrium (**endometritis**), the oviducts (**salpingitis**), the ovary (**oophoritis**), the uterine wall (**myometritis**), or portions of the parietal peritoneum (**peritonitis**).

A. Acute PID mostly involves the tubes and the sequelae, such as destruction of tubal architecture and function and pelvic adhesions.

B. Chronic PID is a misnomer because the chronic problems associated with PID—hydrosalpinx, infertility, adhesions, and pain—are bacteriologically sterile. True chronic PID, such as pelvic tuberculosis and actinomycosis, is rare. *[ˌæktinoˈmaiˈkoʊsis] 放线菌病*

II. EPIDEMIOLOGY OF PID

A. Costs. PID is essentially a sexually transmitted disease, which has become a major health concern.

1. Approximately 1 million cases of acute PID occur each year in the United States.

2. Direct and indirect costs of PID and its sequelae are predicted to be $3.5 billion annually by 1990.

3. In the United States, these costs involve 267,000 inpatient hospital admissions and 119,000 operations annually.

B. Incidence

1. PID is a disease of the young woman. The peak incidence occurs in women in their late teens and early twenties.

2. Acute PID occurs in 1%–2% of young sexually active women annually and is the most common serious infection in women ages 16–25 years of age. Initiation of intercourse at age 15 results in a one in eight chance of PID. Fifty percent of these girls have four or more sexual partners that first year. *[siˈkwiːlə] 后遗症.*

3. Medical sequelae develop in one in four women with acute PID.
  a. Ectopic pregnancy rate increases six- to tenfold in women with PID. Approximately 50% of all ectopic pregnancies are thought to result from the tubal damage caused by PID.
  b. Chronic pain increases fourfold. Both chronic pelvic pain and dyspareunia (90,000 new cases/yr) are related to PID.
  c. Infertility results after acute PID in 6%–60% of cases, depending on the severity and the number of episodes of infection. Tubal obstruction results:
    (1) After one episode of PID: 11.4%
    (2) After two episodes of PID: 23.1%
    (3) After three episodes of PID: 54.3%
  d. Mortality, though rare, does occur, particularly in neglected cases where a ruptured tubo-ovarian abscess can result in septic shock and death.

C. Contraceptive use. Women who are not sexually active and use no contraception do not develop PID. Conversely, women who are sexually active but use no contraception develop 3.42 cases of PID/100 woman years.

1. **Oral contraceptives** appear to protect the user against PID. Only 0.91 cases of PID/100 woman years have been reported among women using the pill. This may be due to:
   a. Decreased menstrual flow
   b. Decreased ability of pathogenic bacteria to attach to endometrial cells
   c. The presence of progesterone

2. **Barrier methods** of contraception (i.e., the diaphragm, condoms, and foam) are also protective against PID. Only 1.39 cases/100 woman years have been reported. Spermicides may also be bactericidal. Any barrier to spermatozoa also acts as a barrier to pathogenic bacteria.

3. **Intrauterine devices** (IUDs) have been linked to an increased risk of PID (5.21 cases/100 woman years), possibly as the result of:
   a. The creation of a sanctuary for bacteria from the body's defenses
   b. The establishment of chronic anaerobic endometritis within the uterine cavity

III. BACTERIOLOGY. Acute PID is usually a polymicrobial infection caused by organisms that are considered normal flora of the cervix and vagina.

A. Organisms cultured from the tube

1. *Neisseria gonorrhoeae*, a gram-negative diplococcus, which now has penicillinase-producing strains that make treatment more difficult.

2. *Chlamydia trachomatis*, an obligate intracellular organism due to its inability to produce adenosine triphosphate

3. Endogenous aerobic bacteria, such as *Escherichia coli*, *Proteus*, *Klebsiella*, and *Streptococcus*

4. Endogenous anaerobic bacteria, such as *Bacteroides*, *Peptostreptococcus*, and *Peptococcus*

5. *Mycoplasma hominis*

6. *Actinomyces israelii*, which is found in 15% of IUD-associated cases of PID, particularly in unilateral abscesses. It is rarely found in women who do not use an IUD.

B. Organism prevalence

1. *Neisseria gonorrhoeae* is the only organism recovered by direct tubal or cul-de-sac culture in one-third of women with acute PID.

2. One-third have a positive culture for *Neisseria* plus a mixture of endogenous aerobic and anaerobic flora.

3. One-third have only aerobic and anaerobic organisms.

4. *C. trachomatis* is found in tubal cultures of approximately 20% of all women with salpingitis.

5. *N. gonorrhoeae* and *C. trachomatis* coexist in the same individual 25%–40% of the time.

IV. PATHOPHYSIOLOGY. There is a multifactorial microbiologic etiology. PID or salpingo-oophoritis is generally preceded by vaginal and cervical colonization of pathologic bacteria, a state that may exist for months or years. An inciting event occurs, which allows bacteria to ascend the uterus to the tubal lumen, usually bilaterally.

A. Inciting events

1. **Menstrual periods.** Degenerating endometrium is a good culture medium. Two-thirds of acute PID cases begin just after menses.

2. **Sexual intercourse.** Bacteria laden fluids may be pushed into the uterus, and uterine contractions may assist their ascent.

3. **Iatrogenic events**
   a. Elective abortion
   b. Dilatation and curettage
   c. IUD insertion or use
   d. Hysterosalpingography
   e. Radium insertion into the endometrial cavity

B. Chronology of salpingo-oophoritis. Infection is usually bilateral, but unilateral infection is possible, especially in association with an IUD. The presence of chronic anaerobic endometritis near one tubal ostia may explain this. The clinical course is as follows:

1. **Endosalpingitis** develops initially with edema and, ultimately, destruction of luminal cells, cilia, and mucosal folds. Bacterial toxins are most likely to be responsible for this.

2. Infection spreads to the tubal muscularis and serosa. It then spreads by direct extension to the abdominal cavity via the fimbriated end of the tube.

3. **Oophoritis** develops over the surface of the ovaries, and microabscesses may develop within the ovary.

4. **Peritonitis** can develop, and upper abdominal infection may result either by direct extension of infection up the abdominal gutters laterally or by lymphatic spread. Development of **peri-hepatitis** with adhesions and right upper quadrant abdominal pain is known as the **Fitz-Hugh–Curtis syndrome**.

5. Low-grade, smoldering, or inadequately treated infections allow less virulent bacteria to contribute to the process, resulting in mixed infections. Anaerobes then play a major role with the development of pelvic abscesses.

6. **Sequelae of PID** are:
   a. Pyosalpinges (tubal abscesses)
   b. Hydrosalpinges (fluid-filled, dilated, thin-walled, destroyed tubes, usually totally obstructed)
   c. Partial tubal obstruction and crypt formation, resulting in ectopic pregnancies
   d. Total tubal obstruction and infertility
   e. Tubo-ovarian abscesses
   f. Peritubular and ovarian adhesions
   g. Dense pelvic and abdominal adhesions
   h. Ruptured abscesses, resulting in sepsis and shock
   i. Chronic pelvic pain and dyspareunia

V. DIAGNOSIS

A. **The signs and symptoms of PID** are relatively nonspecific. Thus, there is both a high false-positive rate and a high false-negative rate of diagnosis. Laparoscopic studies have revealed the inadequacy of diagnosing acute PID via the usual history and physical examinations and laboratory studies (Tables 24-1 and 24-2).

1. Based on symptoms, a high degree of suspicion is essential to make the diagnosis.

2. It is possible that only very mild symptoms will appear in spite of serious infection. Women with *C. trachomatis* may present with few symptoms but then may exhibit a severe inflammatory process when examined by the laparoscope.

B. **Common presenting complaints**

1. Generalized lower abdominal pain

2. Adnexal tenderness

3. Fever or shaking chills

Table 24-1. Laparoscopic Findings in Patients with False-Positive Clinical Diagnosis of Acute Pelvic Inflammatory Disease (PID) with Pelvic Disorders Other than PID

Laparoscopic Finding	No.
Acute appendicitis	24
Endometriosis	16
Corpus luteum bleeding	12
Ectopic pregnancy	11
Pelvic adhesions only	7
Benign ovarian tumor	7
Chronic salpingitis	6
Miscellaneous	15
Total	98

Note.—Reprinted with permission from Jacobson LJ: Differential diagnosis of acute pelvic inflammatory disease. *Am J Obstet Gynecol* 138:1007, 1980.

Table 24-2. Laparoscopy and Laparotomy Diagnoses in Patients with False-Negative Clinical Diagnosis of Acute Pelvic Inflammatory Disease (PID) by Laparoscopy

Clinical Diagnosis	Visual Diagnosis: Acute PID (No.)
Ovarian tumor	20
Acute appendicitis	18
Ectopic pregnancy	16
Chronic salpingitis	10
Acute peritonitis	6
Endometriosis	5
Uterine myoma	5
Uncharacteristic pelvic pain	5
Miscellaneous	6
Total	91

Note.—Reprinted with permission from Jacobson LJ: Differential diagnosis of acute pelvic inflammatory disease. *Am J Obstet Gynecol* 138:1007, 1980.

   4. Nausea and vomiting

   5. Dysuria and urethritis

   6. Foul-smelling vaginal discharge

   7. Adnexal masses or fullness

   8. Elevated white count and sedimentation rate

   9. History of concurrent or just finished menses

C. **Differential diagnosis** when considering PID should include:

   1. Ectopic pregnancy

   2. Ruptured ovarian cyst

   3. Appendicitis

   4. Endometriosis

   5. Inflammatory bowel disease

   6. Degenerating fibroids

   7. Spontaneous abortion

   8. Diverticulitis

D. **Diagnostic techniques**

   1. Cervical Gram stain. If gram-negative intracellular diplococci are present, a presumed diagnosis of gonorrhea (*N. gonorrhoeae*) is made. However, one-half of the gonorrhea cases will be missed by Gram stain alone.

   2. Culdocentesis. If purulent fluid is obtained, a culture may assist in antibiotic selection. However, infections may be secondary to another primary process.

   3. Laparoscopy. If the disease process is not clear, this is the ultimate technique to establish the diagnosis.

   4. Ultrasound. This procedure may be helpful in defining adnexal masses and intrauterine or ectopic pregnancies, especially when a patient has a tender abdomen and will not permit an adequate pelvic examination. Response to therapy can be objectively measured as masses and induration regress.

   5. Serum human chorionic gonadotropin (HCG). A sensitive pregnancy test is important in the differential diagnosis of pelvic pain to rule out the possibility of ectopic pregnancy. Approximately 3%–4% of women admitted with the diagnosis of PID have an ectopic pregnancy.

   6. Blood studies
      a. Leukocytosis is not a reliable indicator of acute PID. Less than 50% of women with acute PID have a white blood cell count of greater than 10,000 cells/ml.

b. An increased sedimentation rate is a nonspecific test and is elevated in approximately 75% of women with laparoscopically confirmed PID.

VI. THERAPY

A. Individualized treatment and a high index of suspicion for infection are mandatory. A decision for outpatient management and thus close follow-up in 48–72 hours or hospitalization must be made. Many experts recommend that all patients be hospitalized. Hospitalization of PID patients should be considered if:

1. The diagnosis is uncertain.

2. Surgical emergencies, such as appendicitis or ectopic pregnancy, must be excluded.

3. A pelvic abscess is suspected.

4. Severe illness precludes outpatient management.

5. The patient is pregnant.

6. The patient has failed an outpatient course of management.

B. Mild PID. An outpatient regimen for patients with mild PID is intramuscular aqueous procaine penicillin G (4.8 million units at two sites) or ampicillin (3.5 g) with oral probenecid (1.0 g), followed by ampicillin (500 mg four times a day for 7 days) or oral tetracycline HCl (500 mg four times daily for 7 days).

1. Advantages. This regimen provides adequate single-dose coverage for gonorrhea, and it is effective against *Chlamydia* and pharyngeal gonococcal infections.

2. Disadvantages
a. The efficacy and side effects of this combined regimen have not been fully evaluated, although it is now recommended by the Centers for Disease Control.
b. Tetracycline is contraindicated for pregnant women. For those who are penicillin allergic, spectinomycin (2.0 g intramuscularly twice a day for 3 days) may be given as replacement therapy, but it is ineffective in the treatment of pharyngeal gonococcal infection.

C. Acute PID

1. The treatment of choice has not been established, as no single agent is effective against all of the possible pathogens. Several combination antibiotic regimens that cover the three major pathogens—*N. gonorrhoeae, C. trachomatis,* and anaerobes—include:
a. Doxycycline (100 mg intravenously twice daily) *plus* cefoxitin (2.0 g intravenously four times daily).
b. Clindamycin (600 mg intravenously four times daily) *plus* gentamicin (2.0 mg/kg intravenously) followed by gentamicin (1.5 mg/kg intravenously three times daily) in patients with normal renal function.
c. Doxycycline (100 mg twice a day) *plus* metronidazole (1.0 g intravenously twice a day).

2. Conservative therapy with intense intravenous antibiotics should be tried first. If clinical improvement results, treatment should continue until the patient is asymptomatic and the masses resolve. This may take 7–14 days.

3. Surgery must be considered if there is no response to antibiotic therapy in 48–72 hours.
a. Colpotomy drainage of a pelvic abscess can be done if:
(1) It is midline.
(2) It dissects the rectovaginal septum.
(3) It is cystic.
b. Laparotomy is often otherwise indicated. Unless there is a well-defined unilateral abscess where a unilateral salpingo-oophorectomy could be done, the treatment of choice is a total abdominal hysterectomy, bilateral salpingo-oophorectomy, and drainage of the pelvic cavity. The patient, regardless of her age, should be prepared for this preoperatively.

VII. OTHER CAUSES OF PELVIC INFECTION

A. Granulomatous salpingitis

1. Tuberculous salpingitis almost always represents systemic tuberculosis (TB). There is a high incidence in indigent countries and a very low incidence in developed countries. It affects women in their reproductive years, but an increased incidence among postmenopausal women has been reported. Primary genital TB is extremely rare in the United States.

    a. Physical findings are variable. Patients usually present with adnexal masses. Induration may be noted in the paracervical, paravaginal, and parametrial tissues. The typical patient is 20–40 years old with known TB and a pelvic mass. Symptoms are related to family history of TB, low level pelvic pain, infertility, and amenorrhea.

    b. Pathology. Grossly, the uterine tube has a classic "tobacco pouch" appearance being enlarged and distended. The proximal end is closed, and the fimbria are edematous and enlarged. Microscopically, there are tubercles with an epithelioid reaction and giant cell formation. There is intense inflammation and scarring.

    c. Treatment involves the standard regimens for disseminated TB, including isoniazid (INH), rifampin, and ethambutol. Prognosis for cure is excellent, but the outlook for fertility is dismal.

2. Leperous salpingitis. The histologic picture is similar to tuberculosis, and it is often difficult to distinguish them on a histologic basis. Langhans' giant cells and epithelioid cells are present. Positive cultures are necessary for a diagnosis of TB.

3. Actinomycosis. *Actinomyces israelii,* the causative agent, is pathogenic for man but not for other mammals. Most gynecologic involvement is infection secondary to appendiceal infection, gastrointestinal tract disorders, or IUD use. There are a total of 100 reported cases annually, and the age range of prevalence is about 20–40 years.

    a. Physical findings. Half the lesions are bilateral and are characterized by adnexal enlargement and tenderness. Presenting symptoms may be confused with appendicitis.

    b. Pathology. Grossly, there is tubo-ovarian inflammation, and on sections of the tube there is copious necrotic material. There may be an adenomatous appearance to the tubal lumen. Microscopically, actinomycotic "sulfur" granules are present. There are club-like filaments that radiate out from the center. There is a monocytic infiltrate, and giant cells may be present.

    c. Treatment. Therapy is a prolonged course of penicillin.

4. Schistosomiasis occurs most commonly in the Far East and Africa.

    a. Physical findings are pelvic pain, menstrual irregularity, and primary infertility. The diagnosis is usually made by histopathology.

    b. Pathology. Grossly, lesions appear as a nonspecific tubo-ovarian process. Microscopically, the ova or schistosome is seen surrounded by a granulomatous reaction with giant and epidermoid cells. An egg within an inflammatory milieu is a very dramatic sight.

5. Sarcoidosis. While very rare, sarcoidosis can lead to a granulomatous salpingitis.

6. Foreign body salpingitis is seen following the use of non–water-soluble dye material for hysterosalpingography; it may also be secondary to medications placed within the vagina, such as starch, talc, and mineral oil.

B. Nongranulomatous salpingitis. This category refers to any other bacterial infection, usually of the peritoneal cavity, which can secondarily cause tubal infection, including:

1. Appendicitis

2. Diverticulitis

3. Crohn's disease

4. Cholecystitis

5. Perinephric abscess

STUDY QUESTIONS

Directions: Each question below contains five suggested answers. Choose the **one best** response to each question.

1. All of the following factors are associated with an increased risk of pelvic inflammatory disease EXCEPT

(A) onset of intercourse at age 15
(B) an elective abortion
(C) oral contraceptive use
(D) hysterosalpingography
(E) use of a copper intrauterine device

2. A unilateral tubo-ovarian abscess is removed from the pelvis of a woman who uses an intrauterine device. Which of the following organisms is most likely to be cultured from that abscess?

(A) *Mycoplasma*
(B) *Chlamydia*
(C) *Actinomyces*
(D) *Bacteroides*
(E) *Peptococcus*

3. A history of acute pelvic inflammatory disease is most commonly associated with which of the following events?

(A) Intrauterine device insertion
(B) Sexual intercourse
(C) Dilatation and curettage
(D) Endometrial biopsy
(E) A recent menstrual flow

4. All of the following procedures can aid in the diagnosis of pelvic inflammatory disease EXCEPT

(A) laparoscopy
(B) ultrasound
(C) culdocentesis
(D) hysterosalpingography
(E) rectal examination

5. All of the following diseases can cause pelvic inflammatory disease EXCEPT

(A) Crohn's disease
(B) syphilis
(C) appendicitis
(D) sarcoidosis
(E) schistosomiasis

Directions: Each question below contains four suggested answers of which **one or more** is correct. Choose the answer

A   if **1, 2, and 3** are correct
B   if **1 and 3** are correct
C   if **2 and 4** are correct
D   if **4** is correct
E   if **1, 2, 3, and 4** are correct

6. Known consequences of pelvic inflammatory disease include

(1) endometriosis
(2) ectopic pregnancy
(3) polycystic ovaries
(4) dyspareunia [dispə 'rɑːnɪə]
                  badly mated

7. The pathogenesis of a tubo-ovarian abscess involves which of the following infections?

(1) Oophoritis
(2) Endometritis
(3) Endosalpingitis
(4) Cervicitis

8. A 21-year-old nulliparous woman presents with a history of lower abdominal pain and bleeding that is 10 days later than her expected menses. On examination her temperature is 99.4°F, her uterus is top normal size and tender, and she has unilateral adnexal fullness. She has a normal white blood cell count. Diagnostic possibilities include

(1) ectopic pregnancy
(2) pelvic inflammatory disease
(3) threatened abortion
(4) appendicitis

9. Which of the following procedures confirm the diagnosis of acute pelvic inflammatory disease?

(1) White blood cell count
(2) Cervical Gram stain
(3) Culdocentesis
(4) Laparoscopy

Directions: The groups of questions below consist of lettered choices followed by several numbered items. For each numbered item select the **one** lettered choice with which it is **most** closely associated. Each lettered choice may be used once, more than once, or not at all.

Questions 10–12

For each of the following clinical situations describing a typical picture of pelvic inflammatory disease, select the organism that is most likely to be responsible for it.

(A) *Staphylococcus aureus*
(B) *Bacteroides fragilis*
(C) *Actinomyces israelii*
(D) *Neisseria gonorrhoeae*
(E) *Chlamydia trachomatis*

10. A sexually active 15-year-old girl comes to the emergency room complaining of acute pain in the lower abdomen that makes walking difficult. She states that the pain began 2 days after her menses ended and that she has a vaginal discharge.

11. A 40-year-old woman has had several admissions to the hospital for pelvic inflammatory disease. On the present admission a tender, fluctuant pelvic mass is noted. She has a temperature of 102°F and looks septic. After 5 days of intravenous antibiotics, there is no response. Exploratory surgery reveals a tubo-ovarian abscess.

12. A 24-year-old woman had an intrauterine device (IUD) inserted after her first delivery 2 years ago. She presents to the emergency room with lower abdominal pain and uterine tenderness. Pelvic examination reveals bilateral adnexal fullness. The IUD is removed and sent to pathology. The patient is started on penicillin.

Questions 13 and 14

For each clinical presentation listed below, select the treatment modality that is most appropriate.

(A) Oral doxycycline
(B) Intramuscular aqueous penicillin G
(C) Cefoxitin and doxycycline in the hospital
(D) Oral isoniazid
(E) Intramuscular spectinomycin

13. A 26-year-old pregnant woman is seen in the clinic for a prenatal checkup. A cervical culture is positive for *Neisseria gonorrhoeae*. She states that 2 years ago when treated with ampicillin for a urinary tract infection, she developed a rash.

14. An 18-year-old nulliparous woman was treated with oral ampicillin for a pelvic inflammatory infection 1 week ago. She continues to experience lower abdominal tenderness bilaterally. She had a positive gonorrhea culture 6 months previously for which she was treated with oral ampicillin. Human chorionic gonadotropin levels are normal.

ANSWERS AND EXPLANATIONS

1. The answer is C. (*II B 2, C 1; IV A 3 a–e*) Oral contraceptive use appears to protect the user against pelvic inflammatory disease (PID) due to decreased menstrual flow, which inhibits the transport of bacteria, decreased ability of bacteria to attach to endometrial cells, and the presence of progesterone. Intrauterine devices (IUDs) have been linked to an increased risk of PID, particularly the Dalkon shield, as has the early initiation of intercourse. Iatrogenic events that may allow bacteria to ascend the uterus to the tubal lumen include elective abortion, hysterosalpingography, dilatation and curettage, and IUD insertion.

2. The answer is C. (*III A 6; IV B; VII A 3*) *Actinomyces israelii* can be found in the 15% of cases of pelvic inflammatory disease that are associated with the use of an intrauterine device (IUD). This is especially true when a unilateral pelvic abscess is present. Microscopically, actinomycotic ''sulfur'' granules are present; in addition, there is a monocytic infiltration, and giant cells may be present. *A. israelii* is rarely found in women who do not use an IUD.

3. The answer is E. (*IV A 1–3*) Pelvic inflammatory disease (PID) is usually preceded by vaginal and cervical colonization of pathologic bacteria. The most common inciting event is a menstrual period; degenerating endometrium is a good culture medium, and two-thirds of acute PID cases begin just after menses. The other answers can also be inciting events, if the pathogens are present at the cervix, but they are less likely to be associated with acute PID than the menses.

4. The answer is D. (*V D 1–6*) The signs and symptoms of pelvic inflammatory disease (PID) are relatively nonspecific; thus, a high degree of suspicion is essential for the diagnosis. Techniques that aid in the diagnosis include laparoscopy, culdocentesis, and ultrasound. A rectal examination should *always* be performed during a pelvic examination to detect pelvic masses. Hysterosalpingography should *never* be performed if PID is suspected as it can disseminate the infection if it is present.

5. The answer is B. (*VII A B*) Bacterial infections that can secondarily cause tubal infection include appendicitis, which often causes pelvic adhesions and perisalpingo-oophoritis, and Crohn's disease, which can cause damage and inflammation of the oviducts. Although rare, schistosomiasis and sarcoidosis can also lead to granulomatous salpingitis. Although syphilis can occur in association with pelvic inflammatory disease (PID), since both are sexually transmitted, it is not a direct cause of PID.

6. The answer is C (2, 4). (*II B 3 a–d*) Six to sixty percent of female infertility is caused by the tubal obstruction from pelvic inflammatory disease (PID), and fifty percent of all ectopic pregnancies are thought to result from the tubal damage caused by PID. Chronic pelvic pain and dyspareunia are related to PID. Endometriosis can cause symptoms similar to those associated with PID and thus must be considered in the differential diagnosis. Polycystic ovaries, which result in oligo-ovulation and enlarged cystic ovaries, is an endocrine disorder.

7. The answer is B (1, 3). (*IV B 1–6*) The offending pathogen initially stimulates an endosalpingitis. The infection spreads to the tubal muscularis and the serosa and by direct extension to the peritoneal cavity and the ovary where an oophoritis usually precedes a tubo-ovarian abscess. Endometritis, inflammation of the endometrium, and cervicitis, inflammation of the cervix, are not necessarily part of the pathophysiology of a tubo-ovarian abscess.

8. The answer is E (all). (*V B, C*) Even though the 21-year-old woman described in the question could certainly have pelvic inflammatory disease (PID) because of the signs and symptoms, the differential diagnosis must include a number of other clinical entities. Her menses could be late because of a pregnancy, although menses can be late for no specific reason. The bleeding and pain could indicate an abortion or an ectopic pregnancy. The adnexal mass could be a corpus luteum of pregnancy or a tubal ectopic pregnancy. Anytime there is lower abdominal pain with any kind of temperature elevation, the possibility of appendicitis cannot be forgotten. The late menses do not exclude PID. The lower abdominal pain, the slight temperature elevation, and the adnexal fullness all point to the possibility of PID.

9. The answer is D (4). (*V D 1–6*) Laparoscopy is the gold standard in terms of diagnosing pelvic inflammatory disease (PID). Direct visualization of the pelvis, tubes, and ovaries confirms or rules out the diagnosis of PID. Most other studies are supportive, but not diagnostic. For example, 50% of cases of *Neisseria gonorrhoeae* PID are missed by cervical Gram stain, and less than 50% of women with PID have a white blood cell count above 10,000 cells/ml. The purulent fluid obtained from the cul-de-sac via culdocentesis may be helpful in making the diagnosis, but that fluid could be coming from an infection elsewhere in the peritoneal cavity.

10–12. The answers are: 10-D, 11-B, 12-C. (*III A 1–6, B 1–5; IV B 5; VII A 3*) The picture of the sexually active teenager is one of acute pelvic inflammatory disease (PID). Initiation of intercourse at age 15 results in a one in eight chance of PID with 50% of these girls having four or more sexual partners in the first year. *Neisseria gonorrhoeae* is thought to be the chief pathogen in the development of acute primary PID. It usually can be cultured from the cervix, especially when there is a discharge present as there is in this case.

The clinical picture of the 40-year-old woman is one of chronic PID with pelvic abscess formation. The pathogens in chronic PID are usually different from those of acute primary PID. There is likely to be a mixture of aerobic and anaerobic organisms. *Hemophilus, Streptococcus,* and *Escherichia coli* are the prominent aerobic organisms found with such abscesses, and *Bacteroides, Peptococcus,* and *Peptostreptococcus* are the prominent anaerobes.

Actinomyces israelii is the organism that has been associated with intrauterine device (IUD) users in 15% of IUD-associated cases of pelvic inflammatory disease. It is not usually found in non-IUD users. The adnexae may be enlarged and tender. "Sulfur" granules are seen microscopically. The therapy is penicillin.

13 and 14. The answers are: 13-E, 14-C. (*VI B 2 b, C 1 a*) Doxycycline should never be given to a pregnant woman as it causes tooth dysplasia and yellowing in the fetus. The 26-year-old pregnant woman appears to have a penicillin allergy so penicillin G would be contraindicated. Spectinomycin is often used as replacement therapy in patients who are penicillin allergic.

Doxycycline, penicillin G, and spectinomycin are outpatient regimens that are inappropriate for this 18-year-old, childless woman. She is at high risk for a missed pelvic infection, future infertility, or ectopic pregnancy unless she is treated aggressively for multiple organisms. Because she has failed at outpatient therapy, she should be treated in the hospital with doxycycline and cefoxitin to cover the major pathogens of pelvic inflammatory disease—*Neisseria gonorrhoeae, Chlamydia,* aerobes, and anaerobes.

I. INTRODUCTION

A. Definition. Endometriosis is the presence of functioning endometrial glands and stroma outside their usual location in the uterine cavity, often resulting in significant pelvic adhesions. It is primarily a pelvic disease with implants or adhesions of the ovaries, fallopian tubes, uterosacral ligaments, rectosigmoid, and bladder. It is rare to find endometriosis outside the pelvis, suggesting a metastatic spread. Although it is a **benign disease** of young women, endometriosis usually affects women in their reproductive years. Endometriosis is often associated with:

1. Crippling dysmenorrhea

2. Severe dyspareunia

3. Chronic pelvic pain

4. Infertility

5. Loss of work

6. Occasionally, early castration

B. Infertility. Pregnancy, with its positive effect on improving endometriosis, is very often difficult to achieve.

1. Infertility among women with endometriosis is approximately 30%–40%.

2. Endometriosis in infertile women has been demonstrated by the laparoscope in 15%–25% of cases.

II. THEORIES OF PATHOGENESIS

A. Retrograde menstrual flow. One theory postulates that the flow of menstrual debris through the fallopian tubes in a retrograde manner causes the spread of endometrial cells into the pelvis where they implant or set up irritative foci, which stimulate coelomic metaplasia and differentiation of the peritoneal cells into endometrial type tissue.

1. **Clinical evidence.** Endometriosis is commonly found in dependent portions of the pelvis. Flow of menstrual blood from the fallopian tubes has been observed during laparoscopy.

2. **Experimental evidence.** Endometrial fragments from the menstrual flow can grow both in tissue culture and following injection beneath the skin of the abdominal wall.

B. Vessel spread. Endometriosis at sites distant from the pelvis may be due to vascular or lymphatic transport of endometrial fragments.

C. Genetic and immunologic influences. Siblings have a relative risk of 7% of having endometriosis compared to 1% in a control group. In addition, it has been suggested that an immunologic deficiency may be involved in the pathogenesis of endometriosis. Monkeys with spontaneous endometriosis were found to have a cell-mediated response to autologous endometrial tissue that was significantly lower than controls. Thus, a genetic influence could manifest through a deficient immunologic system.

III. DIAGNOSIS

A. Signs and symptoms. Endometriosis should be suspected in any woman complaining of **infertility**. Suspicion is hightened when there are also complaints of **dysmenorrhea** and **dyspareunia**.

1. **Dysmenorrhea**. Painful menses are suggestive of endometriosis if they begin after years of relatively pain-free menses.

2. **Pelvic pain**. Pain can be diffuse in the pelvis, or it can be more localized, often in the area of the rectum. The degree of endometriosis often does not correlate with the amount of pain experienced. Many women who have endometriosis are asymptomatic.

3. **Dyspareunia.** Painful intercourse may be due to:
   a. Endometrial implants of the uterosacral ligaments
   b. Endometriomas of the ovaries
   c. Fixed retroversion of the uterus secondary to the endometriosis

4. **Infertility**. The infertility associated with endometriosis is often difficult to understand because of the small amount of endometriosis that is involved. Significant quantities of prostaglandin are reported to be secreted from the endometrial implants near the tubes and ovaries, which may interfere with tubal function and mobility, ovulation, steroidogenesis, and luteal function.

5. **Other signs of endometriosis**. Irregular menses, cyclic rectal bleeding or pain, and hematuria may be signs of endometriosis of the ovaries, rectosigmoid, and bladder, respectively.

B. Examination. The diagnosis of endometriosis combines the findings from the **history**, the **pelvic examination**, and **laparoscopy**.

1. **History**. The symptoms described by the patient are correlated with the physical examination and the diagnostic procedures in arriving at a diagnosis. A history of endometriosis in the patient's mother or sisters is important.

2. **Pelvic examination**. With minimal endometriosis, the pelvic examination may be normal.
   a. **Beading, nodularity,** and **tenderness of the uterosacral ligaments** are characteristic of endometriosis and can be best appreciated on rectovaginal examination,
   b. **Endometriomas** or **chocolate cysts of the ovaries** are palpated as adnexal masses, often fixed to the lateral pelvic walls or posterior to the broad ligament.
   c. **The uterus** is often in a **fixed, retroverted position**.

3. **Laparoscopy**. Visual diagnosis of endometriosis via the laparoscope is essential because ovarian enlargement and nodularity of the cul-de-sac may be produced by metastatic ovarian carcinoma, bowel cancer, or calcified mesotheliomas.

C. Classification of endometriosis. Because both treatment and prognosis of endometriosis are determined to some extent by the severity of the disease, it is desirable to have a uniform system of classification that takes into account both the extent and severity of the disease. Unfortunately, the diversity of the different classification systems precludes accurate comparisons and leaves the question regarding the most efficacious treatment of varying degrees of endometriosis unanswered.

IV. MANAGEMENT. It is important to consider the age of the patient, the extent of the disease, the reproductive plans of the couple, the duration of the infertility, and the severity of the symptoms.

A. Expectant therapy. No therapy has proven to be a logical approach to patients with minimal disease. This is especially appropriate in the young woman with short-term infertility. In a comparison of patients with mild endometriosis, the pregnancy rate in 1 year was 72% in patients managed expectantly and 76% in patients treated with conservative surgery.

B. Medical therapy. Ectopic endometrium responds to cyclic hormone secretion in a fashion similar to normal endometrium; thus, hormonal suppression of a woman's menses constitutes the basis of medical therapy.

1. **Oral contraceptives**. The use of a continuous combination estrogen/progestin pill creates a pseudopregnancy with amenorrhea. The pseudopregnancy causes a decidualization, necrobiosis, and resorption of the ectopic endometrium. This form of treatment is only appropriate in mild endometriosis where there is not a lot of distortion of the pelvic anatomy by adhesions or endometriomas. An oral contraceptive (Enovid, Ovral) with strong progestational properties should be taken continuously for 9 months in the following manner:

a. Dosage. Initially, the patient takes one tablet per day. The dosage is then increased by one to two tablets per day as is necessary to control breakthrough bleeding. The usual dose over the period of 9 months is two to three tablets per day.

b. Pregnancy rate following pseudopregnancy has generally been between 25% and 50%.

c. Recurrence rate. The fact that pseudopregnancy does not cure endometriosis is noted in the recurrence rate of the disease—about 17%–18% in 1 year and higher with extended periods of post-treatment observation.

2. Danazol. The continuous use of this testosterone derivative induces a pseudomenopause. The pseudomenopause transiently reduces ovarian steroid secretion. Any endometrial tissue, including implants, atrophies.

a. Dosage. The effective dose ranges between 400 mg/day and 800 mg/day (200 mg tablets) for 6 months.

(1) **Lower doses** offer mainly symptomatic relief.

(2) **Higher doses** produce a pregnancy rate of 40%–60% after 6 months of pseudomenopause.

b. Side effects are related both to the hypoestrogenic environment it creates and to its androgenic properties.

(1) **Hypoestrogenic properties:** water retention, decreased breast size, atrophic vaginitis, dyspareunia, hot flashes, muscle cramps, and emotional lability

(2) **Androgenic properties:** weight gain, acne, oily skin, deepening of the voice, and growth of facial hair

c. Prognosis with danazol is related to the extent of the endometriosis and the dose of the drug; with the 800 mg/day regimen for 4–9 months, the pregnancy rate is 50%–80%.

d. Recurrence rates are highest (23%) during the first year after stopping the danazol.

e. Cost is a factor that must be considered. Therapy at the 800 mg/day level costs approximately $150/month.

3. Progestogens. Long-acting, intramuscular progestogens (medroxyprogesterone acetate 100–200 mg/month) suppress hypothalamic–pituitary function, leading to amenorrhea and decidual rather than atrophic endometrial changes.

a. Breakthrough bleeding is a nuisance side effect, but weight gain and depression are potential problems for the patient.

b. Prolonged amenorrhea following treatment makes this regimen undesirable in women who desire immediate fertility.

4. Gonadotropin-releasing hormone agonists. With continuous administration, these agents first stimulate gonadotropin release, then suppress pituitary–ovarian function, leading to a "medical hypophysectomy."

a. The drug is administered daily in the form of intranasal spray or subcutaneous injection.

b. Amenorrhea and atrophic endometrial changes occur.

c. Menopausal-type symptoms (i.e., hot flashes, decreased libido, and vaginal dryness) occur due to a hypoestrogenic state.

C. Surgical therapy. If anatomical factors such as tubo-ovarian adhesions or large endometriomas indicative of moderate to severe disease are noted, the treatment is surgical. Medical therapy and hormonal suppression will not dissolve the adhesions or eliminate the endometriomas. The debate over the appropriateness of conservative surgery versus medical therapy in minimal endometriosis is unresolved.

1. Conservative surgery involves the excision, fulguration, or lasar vaporization of endometriotic tissue, the excision of ovarian endometriomas, and the resection of severely involved pelvic viscera, leaving the uterus and at least one tube and ovary in tact. Additional infertility surgery measures for endometriosis include the gentle handling of tissue, lysis of adhesions, precise dissection, and meticulous hemostasis.

a. Reconstruction of all peritoneal surfaces is essential. Covering the raw areas in the pelvis can be achieved with the use of free peritoneal or omental grafts to prevent adhesions.

b. Dextran instillation. As protection against formation of further adhesions, approximately 200 ml of 3% dextran 70 should be instilled and left in the peritoneal cavity at the conclusion of the conservative operation.

c. Suspension of the retroverted uterus also may be a useful adjunct to prevent further adhesion formation by preventing the ovaries from adhering to raw areas in the cul-de-sac.

d. Plication of the uterosacral ligaments following excision of endometrial implants will aid in keeping the uterus in an anterior position.

e. The selective use of danazol following laparoscopy and 6–8 weeks prior to surgery aids surgery by softening implants and making the dissection less difficult.

f. Postoperative use of hormones has been the subject of great controversy because the highest pregnancy rates following conservative surgery occur in the first year after surgery; thus, most physicians are reluctant to use hormones that prevent pregnancy, even for a few months. However, an improved pregnancy rate in patients with severe endometriosis who were treated with danazol for 3–4 months following surgery has been reported. The pregnancy rate for the surgery alone group was 30%, while the pregnancy rate for the surgery/danazol group was 79%.

g. Pregnancy rates. With conservative surgery alone, there has been a conception rate of 62% in patients with mild disease, 55% in patients with moderate disease, and 50% in patients with severe disease.

2. Radical surgery, which involves a total abdominal hysterectomy and bilateral salpingo-oophorectomy, is used in patients who have completed their childbearing or in whom the severity of the endometriosis precludes any attempt at reconstruction. A less than complete pelvic cleanout in these cases guarantees reoperation at a later date. Radical surgery for endometriosis of women in their reproductive years means castration at an early age. In these women, replacement estrogen is essential to prevent problems with loss of calcium from bones, atrophic changes in the pelvis, especially the vagina, and premature aging of the cardiovascular system. However, estrogen replacement can be used with only a small risk of inciting growth of residual endometriosis.

V. MAINTENANCE OF FERTILITY AND SYMPTOMATIC RELIEF. Finding endometriosis by laparoscope in a young woman who has pelvic pain and no immediate interest in pregnancy is a common problem. The goal for this type of patient is the relief of the dysmenorrhea and the prevention of further growth of the endometriosis.

A. Birth control pills. Cyclic birth control pills are appropriate treatment for mild disease because they reduce the amount of endometrial buildup and shedding, thereby preventing further growth of the endometriosis.

B. Nonsteroidal anti-inflammatory drugs (NSAIDs). In women with endometriosis, increased concentrations of prostaglandins in the peritoneal fluid have been noted. The prostaglandin synthetase inhibitors (i.e., NSAIDs) are effective in controlling the endometriosis-related dysmenorrhea.

C. Danazol. Advanced disease should be treated with 6 months of danazol followed by cyclic birth control pills to decrease the risk of future further endometrial seeding and to preserve future fertility.

STUDY QUESTIONS

Directions: Each question below contains five suggested answers. Choose the **one best** response to each question.

1. All of the following conditions have been theorized as factors in the pathogenesis of endometriosis EXCEPT

(A) coelomic metaplasia
(B) endometrial hyperplasia
(C) retrograde menstruation
(D) immunologic deficiency
(E) lymphatic spread of endometrial fragments

2. Medical therapy for endometriosis with oral contraceptives is characterized by all of the following results EXCEPT

(A) disappearance of endometriomas
(B) amenorrhea
(C) pregnancy rate of about 35%
(D) necrobiosis of endometrial implants
(E) continuous use of oral contraceptives

3. Danazol treatment for endometriosis is associated with all of the following signs and symptoms EXCEPT

(A) acne
(B) weight gain
(C) hot flashes
(D) mucoid vaginal discharge
(E) decreased breast size

Directions: Each question below contains four suggested answers of which **one or more** is correct. Choose the answer

A if **1, 2, and 3** are correct
B if **1 and 3** are correct
C if **2 and 4** are correct
D if **4** is correct
E if **1, 2, 3, and 4** are correct

4. Infertility in endometriosis is related to

(1) the extent of the disease
(2) local prostaglandin secretion
(3) the associated hydrosalpinges
(4) altered steroidogenesis

5. Dyspareunia in endometriosis can be caused by

(1) endometriomas
(2) fixed retroversion of the uterus
(3) uterosacral implants
(4) danazol therapy

6. Which of the following findings suggest the diagnosis of endometriosis?

(1) Nodularity of the uterosacral ligaments
(2) Ovarian enlargement
(3) Fixed retroversion of the uterus
(4) Laparoscopic visualization of implants

7. A hypoestrogenic state is associated with which of the following therapies for endometriosis?

(1) Oral contraceptives
(2) Danazol
(3) Progestogens
(4) Gonadotropin-releasing hormone agonists

Directions: The group of questions below consists of lettered choices followed by several numbered items. For each numbered item select the **one** lettered choice with which it is **most** closely associated. Each lettered choice may be used once, more than once, or not at all.

Questions 8–10

For each clinical presentation listed below, select the most appropriate therapeutic modality.

(A) Expectant management
(B) Danazol therapy
(C) Conservative endometriosis surgery
(D) Cyclic oral contraceptives
(E) Radical endometriosis surgery

8. A 26-year-old medical student presents with an established diagnosis of mild endometriosis. She states that she wants to finish a residency program before even thinking of a pregnancy.

9. A 24-year-old woman presents with a 6-month history of infertility. A laparoscopic diagnosis of mild endometriosis with scattered cul-de-sac implants is made. There are no other infertility factors involved with this woman.

10. A 32-year-old lawyer presents with a 5-year history of infertility. A laparoscopic diagnosis of moderate endometriosis is made. Scattered endometrial implants in the pelvis, a 2 cm endometrioma on the left ovary, and adhesions between the tube and ovary on each side are found.

ANSWERS AND EXPLANATIONS

1. The answer is B. (*II A–C*) The classic theory of endometriosis involves the retrograde flow of menstrual debris out through the tubes, resulting in implantation in the pelvis. The fragments are thought to serve as irritative foci, which then stimulate coelomic metaplasia into endometrial-type tissue. Lymphatic spread may explain endometriosis at sites distant from the pelvis. Because endometriosis is found in siblings, a genetic influence could manifest through a deficient immunologic system. Endometrial hyperplasia occurs in anovulatory patients who have unopposed estrogen stimulation of the endometrium and has nothing to do with endometriosis.

2. The answer is A. (*IV B 1 a, b*) Medical therapy for endometriosis with oral contraceptives induces a pseudopregnancy; that is, the continuous use of the estrogen/progestin medication results in amenorrhea for about 9 months. The medication causes a decidualization, necrobiosis, and resorption of the endometrial implants, but it does not eliminate structural abnormalities, such as endometriomas. The pregnancy rate following a pseudopregnancy ranges between 25% and 50%.

3. The answer is D. [*IV B 2 b (1), (2)*] Danazol therapy induces a hypoestrogenic and androgenic state in the treated woman, which manifests as a pseudomenopause. The hypoestrogenic state is responsible for the hot flashes and the decreased breast size. The androgenic state is responsible for the weight gain and the increased sebaceous activity in the skin, resulting in acne. One would not expect a mucoid vaginal discharge in a hypoestrogenic state as it is estrogen that stimulates the secretion of cervical mucus.

4. The answer is C (2, 4). (*I A, B; III A 4*) It has never been possible to correlate the amount of pelvic endometriosis with fertility. At times, only scattered implants are associated with infertility, while more anatomic alterations do not produce infertility. The disease is not usually associated with a blocked tube or hydrosalpinx. The secretion of prostaglandin from the local implants is hypothesized as causing infertility by altering tubal function, by affecting steroidogenesis, or by affecting ovulation.

5. The answer is E (all). [*III A 3, B 2 a–c; IV B 2 b (1)*] Dyspareunia, or painful intercourse, in endometriosis can be caused by those conditions that alter the pelvic anatomy and induce pain with contact to that area. Uterosacral implants or nodules are painful when touched, as is a uterus that is no longer mobile because of fixation to the posterior cul-de-sac. Enlarged ovaries (endometriomas) may be painful when touched during coitus. Danazol induces a hypoestrogenic state that results in an atrophic vagina and dyspareunia.

6. The answer is D (4). (*III B 1–3*) The only way to diagnose endometriosis is by visualization at surgery or laparoscopy or by biopsy of an implant. History and physical examination are suggestive but not diagnostic. The physical findings of cul-de-sac nodularity, fixed retroversion of the uterus, and ovarian enlargement are compatible with endometriosis but could also be found in pelvic or bowel cancer and chronic infection.

7. The answer is C (2, 4). (*IV B 1–4*) Although all four of the therapies for endometriosis [i.e., oral contraceptives, danazol, progestogens, and gonadotropin-releasing hormone agonists (GnRH)] listed in the question suppress hypothalamic–pituitary function so that ovulation does not occur, amenorrhea results, and endometrial implants regress, only danazol and the GnRH agonists induce a hypoestrogenic state. In both cases, the ovaries do not produce estrogen, and none is supplied by the medication. With the birth control pills, there is no estrogen from the ovaries, but estrogen is supplied as one of the two ingredients of the pill. The progestogens suppress ovarian function to variable degrees, thus allowing some estrogen production by the ovaries, which explains the decidual rather than the atrophic nature of the endometrium.

8–10. The answers are: 8-D, 9-A, 10-C. (*IV A, B 1, C 1*) The 26-year-old woman with mild endometriosis who is not infertile does not need any therapy for her endometriosis at the present time. However, because she wants to maintain her fertility, her disease should not be allowed to progress. Cyclic use of oral contraceptives helps prevent progression of the endometriosis by reducing the amount of endometrial shedding (when compared with the endometrial proliferation and shedding of a natural cycle) and further growth of the endometriosis.

The 24-year-old woman with a 6-month history of infertility has mild endometriosis without any anatomic alterations of her pelvis. There is no need for immediate medical or surgical therapy. An expectant approach in a young woman with mild endometriosis should yield a pregnancy rate of 60%–70% within a year.

The woman in her thirties with a 5-year history of infertility has anatomic changes in her pelvis because of the endometriosis. Because of this woman's age and the significant length of her infertility, medical therapy would be inappropriate because it takes 6–9 months and has questionable results in women with anatomic changes, such as endometriomas and pelvic adhesions. Thus, the indicated therapy is conservative surgery to resect the endometrioma, lyse the adhesions, and remove the implants.

26
Vulvovaginitis
John M. Riva

I. INTRODUCTION. Vulvovaginitis is one of the most common gynecologic problems seen by the practicing gynecologist. The spectrum of disorders that create vulvovaginal symptoms is considerable and will be enumerated below.

II. VULVOVAGINAL ANATOMY AND PHYSIOLOGY

A. Vulva. The vulva is made up of the mons pubis, labia majora and minora, clitoris, and the vestibule. The vulva is predominantly covered by a keratinized squamous epithelium with associated hair follicles, sebaceous glands, and sweat glands. The labia minora, although covered with keratinized epithelium, does not have either hair follicles or sebaceous glands. The vestibule is a nonkeratinized mucous membrane. Both the Skene's glands and Bartholin's glands drain into the vestibule and provide lubrication to the vestibule.

  1. Nerve supply. Symptoms of vulvovaginal disorders are frequently due to the irritation of the sensory nerves of the vulva. These nerves include the perineal, genitofemoral, and ilioinguinal nerves.

  2. Lymphatic supply. Many infections or inflammatory conditions of the vulva and distal vaginal wall are accompanied by an increase in lymphatic drainage and tender lymphadenopathy. The vulva is drained by the superficial inguinal lymphatics.

B. Vagina. This structure is a hollow cyclinder approximately 7–8 cm in length. It is covered by a stratified, nonkeratinized mucous membrane that is under the hormonal influence of the ovarian steroids. The nerve supply of the vagina is from the pudendal nerve and is not as rich in the distribution of fine sensory nerves as is the vulva. The vagina is usually resistant to vaginal infection because of the following factors:

  1. Marked vaginal acidity (pH 4.0–5.0), resulting from the production of lactic acid by Döderlein's bacilli

  2. Thick protective epithelium, which is secondary to the normal levels of estrogen circulating in the adult

III. DIAGNOSIS. The medical history is an important and essential step in evaluating the potential causes of vulvovaginal symptoms. It is important to characterize the patient's symptomatology and associated contributing features.

A. Symptomatology

  1. Vulvar symptoms. The three most common symptoms are:
  a. Burning
  b. Itching
  c. Odor

  2. Vaginal discharge. Discharge should be characterized with respect to:
  a. Consistency
  b. Viscosity
  c. Color

B. Contributing features. There are certain factors that can predispose to vulvovaginal infection or irritation, including:

  1. Sexual habits, particularly possible complaints from sexual partners regarding irritation

2. Recent systemic or local infection

3. Use of antibiotics

4. History of diabetes

5. Nutritional habits

6. Previous vulvovaginal infections

7. Vaginal hygienic practices

8. Contraceptive methods

9. Menstrual history

IV. PHYSICAL EXAMINATION. A general physical examination should be performed as part of the workup of any new patient or any patient who has not been seen within a year.

A. Pelvic examination, which is essential in the management of vulvovaginitis, should consist of a thorough evaluation of the following:

1. The external genitalia to detect gross lesions, edema (and discoloration) of the labia, ulceration, condylomata, and to rule out pubic lice

2. The inguinal area, which should be palpated for the presence or absence of lymphadenopathy and any discoloration noted

B. Speculum examination, using water as the only lubricant to avoid interfering with specimen collection and culturing, should reveal:

1. The nature of the vaginal discharge, in particular the consistency, viscosity, color, and odor. When an infectious vaginitis is suspected, a vaginal pH helps to differentiate the various infections. Microscopic inspection of the vaginal secretions in saline and a 10% potassium hydroxide solution is helpful in making a diagnosis. Occasionally, Gram stains and cultures are useful in difficult cases.

2. Evidence of trauma, congenital abnormalities, or characteristic lesions (i.e., "strawberry spots" if *Trichomonas vaginalis* is suspected) of the vaginal walls

3. The presence or absence of cervical abnormalities. A culture of the endocervix will detect gonorrhea, and a Pap smear (Papanicolaou's test) will detect carcinoma or infection.

V. VULVOVAGINAL CONDITIONS. In self-referred, female clinic patients with sexually transmitted disease, vaginitis is the most common diagnosis. Vaginitis is characterized by one or more of the following symptoms: **increased volume of discharge; abnormal yellow or green color of discharge; vulvar itching, irritation, or burning; dyspareunia; and malodor.** Vaginitis may be caused by infectious agents, such as *Candida*, *Gardnerella*, and *Trichomonas*, by atrophic changes, vulvar dystrophies, and trauma. Acute herpes simplex genitalis can cause acute vulvar symptoms necessitating prompt evaluation and treatment.

A. *Candida* **vaginitis (candidiasis or moniliasis)**

1. Etiology. The etiologic agent for this infection is the yeast (fungi) organism, *Candida albicans* or *Monilia*. Since the organism is a common inhabitant of the bowel and perianal region, normal activity and increased moisture in this area often provide a ready pathway to the vagina. The marked increase in the frequency of this disease has been related to:
  a. Changes in contraceptive practices
  b. Increased use of systemic steroids
  c. Widespread and often indiscriminate use of antibiotics
  d. Changes in styles of women's clothing, such as use of synthetic materials
  e. Undiagnosed or uncontrolled diabetes

2. Clinical presentation. Characteristically, monilial vaginitis presents as a thick, white discharge with extreme vulvar pruritus. Symptoms may recur and be most prominent just before menses and frequently during pregnancy. The vulva and vagina have a beefy red appearance often with patches of curd-like, cheesy material that adheres to the vaginal walls.

3. Diagnosis. Vaginal pH is frequently slightly more basic (4.5–4.8) than the normal vaginal pH. Hyphae or pseudohyphae on saline or, more particularly, 10% potassium hydroxide wet mount preparations of the discharge are diagnostic. Gram stain or culture on Nickerson's medium are helpful in diagnosing difficult cases.

4. Treatment. Therapy of monilial vaginitis involves the use of polyene antifungal agents or one of the imidazoles (clotrimazole or miconazole). Treatment in the form of suppositories or cream preparations for 3–7 days is often sufficient to cure over 90% of these infections.

a. A repeat 7-day course often eradicates persistent infections.

b. For chronic or refractory infections, consideration should be given to oral therapy with ketoconizole (200 mg daily). This approach reduces the intestinal source of reinfection. Evaluation and treatment of the male consort have reduced recurrent infections in women with refractory infections.

B. *Trichomonas vaginalis* vaginitis (trichomoniasis)

1. Etiology. The etiologic agent is the motile protozoan, *Trichomonas,* which not only infects the vagina but also involves the urethra and periurethral glands. In addition, almost 70%–80% of the male partners of the infected patient harbor the organism; thus, trichomoniasis should be considered a venereal disease.

2. Clinical presentation. The discharge is often greenish grey and frothy and may be associated with "strawberry spots" on the cervix and vagina. The discharge is often malodorous, profuse, and associated with intense pruritus.

3. Diagnosis. The vaginal pH is often between 5 and 6. Using a saline wet mount of the vaginal discharge, confirmation is made by identifying the highly motile trichomonads under low-power magnification. When examined under high-power magnification, the pear-shaped organisms (twice the size of leukocytes) often are intermixed with numerous clumps of white cells that appear to "jiggle."

4. Treatment. Due to multiple sites of infection and the fact that trichomoniasis is sexually transmitted, vaginal therapy alone is often ineffective; systemic agents are necessary, and both partners may need therapy. The only consistently effective drug has been metronidazole (Flagyl), 250 mg three times a day for 7 days, although an equally effective cure rate and good compliance rates have been demonstrated with the immediate administration of a 2 g dosage regimen. In resistant cases, intravenous metronidazole has proven effective. The potential side effects of metronidazole, including a disulfiram (Antabuse)-like reaction, a reversible neutropenia, and potential teratogenicity, should be considered.

C. *Gardnerella vaginalis* vaginitis

1. Etiology. The vaginal discharge that is not associated with *T. vaginalis, C. albicans,* or uterine infections, is usually attributed to nonspecific vaginitis caused by *G. vaginalis.*

2. Clinical presentation. The discharge is watery and malodorus. It also is homogeneous, low in viscosity, contains fewer leukocytes, and is uniformly adherent to the vaginal walls. Irritation of the vulva and vagina is uncommon.

3. Diagnosis. The vaginal pH in this infection is consistently between 5.0–5.5. Wet mount preparations with saline reveal a "clean" background with minimal or no leukocytes. The "clue" cell is a squamous cell whose sharp borders and cytoplasm are obscured by coccobacillary bacteria. The "clue" cell is diagnostic of *G. vaginalis.* Application of a 10% potassium hydroxide to the wet mount specimen produces a fishy odor and is called a positive "whiff" test.

4. Treatment. Although generally frustrating, the treatment can be effected by using vaginal creams containing sulfonamide or the administration of oral ampicillin (500 mg four times a day for 7 days). The most effective therapy consists of oral metronidazole (500 mg twice daily for 7 days). Sexual partners should be treated to prevent reinfection.

D. Atrophic vaginitis

1. Etiology. Atrophic vaginitis is most often seen in postmenopausal women but may also be found in surgically castrated young women and in women who are breast-feeding (lactating). Atrophic changes in the vulvovaginal tissues result from estrogen withdrawal as the normal protective thickness of the vaginal epithelium is dependent on the estrogen stimulation.

2. Clinical presentation. Without consistent and sufficient estrogen, the vaginal epithelium becomes thin, and the vulvar structures may atrophy. The amount of glycogen is also decreased, and the pH changes to an alkaline state. The vagina is often reddened with punctated hemorrhagic spots throughout the vaginal wall.

3. Diagnosis. One must suspect atrophic vaginitis in any of the above-mentioned women who complain of leukorrhea, pruritus, burning, tenderness, and dyspareunia.

4. Treatment. Topical administration of vaginal cream containing estrogen causes a reversal of symptoms within 1 week of treatment. Vulvovaginal tissues begin to thicken, and the pruritus disappears. A maintenance dose one to three times a week is sufficient to maintain a healthy vaginal epithelium.

E. Vulvar dystrophies

1. Etiology. Vulvar dystrophies are dermatologic conditions of the vulvar skin of uncertain etiology. Most frequently seen in postmenopausal women, there is often a history of chronic candidal vulvovaginitis. The dystrophies can be:
   a. Hyperplastic where the epithelium is markedly thickened
   b. Atrophic (lichen sclerosus et atrophicus)
   c. A mixture of both

2. Clinical presentation
   a. With hyperplastic dystrophy, the most common symptom is constant pruritus. Scratching frequently exacerbates the pruritus.
   b. With lichen sclerosus, pruritus or, more commonly, chronic soreness associated with "vulvar dysuria" frequently occur.

3. Diagnosis. Both vulvar dystrophies are diagnosed by histologic inspection of vulvar biopsies.
   a. Hyperplastic dystrophy presents as very thickened skin ("elephant hide") accompanied by linear excoriations from scratching.
   b. Lichen sclerosus presents as extremely pale, thin skin often with subepithelial hemorrhages. In its severest form, painful contraction of the introitus or clitoral hood are noted.

4. Treatment
   a. Hyperplastic dystrophy responds well to a 6–8 week trial of topical fluorinated steroid cream.
   b. Lichen sclerosus responds to topical testosterone preparations on a chronic basis.

F. Traumatic vaginitis

1. Etiology. Traumatic vaginitis is usually the result of injury or chemical irritation. In adult women, the most common cause of injury to the vagina is a "lost" tampon. In pediatric patients, foreign bodies placed in the vagina serve as sources of infection or trauma (i.e., wads of paper, chewing gum, paper clips, etc.). Chemical irritation can be secondary to douches, deodorants, lubricants, or sexual aids.

2. Treatment. Vulvovaginitis resulting from foreign bodies or chemical irritants respond immediately to withdrawal of the causative agent. For example, the trauma to the vaginal mucosa and secondary infection that result from a tampon left in place for days or weeks is easily reversed by thoroughly cleansing the vaginal mucosa and instilling sulfonamide creams intravaginally for 7–10 days.

G. Neoplasia

1. Etiology. Malignancies can masquerade for months as vulvar lesions, which are often ignored by patients or mistreated by physicians as irritations or infections.

2. Diagnosis. Patients who present with a long-term history of symptoms and treatment failures of vulvar lesions should have a biopsy before further therapeutic trials are instituted. An accurate and definitive diagnosis can be made using a localizing stain of toluidine blue dye, a small amount of local anesthesia, a biopsy punch, and scissors.

3. Treatment is as indicated by the pathology report.

H. Herpes simplex genitalis

1. Etiology. Herpes genitalis, an acute inflammatory disease of the genitalia, is the most widespread venereal disease seen today. Most cases are caused by the herpesvirus (*Herpesvirus hominis*) type 2 (HSV-2); herpesvirus type 1 (HSV-1) is the etiologic agent in only 13% of cases. The majority of patients with primary disease are teenage girls and unmarried women.

2. Clinical presentation
   a. The infection is usually acquired from a sexual contact with symptoms appearing within 3–7 days.
   b. The symptoms consist of hyperesthesia, burning, itching, dysuria, and frequently exquisite pain and tenderness of the vulva; lymphadenopathy is almost always present.
   c. Vulvar dyspareunia makes intercourse unbearable.

    d. Primary lesions persist for 3–6 weeks and usually heal without scarring. The primary lesions:

      (1) May involve the vestibule, labia minora, perianal skin, vagina, and cervix

      (2) Appear as widespread vesicles, which rapidly rupture, leading to ulcer formation

      (3) Often coalesce, forming bullae and large ulcerations

      (4) May be associated with severe inflammatory reactions and varying degrees of edema

    e. Recurrent infections represent flare-ups of a latent infection not a reinfection.

      (1) The dormant herpesvirus resides in the neurons of the sensory ganglia, which supply the areas of cutaneous involvement.

      (2) Healing of recurrent lesions takes 7–10 days.

3. Diagnosis

    a. HSV-2 should be suspected in the presence of superficial ulcerations of the vulvovaginal tissues.

    b. Cytologic studies offer confirmatory evidence of a herpes simplex infection if there is enlargement of the nuclei and displacement of the chromatin against the nuclear membrane.

    c. The virus may be recovered by rubbing the base of the ulcer with a cotton swab and culturing it in Eagle's medium containing 5% fetal calf serum.

4. Treatment

    a. Acyclovir (Zovirax) is an antiviral drug that is effective against herpesvirus.

      (1) It is an acyclic purine nucleoside analogue with in vivo and in vitro activity against herpes simplex.

      (2) It is indicated for the *initial* clinical episode of HSV-2.

      (3) It can be applied topically or taken orally.

    b. Sitz baths, wet dressings, analgesics, and boric acid solutions may offer some symptomatic relief.

5. Dangers of HSV-2

    a. Pregnancy. The herpesvirus may be transmitted to the fetus after rupture of the membranes; fetal herpes can be fatal.

      (1) A patient with active herpes whose membranes have been ruptured for less than 4 hours should be delivered immediately by cesarean section.

      (2) If positive results are obtained by culture within 2 weeks of the onset of labor, even in the absence of a lesion, abdominal delivery is indicated with the onset of labor.

      (3) Abdominal delivery is also indicated in patients with obvious herpetic lesions who are in labor, regardless of previous negative culture results.

    b. Cervical cancer. There appears to be a relationship between infection with HSV-2 and cervical carcinoma (see Chapter 37).

STUDY QUESTIONS

Directions: Each question below contains five suggested answers. Choose the **one best** response to each question.

1. If a woman presents with a chronic yeast infection, it is important to elicit a history of all of the following EXCEPT

(A) diabetes
(B) pregnancy
(C) use of antibiotics
(D) use of oral contraceptives
(E) use of vinegar douches

2. Atrophic vaginitis would be expected in all the following clinical situations EXCEPT

(A) menopause
(B) lactation
(C) oral contraceptive use
(D) surgical castration in a young woman
(E) pseudomenopause during endometriosis therapy

Directions: Each question below contains four suggested answers of which **one or more** is correct. Choose the answer

A   if **1, 2, and 3** are correct
B   if **1 and 3** are correct
C   if **2 and 4** are correct
D   if **4** is correct
E   if **1, 2, 3, and 4** are correct

3. Normal vaginal health depends on which of the following factors?

(1) A pH of 4.5
(2) Döderlein's bacilli
(3) Estrogen
(4) *Escherichia coli*

4. *Candida* vaginitis can be diagnosed by

(1) microscopic examination of vaginal secretions in 10% potassium hydroxide
(2) finding characteristic "strawberry spots" on the cervix and vagina
(3) culture on Nickerson's medium
(4) microscopic examination of vaginal secretions, using a saline wet mount

5. Infection with which of the following organisms results in vaginitis for which both partners must be treated?

(1) *Trichomonas*
(2) *Candida*
(3) *Gardnerella*
(4) *Herpesvirus*

6. Hyperplastic vulvar dystrophy is associated with which of the following?

(1) Treatment is topical testosterone ointment
(2) Marked atrophy of the vulvar structure results
(3) The etiologic agent is herpes simplex virus type 2
(4) It responds well to a short course of fluorinated steroid cream

Directions: The group of questions below consists of lettered choices followed by several numbered items. For each numbered item select the **one** lettered choice with which it is **most** closely associated. Each lettered choice may be used once, more than once, or not at all.

Questions 7–9

For each of the descriptions of vaginitis that follow, select the therapy that would be most appropriate.

(A) Metronidazole
(B) Estrogen cream
(C) Polyene antifungal agent
(D) Vinegar douch
(E) Sulfonamide vaginal cream

7.   A woman states that she has been on ampicillin for a week because of a urinary tract infection. Upon completing the antibiotics, she noted a thick, white vaginal discharge with severe vulvar itching.

8.   A patient states that she has a malodorous discharge and intense itching. She adds that her partner also has a slight discharge. Pelvic examination reveals "strawberry spots" on the cervix.

9.   A patient complains of a watery, malodorous discharge with very little itching or burning. A wet mount preparation in saline of the vaginal secretions reveals "clue cells."

ANSWERS AND EXPLANATIONS

1. The answer is E. (*V A 1 a–e*) Various changes in the vaginal environment contribute to conditions that encourage chronic yeast infections in some women. Antibiotics change the normal vaginal flora. Pregnancy and oral contraceptives alter the vaginal epithelium by hormone-induced changes that reflect a progesterone rather than an estrogen dominance. Douching with a vinegar solution is often used as a prophylaxis against vaginitis because of the acidic nature of the douche; it would not be a predisposing factor to a yeast infection.

2. The answer is C. (*V D 1*) Healthy vaginal epithelium that is resistant to infection is dependent on estrogen stimulation. When there is an estrogen deficiency, atrophic changes in the vulvovaginal epithelium occur with thinning and decreased resistance to infection. All of the answers listed in the question—menopause, lactation, surgical castration, and endometriosis therapy—are associated with markedly reduced or absent circulating estrogen levels except oral contraceptive use. Even though progesterone in the oral contraceptives dominate, there is enough estrogen present to prevent atrophic vaginitis.

3. The answer is A (1, 2, 3). (*II B 1–2*) The vagina is normally resistant to most infections because of certain environmental factors. Normal levels of estrogen generate thick protective epithelium; an atrophic epithelium is present in the absence of estrogen. An acidic pH is also necessary. The acidity (i.e., pH between 4.0 and 5.0) results from the production of lactic acid by the Döderlein's bacilli, which protect the vagina from infection. *Escherichia coli* is a natural inhabitant but does not contribute to vaginal health.

4. The answer is B (1, 3). (*V A 3, B 2–3*) *Candida albicans* can be readily cultured on Nickerson's medium. Microscopic examination of the vaginal secretions in 10% potassium hydroxide permits the visualization of the yeast pseudohyphae because the normal vaginal cells are lysed and pseudohyphae remain. *Trichomonas vaginalis* is easily seen using a saline wet mount. "Strawberry spots" are characteristic of *Trichomonas* not *Candida*.

5. The answer is A (1, 2, 3). (*V A 4, B 4, C 4, H 4*) In both *Trichomonas* and *Gardnerella* vaginitis, the sexual partners of the patient should be treated to prevent reinfection. Treatment of partners with *Candida* vaginitis has reduced recurrent infections in women with refractory infections. Infection with herpesvirus does not result in vaginitis, and to date, treatment is symptomatic only.

6. The answer is D (4). (*V E 1–3*) Hyperplastic dystrophy of the vulva is of uncertain etiology but has been associated with chronic candidal vulvovaginitis, not herpes simplex virus type 2. This disorder is probably due to chronic vulvar irritation, which produces a thickened epithelium resembling elephant skin. It is not associated with atrophy of the vulvar structures as is seen with lichen sclerosus. The most common symptom of hyperplastic vulvar dystrophy is incessant pruritus, which responds nicely to a short course of topical fluorinated steroid cream. Testosterone ointment is used in chronic treatment of lichen sclerosus.

7–9. The answers are: 7-C, 8-A, 9-A. (*V A 1–4, B 1–4, C 1–4*) Antibiotic use is one of the predisposing causes of a yeast infection. A thick, cheesy, white vaginal discharge is characteristic of a yeast infection. Therefore, the treatment of the woman who had been taking ampicillin would involve one of the antifungal medications.

The patient who presents with a malodorous discharge and intense itching has the signs and symptoms of *Trichomonas* vaginitis. *Trichomonas* is associated with a greenish grey, frothy, often malodorous discharge. Approximately 70%–80% of the male partners of infected patients harbor the organism. Characteristic "strawberry spots" can be seen on the cervix and vagina. The organism can be seen microscopically when saline is used to prepare a wet mount of the vaginal secretions. Metronidazole (Flagyl) should be used to treat both the patient and her partner.

When "clue cells" are found on microscopic examination of a vaginal discharge, the diagnosis is *Gardnerella* vaginitis. The most effective therapy for this vaginitis is oral metronidazole with treatment of the sexual partner to prevent reinfection.

27
Dysfunctional Uterine Bleeding
William W. Beck, Jr.

I. DEFINITIONS

A. Dysfunctional uterine bleeding (DUB) is excessive uterine bleeding with no demonstrable organic cause.

　1. It is most frequently due to abnormalities of endocrine origin.

　2. It is most often associated with anovulation but occasionally with poor quality ovulatory cycles.

B. Intermenstrual bleeding is bleeding of variable amounts that occurs between regular menstrual periods.

C. Menometrorrhagia is prolonged uterine bleeding that occurs at irregular intervals.

D. Menorrhagia (hypermenorrhea) is prolonged (more than 7 days) and excessive (greater than 80 ml) uterine bleeding that occurs at regular intervals.

E. Metrorrhagia is uterine bleeding that occurs at irregular but frequent intervals; the amount of uterine bleeding is variable, and the duration of the flow is often prolonged.

F. Polymenorrhea is uterine bleeding that occurs at regular intervals less than 21 days apart.

G. Oligomenorrhea is infrequent uterine bleeding that occurs at intervals more than 40 days apart.

II. ETIOLOGY OF DUB

A. Anovulatory cycles. DUB often occurs in the absence of cyclic hormonal changes that determine the menstrual cycle. Ninety percent of all DUB is thought to be anovulatory in nature.

B. Ovulatory cycles. Abnormal bleeding can be associated with ovulation and characterized by regular cycles of approximately the same duration.

　1. Midcycle spotting is a scanty intermenstrual discharge, which is associated with a decrease in estrogen at midcycle following ovulation.

　2. Frequent menses or polymenorrhea is associated with a short follicular phase.

　3. Luteal phase deficiency, which may be associated with premenstrual spotting, results when the luteal phase is shortened by prematurely decreased progesterone levels.

　4. Prolonged corpus luteum activity is the result of persistent progesterone production in the absence of pregnancy, resulting in prolonged cycles or protracted menstrual bleeding.

III. PHYSIOLOGY OF DUB

A. Anovulatory bleeding. Most DUB is anovulatory and is an example of estrogen withdrawal or estrogen breakthrough bleeding. The anovulatory patient must rely on endogenous estrogen to heal or rehabilitate the endometrium.

　1. The healing is only temporary.

　2. As quickly as it rebuilds, tissue fragility and breakdown recur at other endometrial sites, resulting in a continuation of the bleeding.

B. Bleeding patterns. Bleeding involves random portions of the endometrium at variable times and in an asynchronous manner.

  1. The heaviest bleeding is due to high sustained levels of estrogen and is seen with:
  a. Polycystic ovarian disease
  b. Obesity
  c. Immaturity of the hypothalamic–pituitary–ovarian axis as in postmenarchal teenagers
  d. Late anovulation as seen in the perimenopausal period when a woman is in her late forties

  2. Prolonged and excessive flow
  a. There is a large amount of tissue available for sloughing (and bleeding).
  b. There is no rhythmic vasoconstriction or coiling of the spiral arteries and no orderly vascular collapse to induce stasis, ischemia, and degradation of the endometrium.

C. Endometrial physiology. In the absence of growth-limiting progesterone and periodic desquamation, the endometrium attains an abnormal height without concomitant structural support:

  1. The endometrium displays intense vascularity and back-to-back glandular appearance without an intervening stromal support matrix.

  2. This tissue is fragile and exhibits superficial breakdown and bleeding.

  3. As one site heals, another site breaks down, resulting in continuous bleeding.

IV. MANAGEMENT OF DUB

A. Diagnosis. It is inappropriate to assume that abnormal uterine bleeding is endocrine in origin. Organic disease, such as polyps, endometrial hyperplasia, intrauterine malignancy, pregnancy, and blood dyscrasias, must be ruled out. This may be accomplished by:

  1. Endometrial sampling
  a. Endometrial biopsy
  b. Endometrial aspiration (i.e., VABRA aspiration)
  c. Dilatation and curettage

  2. Hysteroscopy or direct visualization of the endometrial cavity

  3. Blood studies, such as:
  a. Serum human chorionic gonadotropin levels to determine the presence of a pregnancy or a hydatidiform mole
  b. Platlet count and function to determine the presence of von Willebrand's disease or thrombocytopenia
  c. Complete blood count and differential to determine the presence of leukemia

B. Estrogens. The rationale for estrogen therapy is based on the fact that estrogen in pharmacologic doses causes rapid growth of the endometrium.

  1. Bleeding responds to estrogen therapy because a rapid growth of endometrial tissue occurs over the denuded and raw epithelial surfaces.

  2. The use of conjugated estrogen (10 mg/day in divided doses) controls most acute bleeding in 24 hours.
  a. Progestin therapy is also required.
  b. Conjugated estrogen is continued at the same dose and a progestin [e.g., medroxyprogesterone (Provera)] at 10 mg/day is added.
  c. Both hormones are then continued for another 7–10 days before stopping therapy.

  3. Parenteral estrogen is effective in treating acute profuse DUB.
  a. A total of 20 mg of conjugated estrogen is administered intravenously every 4–6 hours.
  b. Bleeding usually stops in 12 hours.
  c. A progestin must be started at the same time.

C. Progestins. These are ultimately the treatment of choice because most women with DUB are anovulatory and have unopposed estrogen in the system.

  1. Progestins do not stop the acute DUB as effectively as estrogen. However, they are warranted for long-term control after the acute episode of DUB is controlled.

  2. Medroxyprogesterone (10 mg/day for 10 days) produces regular withdrawal bleeding in patients with adequate amounts of endogenous estrogen.

3. Progestins acts as antiestrogens.
    a. They diminish the effect of estrogen on target cells by inhibiting estrogen receptor replenishment in the cell.
    b. This antimitotic, antigrowth effect of progestin supports its use in the treatment of unopposed estrogen and endometrial hyperplasia.

4. Progestins support and organize the endometrium so that an organized sloughing of the endometrium occurs after progestin withdrawal.

D. Combined estrogen and progestin (i.e., the oral contraceptives)

1. A convenient way to stop DUB involves the use of the combination oral contraceptives, which contain both an estrogen and a progestin.
    a. Four tablets of an oral contraceptive with 50 μg estradiol in divided doses over 24 hours provides enough estrogen to stop acute bleeding and simultaneously provide progestin.
    b. Treatment is continued for at least a week after the bleeding stops.

2. The oral contraceptives are not as effective in controlling bleeding as are high doses of conjugated estrogen.
    a. The combination of estrogen and progestin does not afford as rapid an endometrial growth pattern as estrogen alone.
    b. The progestin decreases the synthesis of estrogen receptors, thus decreasing the effectiveness of the growth-promoting action of estrogen on the fragmented, bleeding endometrium.

E. Nonsteroidal anti-inflammatory drugs (NSAIDs)

1. The NSAIDs inhibit prostaglandin synthesis.

2. Prostaglandins have important actions on the endometrial vasculature and endometrial hemostasis.
    a. Thromboxane is the platelet proaggregating vasoconstrictor.
    b. Prostacyclin is the antiaggregating vasodilator.

3. The concentration of prostaglandins increase progressively during the menstrual cycle, and prostaglandin synthetase inhibitors (the NSAIDs) decrease menstrual blood loss.
    a. The NSAIDs may work by altering the balance between thromboxane and prostacyclin.
    b. The ideal pharmacologic action would be to block the synthesis of prostacyclin alone without decreasing thromboxane formation.

4. The NSAIDs are primarily effective in reducing menstrual blood loss in women who ovulate.

STUDY QUESTIONS

Directions: Each question below contains five suggested answers. Choose the **one best** response to each question.

1. Dysfunctional uterine bleeding is frequently associated with

(A) endometrial polyps
(B) anovulation
(C) cervicitis
(D) systemic lupus erythematosus
(E) von Willebrand's disease

2. The abnormal pattern of bleeding seen with the short follicular phase is described by the term

(A) menorrhagia
(B) menometrorrhagia
(C) polymenorrhea
(D) anovulatory bleeding
(E) metrorrhagia

3. For women in their thirties and forties with abnormal uterine bleeding, the most accurate diagnostic procedure is

(A) basal body temperature
(B) endometrial biopsy
(C) dilatation and curettage
(D) hysteroscopy
(E) hormone therapy

Directions: Each question below contains four suggested answers of which **one or more** is correct. Choose the answer

  A   if **1, 2, and 3** are correct
  B   if **1 and 3** are correct
  C   if **2 and 4** are correct
  D   if **4** is correct
  E   if **1, 2, 3, and 4** are correct

4. Which of the following diagnoses might be associated with dysfunctional uterine bleeding?

(1) Thrombocytopenia
(2) Endometrial polyps
(3) Hydatidiform mole
(4) Polycystic ovarian disease

5. Postmenarchal bleeding is characterized by

(1) estrogen breakthrough bleeding
(2) midcycle spotting
(3) anovulatory bleeding
(4) progesterone withdrawal bleeding

6. Properties of the progestins include which of the following?

(1) They are used in treating endometrial hyperplasia
(2) They diminish the effect of estrogen on target cells
(3) They have antimitotic activity
(4) They enhance estrogen receptor replenishment in the cell

Directions: The group of questions below consists of lettered choices followed by several numbered items. For each numbered item select the **one** lettered choice with which it is **most** closely associated. Each lettered choice may be used once, more than once, or not at all.

Questions 7–9

For each clinical situation listed below, select the laboratory finding most likely to be associated with it.

(A) Platelet function test
(B) Elevated progesterone
(C) Hematocrit
(D) Positive human chorionic gonadotropin levels
(E) None of the above

7. Anovulation

8. Ectopic pregnancy and hydatidiform mole

9. Von Willebrand's disease

ANSWERS AND EXPLANATIONS

1. The answer is B. (*I A 1–2; IV A*) Dysfunctional uterine bleeding (DUB) is associated with anovulation in 90% of cases. DUB is a diagnosis of exclusion, which is made after organic causes of bleeding, such as endometrial polyps, cervicitis, systemic lupus erythematosus, and von Willebrand's disease, have been ruled out. If another etiology or source can be found for the bleeding, it is not DUB.

2. The answer is C. (*I A–F; II B 2, 3*) Some dysfunctional bleeding is associated with ovulatory cycles, such as polymenorrhea, which is characterized by menses that occur at regular intervals of less than 21 days. Of necessity, these cycles are associated with a short follicular phase. Menorrhagia, menometrorrhagia, and metrorrhagia are characterized by heavy, prolonged, and irregular bleeding. These are usually associated with anovulatory cycles; if ovulation occurs, it is not associated with a short follicular phase.

3. The answer is C. (*IV A 1, 2*) Women in their late reproductive years have a significant risk of a pathologic cause for abnormal uterine bleeding, such as endometrial hyperplasia or carcinoma. The most thorough method of endometrial sampling to exclude pathology is a dilatation and curettage. An endometrial biopsy may miss a lesion. Hysteroscopy can aid in the diagnosis of a gross endometrial pathology, but not a microscopic diagnosis. A hormonal assay for estrogen or progesterone cannot diagnose an endometrial pathology.

4. The answer is D (4). (*I A 1–2; III A, B 1*) Dysfunctional uterine bleeding (DUB) is usually anovulatory in nature and due to estrogen breakthrough bleeding. Polycystic ovarian disease is characteristically an anovulatory state with sustained estrogen secretion. Thrombocytopenia, polyps, and hydatidiform mole are organic causes of uterine bleeding, and, therefore, not DUB, which is a diagnosis that excludes organic causes for bleeding.

5. The answer is B (1, 3). (*II A, B 1; III A, B 1 a–d*) Uterine bleeding during the first few years after the menarche is often both irregular and anovulatory due to an immaturity of the hypothalamic–pituitary–ovarian axis. The irregular bleeding that does occur is due to sustained estrogen secretion with breakthrough bleeding. Both midcycle spotting and progesterone withdrawal bleeding are associated with ovulatory cycles and are not, therefore, compatible with the anovulatory nature of the postmenarchal bleeding.

6. The answer is A (1, 2, 3). (*IV C 1–4*) Progestins are one of the synthetic steroids (i.e., they have a progesterone-like quality) that are used in treating dysfunctional uterine bleeding (DUB). DUB is most frequently associated with anovulation and continuous or unopposed estrogen secretion. Thus, a progesterone-like compound is an excellent substance to use in treating DUB because it is basically an antiestrogen. The progestins diminish the effect of estrogen on target cells by inhibiting, not enhancing, estrogen receptor replenishment in the cell. The progestins are antimitotic and antigrowth in character as they oppose the effects of estrogen at the cellular level. Thus, they are effective agents in treating endometrial hyperplasia, which is usually the result of unopposed estrogen.

7–9. The answers are: 7-E, 8-D, 9-A. (*I A 1–2; II A; IV A 3*) None of the laboratory findings listed in the question would be useful in diagnosing anovulation, which can be diagnosed by an endometrial biopsy that reveals a proliferative endometrium. Human chorionic gonadotropin (HCG) is the hormone secreted by any conceptus from the trophoblastic tissue; thus, elevated HCG levels indicate pregnancy or a pregnancy-related complication, such as hydatidiform mole. Von Willebrand's disease is associated with a factor VIII deficiency and platelet dysfunction, but not with abnormal platelet counts. An elevated progesterone level indicates ovulation and, thus, is not present in an anovulatory cycle.

William W. Beck, Jr.

I. INTRODUCTION

A. Rape. Sexual assault is a term used to describe manual, oral, or genital contact with the genitalia of the victim without the victim's consent. Rape and incest are coital forms of sexual assault. The primary motive of rape is aggression. Three basic components of rape are:

1. The offender's genitalia must contact the genitalia of the victim.

2. The act must be accomplished against the victim's will.

3. There must be an element of force or threat of physical harm.
   a. Force is often accomplished with a weapon that may injure or kill.
   b. Resistance to force is no longer required to prove rape.

B. Statutory rape. Sexual activity with individuals who are unable to consent either because they are below the age of consent or because their consciousness has been altered by illness, sleep, drugs, or alcohol is considered statutory rape.

II. EPIDEMIOLOGY

A. Although rape is one of the least reported crimes, as victims fear being further victimized by the attitudes of society, reported rape is increasing by an annual rate of 9%. The number of rapes peaks in the summer and is more frequent in the more highly populated Southern states and in lower socioeconomic groups.

B. The offenders are typically young men between the ages of 16 and 25 years, who are of low social status, poorly educated, single, and black.

C. Rape is a crime of violence.

1. In 86% of all rapes, the assailant either carries a weapon or threatens the victim with death.

2. Victims experience violence as roughness (29%), nonbrutal beatings (25%), and brutal beatings (20%).

3. Approximately 0.5% of rapes terminate in death.

III. MEDICAL EVALUATION

A. Initial contact. It is important for the physician to help the victim overcome feelings of helplessness created by the experience of rape. The victim may object to being examined, especially by a male physician as she may perceive the examination as a continuation of the violation. If there are no threatening injuries, it is appropriate for the physician to delay the examination until a family member, a friend, a member of a woman's support organization, or a female nurse has comforted the patient. The physician must remain objective while offering reassurance and emotional support.

B. History. Both the victim's history and the physical examination are important in evaluating the actual and potential harm and in providing information for possible future legal action.

1. A precise description of all forms of sexual activity, including the areas of the body involved, is mandatory.

2. The physician must note whether or not the victim has changed clothes, urinated, bathed, showered, douched, or brushed her teeth since the alleged attack.

3. The time of the most recent sexual intercourse before the assault must be noted.

4. The date of the victim's last menstrual period and her birth control status are important.

C. Physical examination. Sketches or photographs made during the physical examination are ideal for documentation and notation of the precise location of any cuts or bruises sustained by the victim.

1. Signs of resistance—choke marks on the neck, bites, or scratches—should be described. Since the signs of blunt trauma—ecchymoses and hematomas—often do not appear for some time after injury, the victim should be asked to return later for documentation when such marks appear.

2. Evidence of semen. Semen, which is high in histone, will fluoresce when exposed to Wood's light in a darkened room. This is an effective means of localizing moist or dried semen during the physical examination or examination of the clothing.

3. A complete neurologic examination, including a mental status evaluation, is mandatory.

4. Pelvic examination. This is the most critical part of the entire physical examination because of the legal implications of the findings and their documentation.
   a. The perineum is examined for bruising and laceration.
   b. The presence or absence of blood and moist or dried secretions on the mons pubis, vulva, perineum, rectum, buttocks, or thighs are noted.
   c. The status of the hymen is observed and recorded, remembering that:
      (1) Penetration by a penis through an elastic hymen may occur without lacerations.
      (2) The hymen may be ruptured by trauma other than sexual intercourse, including masturbation or introduction of foreign bodies into the vagina.
   d. Speculum examination
      (1) The vaginal mucosa is carefully inspected for abrasions, lacerations, or ecchymoses.
      (2) Swabs of the cervix and vagina should be taken for a gonococcal culture.
      (3) A wet mount is obtained from the vaginal pool to determine the presence or absence of spermatozoa and sperm motility.
      (4) Swabs of the vaginal pool are obtained, smeared on two glass slides, and allowed to air dry to test for the presence of acid phosphatase and the ABO antigen.

D. Laboratory studies

1. Spermatozoa. At the time of the rape examination, a wet mount is obtained from the vaginal pool to determine the presence or absence of spermatozoa.
   a. The presence of motile spermatozoa suggests sexual intercourse within the previous 24 hours.
   b. The presence of nonmotile spermatozoa has little significance.
   c. The absence of spermatozoa does not disprove recent sexual intercourse; the rapist may be azoospermic, severely oligospermic, or may have had a vasectomy.

2. Acid phosphatase. While all ejaculates contain acid phosphatase, it is not unique to semen; it is found in urine, normal vaginal fluid, and all tissues of the human body. However, the concentration of acid phosphatase in semen is important; a fresh ejaculate contains between 400 and 8000 King-Armstrong units/ml. Thus, identification of significant quantities of acid phosphatase in specimens from the vagina, anus, or mouth is strong evidence of recent ejaculation in these areas.

3. ABO antigen. Approximately 80% of men secrete ABO antigens into body fluids, including semen. Thus, ABO typing is excellent confirmatory evidence for the identity of the assailant. If no vaginal fluid is available, the vagina can be washed with sterile saline, which then can be saved for ABO antigen testing.

4. Other studies. Blood should be drawn for a complete blood count and a serum test for syphilis, and urine should be sent for urinalysis.

IV. PROTECTION OF THE VICTIM

A. Venereal disease. Prophylaxis against venereal disease should be administered to all victims at the time of the initial examination. Pediatric doses should be administered to children weighing less than 100 lbs after consultation with a pediatrician.

1. **Antibiotic regimens** include:
   a. 4.8 million units of procaine penicillin intramuscularly with 1 g of oral probenecid or 3.5 g of ampicillin orally with 1 g of probenecid
   b. 2 g of spectinomycin intramuscularly or 1.5 g of tetracycline orally at once followed by 500 mg 4 times daily for 4 days for patients with penicillin allergies
2. **Efficacy.** Because of the emergence of resistant strains of gonorrhea, all victims should be re-cultured in 4 weeks. Penicillin will attack incubating syphilis, whereas spectinomycin will not; if spectinomycin is used, the victim should have a repeat serum test for syphilis in 6 weeks.

B. **Pregnancy.** Human chorionic gonadotropin (HCG) β-subunit determination, if initially negative, should be repeated weekly until it becomes positive or until the onset of menses. Although pregnancy as a result of rape is uncommon, pregnancy prophylaxis should begin within 72 hours of the assault to be effective.

1. The standard dose of diethylstilbestrol (DES) is 25 mg twice a day for 5 days; the extreme nausea that can accompany this therapy can be helped with prochlorperazine (Compazine). Because of the teratogenic effects of DES, a therapeutic abortion is recommended if the therapy fails.
2. Insertion of an intrauterine device is also effective in preventing pregnancy and should be offered as an alternative.

C. **Psychological sequelae**

1. **Support groups.** It is important to encourage victims to contact support organizations as they provide:
   a. Immediate postevaluation counseling and an ongoing relationship with the victim
   b. Group sessions with other victims, providing opportunities for the patient to re-enact the traumatic episode with understanding, objective individuals
   c. Assistance in helping victims convert feelings of rage and shame to healthy anger
2. **Reactions to rape** typically involve three phases:
   a. **The first phase**, which lasts several days or weeks, is an **acute reaction**, in which the patient has difficulty talking about the assault. Shock and dismay are usually replaced by anxiety. Recall of the event may so affect the patient that she becomes totally nonfunctional in her everyday activities. The victim typically suffers from feelings of anger and self-recrimination and fear of the reactions of others.
   b. **The second phase** represents a **pseudoadjustment** period. Anxiety and anger in this stage are managed by denial, repression, and rationalization; the victim frequently withdraws from group sessions and therapeutic efforts.
   c. **The third phase** is marked by **depression**. In attempting to resolve her feelings about the event, the patient may require extensive counseling or psychotherapy.
3. **Psychological problems** may be more complex and intense in pediatric victims.
   a. Acquisition of relevant information may be difficult because of severe anxiety and the inability to communicate clearly.
   b. Parents of assaulted children frequently display considerable anxiety about the psychological and physical well-being of the child. Their irrational behavior toward medical personnel should be seen as an expression of their anger, guilt, and helplessness.

V. **SEXUAL ABUSE OF CHILDREN.** In addition to rape, sexual abuse of children includes fondling, oral and anal sodomy, incest, pornography, and prostitution. Often there is no physical evidence of what has occurred or of force being exerted, but there may be other means used, such as threats, bribery, or coercion.

A. **Incidence.** As with rape, the incidence of sexual abuse of children is an underreported problem, due in part to its perception as a social taboo.

1. It occurs in families of every racial and ethnic background and at every educational and income level.
2. No age-group of children is spared.
3. It is estimated that 1 in 5 girls and 1 in 10 boys are sexually abused prior to their eighteenth birthday.
4. Most sexually abused children are victims of someone they know.

B. Predisposing factors. Social risk factors include children:
1. Who are born to single-parent families
2. Whose mothers and fathers are divorced or separated
3. Who are born into families with mental illnesses
4. Who have a history of abusive parents
5. Who live with homeless families or reside in overcrowded units
6. Whose parents work and leave them home alone
7. Who return to an empty house after school

STUDY QUESTIONS

Directions: Each question below contains five suggested answers. Choose the **one best** response to each question.

1. When taking a history from a rape victim, all of the following information is relevant EXCEPT

(A) the last menstrual period
(B) bathing since the assault
(C) the most recent intercourse before the assault
(D) previous pregnancies
(E) birth control status

2. Supportive evidence in a rape case includes all of the following EXCEPT

(A) motile spermatozoa found on a wet mount 2 hours after the assault
(B) acid phosphatase found on a dried slide taken from the vaginal pool
(C) a lacerated hymen
(D) positive Wood's light examination of dried vulvar secretions
(E) a positive gonococcal culture

3. A victim experiencing the second phase of the psychological reaction to rape typically exhibits

(A) shame and dismay
(B) denial and rationalization
(C) anger and self-recrimination
(D) acute anxiety
(E) none of the above

4. Risk factors that predispose children to sexual abuse include all of the following family patterns EXCEPT

(A) families with divorced or separated parents
(B) families in which the mother works and the father stays home
(C) families with mental illness
(D) single-parent families
(E) families below the poverty level

Directions: Each question below contains four suggested answers of which **one or more** is correct. Choose the answer

A   if **1, 2, and 3** are correct
B   if **1 and 3** are correct
C   if **2 and 4** are correct
D   if **4** is correct
E   if **1, 2, 3, and 4** are correct

5. Sexual assault includes which of the following?

(1) Incest
(2) Genital contact
(3) Rape
(4) Oral sex

6. Correct statements about rape include which of the following?

(1) Rape is a crime of violence
(2) Beatings occur in the majority of rape cases
(3) Aggression is the primary motive of sexual assault
(4) The frequency of rape is higher in Northeastern cities

7. Which of the following factors must be present in order for assault to be designated as rape?

(1) Genital contact
(2) Force
(3) Threat of physical harm
(4) Resistance

8. The occurrence of statutory rape usually involves which of the following factors?

(1) Alcohol
(2) Drugs
(3) Children
(4) Mental retardation

ANSWERS AND EXPLANATIONS

1. The answer is D. *(III B 1–4)* It is important to determine the exact time of the last menstrual period and method of birth control, if any, because of the possibility of pregnancy following rape. Questions about bathing and previous intercourse are important when collecting evidence that may be used in the prosecution of the rapist. A woman's reproductive history is not relevant.

2. The answer is E. *(III C 2, 4 a, D 1 a, 2)* In an alleged rape, anything that suggests intromission and ejaculation is positive evidence. A lacerated hymen can indicate forceful intromission. A positive Wood's light examination and the finding of acid phosphatase suggest the presence of semen. Motile spermatozoa indicate intercourse within 24 hours. A positive gonococcal culture is not evidence of rape because the gonococcus organism could have been acquired prior to the rape from a different source.

3. The answer is B. *(IV C 2 a–c)* Shame, dismay, anxiety, anger, self-recrimination, and the inability to function in everyday activities are characteristic of the first phase of the reaction to rape. The second phase is characterized by a pseudoadjustment period, which is marked by denial, repression, and rationalization.

4. The answer is B. *(V B 1–5)* There are a number of factors that predispose children to sexual abuse. Children who are left alone while parents work or who return home to an empty house after school are at risk. Children from broken homes, families with mental illness, single-parent families, families with histories of abuse, families below the poverty level, and homeless families are also at risk. However, there is no evidence to suggest that children of families in which the mother works and the father does not are at risk.

5. The answer is B (1, 3). *(I A)* Rape and incest are the coital forms of sexual assault. Sexual assault also includes manual, oral, or genital contact with the genitalia of the victim *without the victim's consent*. Therefore, genital contact and oral sex by themselves cannot be considered sexual assault.

6. The answer is B (1, 3). *(I A; II B, C 1–3)* Rape is a crime of violence, the major motive of which is aggression. Beatings occur with great frequency but in less than 50% of reported cases. The occurrence of rape peaks during the summer months and is more frequent in highly populated Southern states. Offenders are typically single, young, poorly educated, black males.

7. The answer is A (1, 2, 3). *(I A 1–3)* For an assault to be designated as rape, there must be contact between the genitalia of the offender and the victim. In addition, there must be an element of force or threat of physical harm. It is no longer necessary to demonstrate resistance by the victim in order to prove rape.

8. The answer is E (all). *(I B)* Statutory rape is defined as sexual activity with individuals who are unable to consent because their consciousness is altered by drugs, alcohol, sleep, or illness (e.g., mental retardation) or because they are below the age of consent (e.g., children).

[handwritten: implantation / nidation]

29
Ectopic Pregnancy
William W. Beck, Jr.

[handwritten: fallopian tube / ovary / cervix / abdominal cavity]

I. INTRODUCTION

A. Definition. An ectopic pregnancy is any gestation occurring outside the uterine cavity. The most usual site for an ectopic pregnancy is the fallopian tube (95%), but it can occur in the ovary, cervix, or abdominal cavity.

B. Incidence. The frequency of ectopic pregnancy is about 1 in 200 pregnancies. In urban centers, which serve high indigent populations, the frequency of ectopic pregnancy is 1 in 80 pregnancies.

C. Significance. There is still a substantial maternal mortality with ectopic pregnancy due to the rapidity with which hemorrhage and shock occur and the elusiveness of the prerupture diagnosis with a consequent delay in surgical treatment.

[handwritten: (1) pelvic infection (2) narrowing of the tube (3) transmigration of the fertilized ovum (4) Intrauterine device usage]

II. ETIOLOGY OF ECTOPIC PREGNANCY

A. Pelvic infection. Chronic salpingitis is a common finding (30%–50%) in a fallopian tube with an ectopic pregnancy. The high incidence of ectopic pregnancy in indigent populations, where pelvic inflammatory disease is endemic, supports this observation.

1. Infection of the tube leads to fibrosis and scarring of intraluminal structures, which may result in transport dysfunction because of constriction of the tube, false passage formation, altered cilia, and abnormal tubal muscular action. All of these features retard the progress of the fertilized ovum on its way through the tube to the uterus, fostering nidation in the tube.

2. Chronic pelvic infection usually involves both tubes. The fact that there is a 10%–15% recurrent ectopic pregnancy rate in the contralateral tube confirms the relationship between pelvic infection and ectopic pregnancy.

B. Narrowing of the tube. Conditions causing significant narrowing of the passageway for the fertilized ovum and, thus, resulting in an increased incidence of ectopic pregnancy include:

1. Congenital defects of the tube, such as diverticuli and sacculations

2. Benign tubal tumors and cysts

3. Uterine fibroids at the uterotubal junction

4. Endometriosis of the tube, which has the capacity to undergo early decidua-like changes

5. Peritubal adhesions secondary to appendicitis or pelvic or abdominal surgery

6. Surgical repair of the tube. Ectopic pregnancy is seen with increased frequency in patients who undergo repair of the tube after previous inflammatory disease or tubal anastomosis following a previous tubal ligation.

C. Transmigration of the fertilized ovum. A significant number of patients \ nancy have been found to have the corpus luteum in the contralateral

1. The delay in transport of the fertilized ovum due to the external tra ovary to the contralateral tube within the peritoneal cavity) could allov tocyst to enlarge to a point at which it will be unable to pass through t the tube.

2. The fertilized ovum could also pass through the uterus (internal transmigration) and pass into the contralateral tube by a reflux mechanism.

D. **Intrauterine device (IUD) usage.** A high percentage of pregnancies conceived with the IUD in place are ectopic. This is probably due to the relative efficiency of the device in preventing intrauterine pregnancies rather than from a specific relationship of the IUD to ectopic pregnancy.

III. SIGNS AND SYMPTOMS OF ECTOPIC PREGNANCY

A. **Bleeding.** The most common symptom is abnormal uterine bleeding or spotting, which usually begins 7–14 days after the missed menstrual period.

1. Abnormal bleeding may occur at the time of the expected menses and be interpreted by the patient as a menses.

2. Major hemorrhage is uncommon, but menstrual-type bleeding occurs in 25% of ectopic pregnancies and may be considered a delayed menses by the patient or the physician.

3. The amount, timing, and character of the bleeding should not obviate the possibility that ectopic pregnancy could be the diagnosis.

B. **Pain.** Unilateral pelvic pain, which may be knife-like and stabbing or dull and less well-defined, is the next most common symptom.

C. **Clinical picture.** Few patients actually present with the classic picture of ectopic pregnancy, which entails amenorrhea and signs of early pregnancy followed by abnormal bleeding, abdominal pain, and fainting (due to hypotension from an intraperitoneal bleed).

1. Ectopic pregnancy can occur with an acute, subacute, or chronic presentation.

2. The mass of the unruptured ectopic pregnancy may be small and not palpable.

3. The uterus is usually enlarged to a 6-week size and is soft. The palpable, only slightly tender tubal ectopic may be confused with an ovary that contains a corpus luteum of pregnancy.

4. Standard urine pregnancy tests are negative in 50% of patients with ectopic pregnancy.

5. The bleeding and pain may be interpreted as a threatened abortion.

IV. DIAGNOSIS OF ECTOPIC PREGNANCY

A. **Index of suspicion.** The possibility of ectopic pregnancy must be suspected in pregnant patients who present with abnormal bleeding and pelvic pain or who give a history of pelvic inflammatory disease or pelvic surgery as this history places them at an increased risk.

B. **Differential diagnosis.** The diagnosis of ectopic pregnancy is usually straightforward as may be seen in a patient with amenorrhea, symptoms of pregnancy, pelvic pain, and bleeding. However, there are other clinical entities that may seem more appropriate.

1. **Adnexal torsion or acute appendicitis.** Although these conditions are suggested by unilateral pelvic pain, they do not produce amenorrhea, syncope, anemia, and early shock.

2. **Aborting intrauterine pregnancy.** In an aborting intrauterine pregnancy, the external bleeding is much more severe than the pain, whereas the reverse is true with an ectopic pregnancy.

3. **Bleeding corpus luteum of a normal intrauterine pregnancy.** The bleeding corpus luteum usually does not produce the severity of pain or shock typical of ectopic pregnancy. In addition, uterine bleeding is usually absent. When heavy internal bleeding is accompanied by shock, there is no other option than to observe the process directly by laparoscopy or laparotomy.

C. **Tests helpful in diagnosing ectopic pregnancy**

1. **Serial testing of the human chorionic gonadotropin (HCG) β-subunit.** Serum HCG β-subunit testing is positive in 100% of ectopic pregnancies, while the urine pregnancy tests for HCG are positive in only about 50% of cases with proven ectopic pregnancy.
   a. The rate of rise of serum HCG can help to differentiate normal from abnormal pregnancies (i.e., ectopic and blighted ovum pregnancies); in a normal pregnancy, the serum HCG level will *double every 2 days*.
   b. At a threshold level of 6000 mIU/ml of HCG, an intrauterine pregnancy should be seen by

ultrasound. Failure to detect fetal echoes within the uterus should suggest the possibility of an ectopic pregnancy.

2. Pelvic ultrasound. Ultrasound is only helpful in ruling out ectopic pregnancy by positively identifying a clearly defined intrauterine sac within the uterus at 7 weeks from the last menstrual period (but not earlier). The ultrasonic presence of an enlarged uterus and an adnexal mass is not helpful since this may simply represent an early intrauterine pregnancy and a corpus luteum.

3. Vaginal ultrasound. Ultrasound performed through the vagina with a vaginal probe can identify the intrauterine sac earlier than pelvic ultrasound.
   a. The intrauterine sac can be detected at HCG levels of 1500–2000 mIU/ml.
   b. An ectopic pregnancy can, therefore, be ruled out 4–6 days earlier with vaginal ultrasound than with pelvic ultrasound.

4. Culdocentesis. This test is useful in patients presenting acutely with pelvic pain, abnormal bleeding, syncope, or shock to determine whether or not there is free blood in the peritoneal cavity.
   a. An 18-gauge needle is inserted behind the uterus into the cul-de-sac.
   b. Aspiration of the cul-de-sac should produce some fluid material.
   c. The normal contents are slightly yellowish and clear with a volume of 3–5 ml. The presence of nonclotting blood in the syringe is diagnostic of free blood in the peritoneal cavity and supportive of the diagnosis of ectopic pregnancy.

5. Laparoscopy. If there is any doubt about the diagnosis, laparoscopy should be performed. It allows the direct visualization of the tubes and ovaries. The risk of a laparoscopy showing a normal pelvis is far less than the risk of a missed ectopic pregnancy.

6. Endometrial histology. In patients undergoing a dilatation and curettage (D and C) for abnormal uterine bleeding, such as in a suspected spontaneous abortion, the finding of decidua in the endometrial sample without chorionic villi indicates an ectopic pregnancy until proven otherwise. An additional finding in such an endometrium may be the Arias-Stella reaction, which is an endometrial response to the hormonal stimulation of pregnancy, producing a patchy, hyperactive, often hypersecretory pattern.

V. TREATMENT OF ECTOPIC PREGNANCY

A. Salpingo-oophorectomy. Surgical managment (removal of the affected ovary) was formerly advocated in cases in which the other adnexa appeared normal and pregnancy was desired.

1. The rationale for this management was based on the fact that all subsequent ovulations would occur from an ovary with an adjacent tube, thereby increasing the patient's potential pregnancy rate per cycle.

2. The removal of a normal ovary is no longer justifiable, despite the need for removing the ipsilateral tube, because of the possibility of in vitro fertilization at a later date and the need for maximum potential in terms of ovum production.

B. Salpingectomy. This is the most common treatment of ectopic pregnancy. The salpingectomy is performed by cross-clamping the broad ligament and removing the whole tube. This form of surgical management is most appropriate in the ruptured ectopic pregnancy where there is considerable bleeding.

C. Unruptured ectopic pregnancy. The frequency with which the diagnosis of unruptured ectopic pregnancy can be made has increased significantly with the combined use of serial testing of the HCG β-subunit, pelvic ultrasound, and laparoscopy. With the unruptured tubal ectopic pregnancy, a more conservative approach to the tube is possible.

1. In the patient with an unruptured tubal pregnancy, **the pregnancy may be milked from the fimbriated end of the tube**. If there is no undue bleeding after the products of conception have been milked from the tube, no further surgery is necessary.

2. Salpingostomy. If the pregnancy is at the midpoint of the tube, a linear salpingostomy—an opening up of the tube—may be performed with removal of the ectopic pregnancy and closure of the tube.

3. Segmental resection of the tube. The segment of the tube involved in the ectopic pregnancy may be removed and an anastomosis of the tubal ends performed. Alternatively, the cut ends of the tube could be ligated with anastomosis at a later date.

D. Prognosis. Patients with ectopic pregnancies must be told of the prognosis for future fertility—that is, approximately 40% of patients never conceive again. Of the 60% who do achieve another pregnancy, 12% will have another ectopic pregnancy, and 15%–20% will abort spontaneously. Because of the high risk in women with previous ectopic pregnancies, the patient should be instructed to notify her physician as soon as she has missed her menses so that the location of the new pregnancy can be detected by serial testing of the serum HCG β-subunit and ultrasound. If it is another tubal pregnancy, early surgical management to preserve the remaining tube is still a possibility at this early stage.

40% never conceive again

60% conceive ⎰ 12% another ectopic pregnancy

⎱ (5-20%) spontaneous abortion

STUDY QUESTIONS

Directions: Each question below contains five suggested answers. Choose the **one best** response to each question.

1. Chronic salpingitis is thought to enhance the possibility of ectopic pregnancy by all of the following EXCEPT

(A) intraluminal fibrosis
(B) altered cilia action
(C) distal tubal closure (hydrosalpinx)
(D) constriction of the tube
(E) false passage formation

2. All of the following are likely reasons for the establishment of a tubal ectopic pregnancy EXCEPT

(A) pelvic infection
(B) peritubal adhesions
(C) tubal anastomosis
(D) transmigration of the fertilized ovum
(E) uterine myoma

3. What percentage of women with a previous ectopic pregnancy can expect to have another ectopic pregnancy, if they conceive again?

(A) 3%
(B) 6%
(C) 12%
(D) 20%
(E) 25%

Directions: Each question below contains four suggested answers of which **one or more** is correct. Choose the answer

A   if **1, 2, and 3** are correct
B   if **1 and 3** are correct
C   if **2 and 4** are correct
D   if **4** is correct
E   if **1, 2, 3, and 4** are correct

4. An ectopic pregnancy in the tube on the contralateral side of the ovary with the corpus luteum means that

(1) external migration of the blastocyst can occur
(2) the ipsilateral tube is blocked
(3) internal migration of the blastocyst is possible
(4) the uterotubal junction of the ectopic tube is blocked

5. Which of the following tests would be helpful in a suspected tubal ectopic pregnancy 6 weeks from the last menstrual period?

(1) Pelvic ultrasound
(2) Serial human chorionic gonadotropin titers
(3) Culdocentesis
(4) Vaginal ultrasound

6. Dilatation and curettage was performed in a patient with a known ectopic pregnancy. Endometrial findings compatible with an ectopic pregnancy include

(1) decidua without villi
(2) hypersecretory endometrial pattern
(3) Arias-Stella reaction
(4) proliferative endometrium

Directions: The group of questions below consists of lettered choices followed by several numbered items. For each numbered item select the **one** lettered choice with which it is **most** closely associated. Each lettered choice may be used once, more than once, or not at all.

Questions 7–9

For each of the clinical presentations listed below, select the diagnosis most likely to be associated with it.

(A) Ectopic pregnancy
(B) Torsion of an ovarian cyst
(C) A threatened abortion
(D) A bleeding corpus luteum
(E) None of the above

7. A 25-year-old woman whose last menses were 6 weeks ago presents with acute left lower quadrant pain. Serum human chorionic gonadotropin (HCG) β-subunit levels are positive. Pelvic ultrasound reveals no sac in the uterus and a 3 × 3 cm left adnexal mass.

8. A 30-year-old woman whose last menses were 8 weeks ago presents with heavy vaginal bleeding and lower left quadrant pain. Serum HCG β-subunit levels are low for dates. Pelvic ultrasound reveals an intrauterine sac without fetal parts.

9. A 35-year-old woman whose last menses were 6 weeks ago presents with acute lower left quadrant pain but no vaginal bleeding. Serum HCG β-subunit levels are appropriate for dates. Culdocentesis reveals nonclotting blood. There is a tender left 3 × 4 cm adnexal mass on pelvic examination. Pelvic ultrasound reveals no gestational sac in the uterus.

ANSWERS AND EXPLANATIONS

1. The answer is C. (*II A 1, 2*) Chronic salpingitis leads to fibrosis and scarring of intraluminal structures, which, in turn, result in transport dysfunction because of constriction of the tube, false passage formation, altered cilia action, and abnormal tubal muscular action. These intraluminal impediments to the passage of the fertilized ovum cause arrest of migration and implantation in the tube. Distal tubal closure (hydrosalpinx) does not cause ectopic pregnancy formation because the egg cannot enter the tube to be fertilized.

2. The answer is E. (*II A 1, B 3–6, C 1*) Chronic salpingitis with scarring and fibrosis of intraluminal structures is a predisposing cause in 50% of ectopic pregnancies. Peritubal adhesions, the result of appendicitis, pelvic surgery, or pelvic infection, have also been associated with ectopic pregnancies. Transmigration of the fertilized ovum with the enlarging blastocyst unable to pass through the isthmus of the contralateral tube is one explanation for an ectopic pregnancy on the contralateral side of the ovary with the corpus luteum. Surgical repair of the tube, especially anastomosis of previously ligated tubes with narrowing of the tubal lumen, is a significant reason for a tubal pregnancy. Uterine myomas rarely cause infertility or tubal blockage; this entity is more likely to be associated with a pregnancy loss than an ectopic pregnancy.

3. The answer is C. (*V D*) There is significant infertility in patients who have had an ectopic pregnancy. Of the 60% of women who will get pregnant again, 12% will have a repeat ectopic pregnancy, and 15%–20% will abort spontaneously.

4. The answer is B (1, 3). (*II C 1–2*) The finding of a tubal ectopic pregnancy on one side and a corpus luteum in the contralateral ovary demonstrates that migration, either external or internal, of the blastocyst must occur. As the blastocyst enters the contralateral tube, it may have attained a size that prevents its passage into the uterus. Likewise, the fertilized ovum may pass in a retrograde fashion from the uterus into the contralateral tube and not be able to pass back into the uterus. The external migration occurs naturally and is not dependent on a blocked ipsilateral tube, which, in fact, is usually patent. The establishment of the ectopic pregnancy in the contralateral tube is not dependent on a blocked uterotubal junction; the blastocyst may just be too large at that point to pass through.

5. The answer is C (2, 4). (*IV C 1–4*) The demonstration that human chorionic gonadotropin (HCG) titers do not rise at the usual rate (doubling every 2 days) in abnormal pregnancies has been helpful in diagnosing ectopic and blighted ovum pregnancies. At 6 weeks from the last menstrual period, a pregnancy is too early to be diagnosed by pelvic ultrasound. Vaginal ultrasound, on the other hand, may pick up the gestational sac at 6 weeks—that is, up to a week before pelvic ultrasound is helpful. Culdocentesis would not be useful at 6 weeks, because few ectopic pregnancies are symptomatic or have ruptured by that time.

6. The answer is A (1, 2, 3). (*IV C 6*) In an ectopic pregnancy, there are no products of conception (i.e., villi) in the endometrial cavity. Decidual tissue and a hypersecretory endometrial pattern (the Arias-Stella reaction) without evidence of chorionic villi are common. A proliferative endometrium is a preovulatory finding and is incompatible with pregnancy.

7–9. The answers are: 7-D, 8-C, 9-D. (*IV B 2, 3, C 1, 2, 4*) The 25-year-old woman described in the question presents with no bleeding, which is unusual with an ectopic pregnancy. The fact that there is no sac in the uterus on pelvic ultrasound is of no significance because pelvic ultrasound does not pick up a sac until after 6 weeks gestation. The adnexal mass is the corpus luteum and not an ectopic pregnancy.

With the low-for-dates human chorionic gonadotropin (HCG) levels, the diagnosis in this 30-year-old woman could be either a threatened abortion or an ectopic pregnancy. Both conditions present with vaginal bleeding, but more bleeding is likely with a threatened abortion. The diagnosis is made by ultrasound, which reveals an intrauterine sac that would be absent in an ectopic pregnancy.

In the 35-year-old woman, whose last menses were 6 weeks ago, the HCG level is appropriate, and there is no vaginal bleeding, suggesting an intrauterine pregnancy. Neither nonclotting blood on culdocentesis nor the absence of a sac in the uterus on pelvic ultrasound at six weeks is diagnostic of an ectopic pregnancy. Therefore, the normal HCG levels, the lack of external bleeding, the tender mass on pelvic examination, and the intra-abdominal bleeding all point to an intrauterine pregnancy with a bleeding corpus luteum.

30
Sexually Transmitted Diseases
John M. Riva

I. INTRODUCTION. With the advent of the sexual revolution over 2 decades ago, there has been a broadened focus beyond the five classic venereal diseases of gonorrhea, syphilis, chancroid, lymphogranuloma venereum, and granuloma inguinale. With the exception of the human immunodeficiency virus (HIV), the spectrum of "new" sexually transmitted diseases (STDs) has expanded with the recognition of the venereal nature of these infectious agents by means of sophisticated epidemiologic and diagnostic techniques.

II. SEXUALLY TRANSMITTED DISEASES

A. Bacterial STDs. This group includes *Neisseria gonorrhoeae*, *Hemophilus ducreyi*, *Calymmatobacterium granulomatis*, and *Gardnerella vaginalis*.

1. **N. gonorrhoeae.** A gram-negative diplococcus, gonorrhea is the most commonly reported communicable disease in the United States. Its only natural host is man. The organism has a predilection for columnar epithelium. In nonpregnant women, it causes cervicitis, urethritis, pelvic inflammatory disease (PID), and acute pharyngitis. In men, it causes urethritis, prostatitis, and epididymitis. Disseminated gonococcal arthritis occurs in both men and women. In the newborn, gonococcal ophthalmia neonatorum is a known consequence of maternal infection.

   a. **Epidemiology.** The incidence is at epidemic levels with nearly 400 cases/100,000 population in the United States. Over 80% of reported cases occur in the 15–29-year-old age-group. In annual screening programs for non-STD clinics, the average gonorrhea detection rate is 2.7%. Transmission by sexual contact from the man to the woman is likely to result in infection after a single exposure. Risk factors include:

   (1) Young age
   (2) Multiple sexual partners
   (3) Failure to use barrier contraception

   b. **Clinical presentation.** *N. gonorrhoeae* has a short incubation time of 3–5 days. About 40%–60% of women with gonorrhea develop symptoms, including:

   (1) Purulent cervical discharge as in acute cervicitis
   (2) Lower abdominal pain, anorexia, and fever as is characteristic of acute pelvic inflammatory disease (PID)
   (3) Onset at the end of menstruation, particularly gonococcal PID

   c. **Diagnosis.** The diagnostic tests commonly employed include:

   (1) Gram stain of cervical secretions, looking for gram-negative diplococci or polymorphonuclear cells
   (2) Thayer-Martin culture medium
   (3) The Gonozyme test, a solid-phase immunoassay for detecting gonococcal antigens.

   d. **Treatment**

   (1) Uncomplicated gonococcal infections can be treated with aqueous penicillin G (4.8 million units intramuscularly at two sites) with probenecid (1 g orally); amoxicillin (3.5 g orally) with probenecid; or doxycycline (100 mg orally twice a day for 7 days).
   (2) In resistent infections or penicillinase-producing *N. gonorrhoeae*, spectinomycin (2 g intramuscularly) can be used. Follow-up cultures in 4–7 days should be obtained, and sexual consorts should be treated.
   (3) Patients with acute PID may require hospitalization and broad-spectrum antibiotics.

2. **H. ducreyi (chancroid).** One of the ulcerative genital diseases, *H. ducreyi* is a small nonmotile, gram-negative rod that has a characteristic "chaining" appearance on Gram stain.

   a. **Epidemiology.** *H. ducreyi* is rare in the United States, but common worldwide. In the United States, this STD is seen most frequently in young sexually active men who visit prostitutes. Trauma facilitates entry into mucosal vulvar tissues in women. The incubation time is 3–5 days.

   b. Clinical presentation. The classic lesion of chancroid is a soft sore or chancre with a superficial, necrotic ulcer base surrounded by a red halo. The lesion is tender and, in nearly 50% of cases, is accompanied by inflammatory inguinal adenopathy (bubo).

   c. Diagnosis. The most common diagnostic techniques, which demonstrate "school of fish" or "chaining" of gram-negative rods, are:

   (1) Gram stain of exudate from the chancre

   (2) Gram stain of the aspirate of the bubo

   d. Treatment. Traditional treatment has been a 10-day course of oral sulfonamides or tetracyclines.

3. *C. granulomatis*. This pleomorphic gram-negative rod is responsible for granulomatous and ulcerative lesions of the lower genital tract.

   a. Epidemiology. This STD is rarely reported in the United States. Although predominantly sexually transmitted, an intestinal reservoir for *C. granulomatis* has been suggested. The incubation time is 1 month.

   b. Clinical presentation

   (1) The initial lesion is an indolent, irregular ulcer with a pink to beefy red base.

   (2) The secondary phase of the disease involves beefy red exuberant granulation tissue with scar formation. Inguinal swelling and suppurative abscess may occur secondary to granulomatous tissue formation.

   (3) Advanced lesions become markedly hypertrophic. Fistulas of the adjacent structures of the vagina, bladder, and rectum may occur. Elephantiasis of the external genitalia may occur. Hematogenous spread to distant sites has been demonstrated.

   c. Diagnosis

   (1) Gram stain of the lesion reveals the pathognomonic cells—the mononuclear cells with intracytoplasmic inclusion cysts containing the pleomorphic rod-like organism. These inclusion cysts are called Donovan's bodies.

   (2) Tissue biopsies demonstrate Donovan's bodies on Wright's or Giemsa stains.

   d. Treatment. Tetracycline (500 mg orally four times a day for 3 weeks) is effective therapy. Reconstructive vulvar or pelvic surgery may be required in advanced cases.

4. *G. vaginalis* (formerly, *Hemophilus vaginalis*). *G. vaginalis* is a sexually transmitted bacterium, which acts in concert with vaginal anaerobic bacteria to produce vulvovaginitis.

   a. Epidemiology. Formerly referred to as nonspecific vaginitis, this infection accounts for approximately 25% of all cases of infectious vulvovaginitis.

   b. Clinical presentation. The vaginal discharge has a greyish, homogeneous nature with low viscosity. Postcoital odor is a common symptom.

   c. Diagnosis

   (1) Wet mount preparations are the main diagnostic tools. Saline preparations of vaginal secretions reveal a "clean" background with squamous cells whose borders are obscured by coccobacillary forms. These are known as the clue cells.

   (2) Application of 10% potassium hydroxide to the slide produces a fishy odor and is called the "whiff test."

   (3) Vaginal pH is between 5.0–5.5 (normal vaginal pH, 4.0–4.5).

   d. Treatment. Intravaginal sulfa-based creams, ampicillin, and metronidazole are effective treatments.

B. Spirochetal STDs. The predominant member of this group is ***Treponema pallidum***, which causes syphilis, a venereal disease that is disseminated by sexual intercourse or intrauterine transmission (congenital syphilis). Disease stages include primary, secondary, and tertiary syphilis.

1. Epidemiology. Approximately 30,000 new cases of primary and early latent syphilis are reported each year in the United States. However, it has been estimated that there are four- to ten-fold more new cases, many of which occur in the male homosexual population. The incubation period ranges from 10–90 days.

2. Clinical presentation

   a. The initial lesion of primary syphilis is a painless, ulcerated, hard chancre usually on the external genitalia, although vaginal and cervical lesions are also detected. The primary lesions resolve in 2–6 weeks.

   b. In untreated patients, this chancre is followed in 6 weeks to 6 months by a secondary or bacteremic stage in which the skin and mucous membranes are affected. Maculopapular rash of the palms and soles and mucous membranes occur. Condyloma latum and generalized lymphadenopathy are seen as well. These lesions usually resolve within 2–6 weeks.

c. Approximately 33% of untreated patients progress to tertiary syphilis with multiple organ involvement. Endarteritis leads to aortic aneurysm and aortic insufficiency, tabes dorsalis, optic atrophy, and meningovascular syphilis.

3. **Diagnosis.** Dark field examination of fresh specimens detects spirochetes in the primary and secondary stages of the disease. Serologic tests are helpful in diagnosing syphilis in patients who do not have primary disease. In the primary stage, the infected individual has not had sufficient time to develop an immune response that can be serologically detected. The two types of serologic tests are:
   a. Nonspecific reagin-type antibody tests (RPR and VDRL)
   b. Specific antitreponemal antibody tests (TPI, FTA-ABS, and MHA). These tests are employed if the nonspecific reagin-type antibody tests are positive.

4. **Treatment.** Patients with either a history of sexual contact with a person with documented syphilis, a positive dark field examination, or a positive antibody specific antitreponemal test should be treated. A fourfold rise in a quantitative antitreponemal test implies reinfection, and these patients should be treated. Penicillin is the mainstay of treatment with tetracycline and erythromycin as suitable alternatives for those patients who are allergic to penicillin.

C. **Chlamydial STDs.** There is a broad spectrum of sexually transmitted disorders caused by this species of obligatory intracellular bacterium. The major pathogen is *C. trachomatis*.

1. **C. trachomatis**, serotypes L_1, L_2, and L_3, are responsible for lymphogranuloma venereum, which produces a wide spectrum of local and regional ulcerations and destruction of genital tissues.
   a. Epidemiology. More commonly seen in tropical countries, there are less than 500 cases/yr reported in the United States with the majority of new cases found in men. The disease progresses through primary, secondary and tertiary stages. Incubation time is between 4 and 21 days.
   b. Clinical presentation
      (1) In women, the lesion occurs on the vulva as a painless vesicular or papular lesion. It generally resolves in a week. The secondary stage involves the development of inguinal adenopathy, which occurs 2–4 weeks after the resolution of the primary lesion.
         (a) The inguinal nodes enlarge and can create a linear refraction of the overlying subinguinal skin, creating a linear groove or ''groove sign.''
         (b) Suppuration of the nodes with sinus tract formation ensues and is accompanied by generalized symptoms of fevers, myalgias and arthralgias.
      (2) In untreated patients, locoregional destruction of anogenital tissues accompanied by lymphatic obstruction and elephantiasis have been reported.
   c. Diagnosis. Complement fixation is the test of choice. Complement fixation titers more than 1:64 are indicative of active infection.
   d. Treatment
      (1) Oral erythromycin or tetracycline over 3–6 weeks is effective therapy. *C. trachomatis* is resistant to penicillin.
      (2) Surgical reconstruction may be required for those patients with considerable tissue destruction in the tertiary stage.

2. **C. trachomatis**, serotypes D, E, F, G, H, I, J, and K, are responsible for acute urethritis, cervicitis, and acute PID.
   a. Epidemiology. Approximately 5% of sexually active women harbor this organism in their cervices. This organism is more commonly recovered from the cervix in both asymptomatic and symptomatic women than gonorrhea. Women at risk are similar to those who contract gonorrhea. It is common to recover *Chlamydia* in women whose partners have nongonococcal urethritis.
   b. Clinical presentation
      (1) Symptoms of urethritis, pyuria, and a negative urine culture in sexually active women is suggestive of a chlamydial infection.
      (2) In symptomatic women, micropurulent cervicitis (more commonly found in women with eversion of the endocervix) can be demonstrated.
      (3) *Chlamydia*-related acute PID accounts for approximately 30% of cases of acute PID. The symptoms are more insidious than gonococcal PID. Fever and lower abdominal pain are not as pronounced but are more protracted in duration.
   c. Diagnosis. The direct immunofluorescence test, using fluorescent tagged monoclonal antibodies against chlamydial surface antigens in the form of a slide test smeared with a swab of endocervical cells, is a rapid diagnostic test of choice.
   d. Treatment. Oral tetracycline, doxycycline, or sulfisoxazole over 7–10 days is effective in uncomplicated cases of urethritis, cervicitis, and acute PID.

D. Viral STDs. The principle viruses associated with STDs include human papillomavirus (HPV), herpes simplex virus (HSV), molluscum contagiosum, and human immunodeficiency virus (HIV).

1. **Human papillomavirus (HPV).** The genital virus in this double-stranded DNA family is responsible for a variety of mucocutaneous genital lesions, affecting both men and women.
   a. **Epidemiology.** More than 40 million sexually active adults in the United States harbor these viruses. The predominant means of transmission is through sexual intercourse, although recent evidence indicates that transmission to the neonate at the time of vaginal birth also occurs. The risk of contracting warts for women whose sexual partners have obvious genital warts is 60%–85%. Incubation time is between 6 weeks to 18 months with a mean time of 3 months. Subclinical or latent papillomaviral lesions have been associated with an increased risk of lower genital pre- and invasive neoplastic lesions of the lower genital tract.
      (1) Viral HPV types 6 and 11 are considered to be low-risk oncoviruses.
      (2) HPV types 31, 33, 35, and 42 are intermediate-risk oncoviruses.
      (3) HPV types 16 and 18 are believed to be high-risk oncoviruses.
   b. **Clinical presentation.** Lesions include overt anogenital warts (condyloma acuminatum), subclinical or latent lesions, and dysplastic lesions. In overt warty disease of the lower genital tract, visual inspection suffices to detect these obvious lesions, which are often multifocal in distribution. Subclinical lesions are not visible to the naked eye.
   c. **Diagnosis**
      (1) In overt warts, direct inspection discerns these lesions. Their nature is confirmed by biopsy.
      (2) Approximately 1% of Pap smears demonstrate the pathognomonic cell, the koilocyte or halo cell. This exfoliated squamous cell has a wrinkled, somewhat pyknotic nucleus surrounded by a perinuclear clear zone or halo.
      (3) Colposcopy, the magnified inspection of lower genital tissues after staining with a weak acetic acid solution, is helpful in detecting latent or associated precancerous lesions caused by HPV. Their appearance is that of small acetowhite flat lesions with vascular punctation or mosaicism. The histologic appearance of these lesions reveals koilocytosis, acanthosis, and variable nuclear atypia.
      (4) Recently, DNA hybridization techniques have been employed not only to detect HPV but to ascertain viral type.
   d. **Treatment**
      (1) For overt genital condyloma, there are a variety of acceptable treatment modalities, including:
         (a) Chemical destructive techniques
         (b) Cryotherapy
         (c) Electrocautery
         (d) Laser vaporization
         (e) 5-Fluorouracil cream
         (f) Interferon
      (2) For HPV-related precancerous conditions, treatment modalities include:
         (a) Cryotherapy
         (b) Laser vaporization
         (c) Surgical excision
      (3) The treatment of latent HPV infections is controversial.

2. **Herpes simplex virus (HSV).** A double-stranded DNA virus, HSV-2, is the predominant genital pathogen, although HSV-1 is seen in approximately 15% of herpetic genital infections. These viruses have an affinity for infecting mucocutaneous tissues of the lower genital tract. The virus is maintained in pelvic ganglion as a latent reservoir for recurrent herpetic genital infection. It most commonly produces recurrent vesiculoulcerative genital lesions. It is responsible for the highly lethal neonatal meningitis in neonates delivered through an actively infected cervix. HSV-2 has been associated with cervical cancer.
   a. **Epidemiology.** Estimates of the prevalence of HSV genital infections suggest that 20 million sexually active adults in the United States are afflicted with this disorder. The predominant mode of transmission is sexual intercourse. The incubation time is between 3 and 7 days.
   b. **Clinical presentation.** Primary genital herpetic infections are both a local and systemic disease. Vulvar paresthesia precedes the development of multiple crops of vesicular lesions.
      (1) Primary lesions become shallow coalescent painful ulcers in a few days and can last for 2–3 weeks. These lesions can be accompanied by severe dysuria with urinary retention, mucopurulent vaginal discharge, painful inguinal adenopathy, generalized myalgias, and fever.
      (2) Recurrent lesions are very similar but less severe in intensity, duration of illness, or sys-

temic side effects. Menses and stressful life situations are associated with recurrent out-breaks.

   c. Diagnosis. Herpes cultures obtained from the vesicular fluid or the edge of the ulcerative lesion gives the best results. Cytologic demonstration of multinucleated epithelial cells with intranuclear inclusions are helpful in the diagnosis.

   d. Treatment. Oral and topical acyclovir are effective in decreasing the severity and duration of painful eruptions. Continuous use of acyclovir on a prophylactic basis may reduce the frequency of eruptions in some patients with frequent recurrent episodes.

3. **Molluscum contagiosum (MC)**

   a. Epidemiology. MC is mildly contagious as an STD. It is a double-stranded DNA poxvirus. The incubation period is several weeks.

   b. Clinical presentation. This virus creates small (1–5 mm) umbilicated papules in the cutaneous genital region of sexually active individuals.

   c. Diagnosis. The lesion itself is pathognomonic of MC, but the diagnosis can be confirmed on histologic demonstration of a papule with a hyperkeratotic plug arising from an acanthotic epidermis. There are intracytoplasmic molluscum bodies noted on Wright's stain.

   d. Treatment. Local excision, cryotherapy, electrocautery, or laser vaporization are suitable treatment modalities.

4. **Human immunodeficiency virus (HIV).** Originally diagnosed in 1981, this unique retrovirus is believed to be responsible for severe deficiencies in cell-mediated immunity, leading to unusual opportunistic infections, malignancy, and eventually death. HIV is also known as acquired immune deficiency syndrome or AIDS.

   a. Epidemiology. Exhaustive epidemiologic studies have demonstrated male homosexuals and bisexuals, intravenous drug abusers, female heterosexual consorts of infected males, recipients of tainted blood or concentrated blood products, and neonates born to infected women are the predominant populations at risk. At the end of 1986, it was estimated that between 1 and 2 million Americans were infected with HIV. Transmission is both horizontal and vertical. Incubation or latency time is between 2 months and 5 years. The prevalence in the general population is estimated to be 9/100,000 people. Men are affected more commonly than women.

   b. Clinical presentation. Approximately 80%–90% of infected individuals are asymptomatic carriers; approximately 10%–20% of these carriers develop symptomatic disease each year, and of these, 80%–90% will die within 2 years of the onset of symptoms.

      (1) Pre-AIDS, or AIDS-related complex, is a prodromal illness to AIDS in seropositive individuals, which is manifested by generalized lymphadenopathy, diarrhea, malabsorption, and weight loss.

      (2) AIDS is manifested by severe alterations of cell-mediated immunity (reversal of the T_4 helper cell to T_8 suppression cell ratio), lymphadenopathy, Kaposi's sarcoma, opportunistic infections (principally *Pneumocystis carinii*), malaise, diarrhea, weight loss, and death.

   c. Diagnosis

      (1) Serologic screening with enzyme-linked immunosorbent assay (ELISA) for individuals at risk can be performed.

      (2) Western blot analysis of persistently positive ELISA is a more specific assay at detecting truly infected individuals.

   d. Treatment. There is no effective prophylactic therapies for preventing infection in high-risk individuals. Current clinical trials are underway, using antiviral and immunomodulating agents in infected patients in an attempt to effect remissions or cures; however, success has not been forthcoming.

E. **Protozoal STDs.** *Trichomonas vaginalis* is the most common sexually transmitted protozoal infection. This organism is responsible for acute vulvovaginitis.

1. **Epidemiology.** This protozoan is transmitted by sexual intercourse. There are approximately 2.5 million infections annually in the United States caused by this organism. It accounts for nearly one-third of all office visits for infectious vulvovaginitis.

2. **Clinical presentation.** *T. vaginalis* characteristically produces a profuse, yellowish-grey, frothy discharge of low viscosity. It is often accompanied by vulvar pruritus. Inspection of the vulvar and vaginal tissues reveal variable erythema. Intense erythematous mottling of the cervix can occasionally be seen and is denoted as the classic "strawberry" cervix.

3. **Diagnosis.** Vaginal pH is between 5 and 6. On wet mount preparations, there is an intense inflammatory response and motile trichomonads. These organisms are twice the size of leukocytes. Cultures for *Trichomonas* are available but are usually reserved for resistant cases where antimicrobial testing can be employed.

4. Treatment. The mainstay of therapy is oral metronidazole in 1–7-day courses. Intravenous metronidazole for 10–14 days may be necessary for highly resistant cases.

F. Ectoparasites. This group of STDs include pediculosis pubis and scabies.

1. **Pediculosis pubis (*Phthirus pubis*).** The crab louse is an insect approximately 1 mm long. It is generally confined to the hair-bearing regions of the vulva. A slow mover, the crab louse has 6 pairs of legs with one pair adapted to grasping hair follicles. It lays its eggs (nits) at the base of hair follicles. After 7 days, nymphs arise from the nits and progress to the adult stage in 2–3 weeks. Adult life expectancy is 30 days.
   a. **Epidemiology.** Pediculosis pubis is a highly contagious STD of young sexually active adults.
   b. **Clinical presentation.** Intense vulvar pruritus secondary to an allergic sensitization is the presenting symptom.
   c. **Diagnosis.** Identification of the crab louse attached to hair follicles or nits at the base of the hair follicle can be made with a hand lens inspection of the hair-bearing pubic region.
   d. **Treatment.** A 1% Lindane solution applied to the infested area and washed off in 8–12 hours is effective treatment.

2. **Scabies (*Sarcoptes scabiei*).** This mite is 0.4 mm in length. Unlike the crab louse, this mite is relatively quick in movement and can be found anywhere on the skin where it burrows a 5 mm tunnel to lay its eggs. Its life span is approximately 30 days.
   a. **Epidemiology.** Scabies can be transmitted by close sexual contact but also by nonsexual contact, such as sharing clothing or bedding.
   b. **Clinical presentation.** The predominant symptom is severe intermittent itching. Hands, wrists, breasts, and buttocks are the most commonly affected sites.
   c. **Diagnosis.** Demonstration of linear burrows with a hand lens is frequently seen. Microscopic slides prepared from scrapings of suspected lesions in mineral oil often demonstrate adult mites, eggs, and fecal pellets.
   d. **Treatment.** Disinfecting clothing, bedding, and the home environment is helpful. A 1% Lindane solution applied to infested areas of the body over 12 hours and washed off is effective treatment.

STUDY QUESTIONS

Directions: Each question below contains five suggested answers. Choose the **one best** response to each question.

1. Which of the following is a diagnostic test for *Hemophilus ducreyi* (chancroid)?

(A) Dark field examination of specimens from the lesion
(B) Nonspecific reagin-type antibody test
(C) Gram stain of the exudate from the ulcer base
(D) Thayer-Martin culture medium
(E) None of the above

2. Which of the following screening tests should be used in evaluating a patient at risk for human immunodeficiency virus?

(A) VDRL
(B) Eastern blot analysis
(C) Southern blot DNA hybridization
(D) Gonozyme test
(E) None of the above

Directions: Each question below contains four suggested answers of which **one or more** is correct. Choose the answer

A if **1, 2, and 3** are correct
B if **1 and 3** are correct
C if **2 and 4** are correct
D if **4** is correct
E if **1, 2, 3, and 4** are correct

3. Correct statements about *Phthirus pubis* include which of the following?

(1) It is a fast-moving insect
(2) It is generally confined to hair-bearing regions of the body
(3) It has a tendency to burrow to lay its nits
(4) It is highly contagious

4. Characteristics of secondary syphilis include

(1) palmar and plantar maculopapular rashes
(2) condyloma acuminatum
(3) a positive FTA-ABS
(4) painless chancres

Directions: The group of questions below consists of lettered choices followed by several numbered items. For each numbered item select the **one** lettered choice with which it is **most** closely associated. Each lettered choice may be used once, more than once, or not at all.

Questions 5–7

For each sexually transmitted disease listed below, select the lesion that is most apt to be associated with it.

(A) Small umbilicated papule
(B) Condyloma acuminatum
(C) Condyloma latum
(D) Soft chancre
(E) Painless hard chancre

5. *Hemophilus ducreyi*

6. Molluscum contagiosum

7. Human pápillomavirus, types 6 or 11

ANSWERS AND EXPLANATIONS

1. The answer is C. (*II A 1 c, 2 c, B 3*) Chancroid is best diagnosed by a Gram stain of the exudate obtained from the base of a chancre. The pathognomonic findings are gram-negative rods that form chains or a "school of fish" pattern. Dark field examination and nonspecific reagin-type antibody test diagnose syphilis. Thayer-Martin medium is the preferred culture media in diagnosing *Neisseria gonorrhoeae*.

2. The answer is E. (*II A 1 c, B 3, D 4 c*) An enzyme-linked immunosorbent assay (ELISA) is the screening test of choice for human immunodeficiency virus. Western blot analysis is a more sensitive test that will differentiate the true-positive from the false-positive on the ELISA test. VRDL is a nonspecific reagin-type antibody test for syphilis. The Gonozyme test is a solid-phase immunoassay for detecting gonococcal antigens. DNA hybridization techniques have recently been employed to detect human papillomavirus and to ascertain the viral serotype.

3. The answer is C (2, 4). (*II F 1 a*) *Phthirus pubis*, or pediculosis pubis (crab louse), is a highly contagious sexually transmitted disease where a single exposure results in transmission 95% of the time. It is a slow-moving insect in comparison to the ectoparasites, such as scabies. It is generally found attached to hair follicles where it lays its nits at the base of the hair follicle.

4. The answer is B (1, 3). (*II B 2 b, 3 b*) Palmar and plantar rashes are one of the pathognomonic mucocutaneous lesions of secondary syphilis. Condyloma latum are exuberant "fig-like" lesions of mucocutaneous tissue seen in secondary syphilis and need to be distinguished from condyloma acuminatum, which is caused by human papillomavirus. The FTA-ABS is a specific antitreponemal antibody test, which is positive in patients with secondary syphilis. A painless chancre is the initial lesion of primary syphilis.

5–7. The answers are: 5-D, 6-A, 7-B. (*II A 2 b, D 1 a–c, 3 b, c*) The soft chancre is associated with *Hemophilus ducreyi* or chancroid. The classic lesion of chancroid is a soft sore with a superficial ulcer crater surrounded by a red halo. This lesion is accompanied in nearly 50% of cases with flocculent inguinal adenopathy or bubo.

The lesion of molluscum contagiosum is very characteristic of the poxvirus infection. This virus creates small, umbilicated papules in the cutaneous genital skin. This lesion by itself is diagnostic.

Human papillomavirus, serotypes 6 or 11, is characterized by fig-like lesions (warts or condyloma acuminatum) in the anogenital region. In overt warty disease, visual inspection will detect these obvious lesions, which may form in clusters. Approximately 60%–85% of women who have sexual intercourse with a male consort with overt warts will develop genital condyloma.

I. INTRODUCTION

A. Definition. Uterine leiomyomas are circumscribed, benign tumors composed of muscle with fibrous connective tissue elements; they are also referred to as fibroids, myomas, or fibromyomas.

1. They are the most common masses of uterine origin and are one of the most frequent abnormalities palpated within the pelvis.

2. Tumors may occur singly but are usually multiple; as many as 100 or more have been found in one uterus.

3. They are present in 20% of white women and 50% of black women by 30 years of age.

4. They may be found in organs outside the uterus, including the fallopian tubes, vagina, round ligament, uterosacral ligaments, vulva, and gastrointestinal tract.

B. Etiology. A leiomyoma is a localized proliferation of smooth muscle cells. As a leiomyoma grows, there is a gradual addition of fibrous material.

1. Leiomyomas arise from immature muscle cells and cell nests. The original cell is in the myometrium, and it may be undifferentiated from mesenchymal myometrial cells.
   a. Contractions of the uterine muscles, which result in points of stress within the myometrium, could act as a growth stimulus to these cell nests.
   b. The multiple points of stress within the myometrium are consistent with the multiple nature of myomas.

2. Evidence suggests that myomas are dependent on estrogen for growth.
   a. Myomas are rarely found before puberty and stop growing after menopause.
   b. New myomas rarely appear after menopause.
   c. There is often rapid growth of myomas during pregnancy.
   d. Myomas are frequently found in conditions of hyperestrogenism, including anovulation, endometrial polyps, and endometrial hyperplasia.

3. Myomas also are found in women with normal cycles who exhibit no hormonal imbalance.

II. CHARACTERISTICS OF MYOMATA UTERI

A. Types of myomas. Three types of leiomyomas occur: intramural, submucous, and subserous.

1. **Intramural myomas** are the most common variety, occurring within the walls of the uterus as isolated, encapsulated nodules of varying size. When myomas extend into the broad ligament, they are known as intraligamentary leiomyomas.

2. **Submucous myomas** are located beneath the endometrium. These tumors grow into the uterine cavity, maintaining attachment to the uterus by a pedicle. The pedunculated myomas may protrude to or through the cervical os. These tumors are often associated with an abnormality of the overlying endometrium, resulting in a disturbed bleeding pattern.

3. **Subserous myomas** grow out toward the peritoneal cavity and cause the peritoneal surface of the uterus to bulge. These tumors may also develop a pedicle, become pedunculated, and reach a large size within the peritoneal cavity without producing symptoms. These potentially mobile tumors may present in such a manner that they need to be differentiated from solid adnexal lesions. A pedunculated myoma may attach to the omentum or mesentery of the small bowel.

a. The myoma may gain an additional blood supply from its secondary attachment, which becomes its main nutritional source.

b. With degeneration of the uterine pedicle, possibly due to intermittent torsion, the myoma becomes dependent on the secondary blood supply, resulting in a parasitic myoma.

B. Pathology

1. **Gross pathology.** Leiomyomas are encapsulated in the sense that they do not invade adjacent tissue, although no real capsule exists. The pseudocapsule is composed of fibrous and muscle tissue that has been flattened by the tumor. Since the vasculature is located on the periphery, the central part of the tumor is susceptible to degenerative changes. On cut surface, the tumors are smooth, solid, and usually pinkish white, depending on the degree of vascularity. The surface typically has a trabeculate, whorl-like appearance.

2. **Microscopic pathology.** The leiomyoma is composed of groups and bundles of smooth muscle fibers in a twisted, whorled fashion. The spindle-shaped smooth muscle cells invariably contain some connective tissue elements.

C. Degenerative changes. A variety of degenerative changes occur in a myoma, which alter the gross and microscopic appearance of the tumor. Degeneration may be related to alterations in circulation, either arterial or venous, secondary to infection, or malignant transformation.

1. **Hyaline degeneration**, the most common type of degeneration, is present in almost all leiomyomas. It is caused by an overgrowth of the fibrous elements, which leads to a hyalinization of the fibrous tissue and, eventually, calcification.

2. **Cystic degeneration** may occasionally be a sequel of necrosis, but cystic cavities are usually a result of liquefaction following hyaline degeneration.

3. **Necrosis** is commonly caused by impairment of the blood supply or severe infection. A special kind of necrosis is the red or **carneous degeneration**, which occurs most frequently in pregnancy. The lesion has a dull, reddish hue and is believed to be caused by aseptic degeneration associated with local hemolysis. Clinically, carneous degeneration during pregnancy must be differentiated from a variety of acute accidents that occur within the abdomen involving the adnexa and other nongenital organs.

4. **Mucoid degeneration.** When the arterial input is impaired, particularly in large tumors, areas of hyalinization may convert to a mucoid or myxomatous type of degeneration; the lesion has a soft gelatinous consistency. Further degeneration can lead to liquefaction and cystic degeneration.

5. **Sarcomatous degeneration.** Malignant degeneration occurs in less than 1% of leiomyomas. Finding a leiomyosarcoma within the core of an apparently benign pseudoencapsulated myoma is suggestive of such a degenerative process. This type of sarcoma is usually of a spindle cell rather than a round cell type. The 5-year survival rates of a leiomyosarcoma arising within a myoma are much better than for a true sarcoma of the uterus when there is no extension of the sarcomatous tissue beyond the pseudocapsule of the myoma.

III. SYMPTOMS AND SIGNS OF MYOMATA UTERI

A. Symptoms. The symptoms of leiomyomas vary greatly, depending on their size, number, and location.

1. **Abnormal menstrual bleeding** is the most common characteristic associated with myomata uteri. This bleeding is typically hypermenorrhea—that is, characterized by an excessively long menstrual period or by excessive bleeding during the normal period. The increase in flow usually occurs gradually, but the bleeding may result in a profound anemia. Bleeding results from necrosis of the surface endometrium overlying the submucous myoma or from disturbance in the hemostatic contraction of normal muscle bundles when there is extensive intramural myomatous growth. Frequently myomas are associated with polyps and endometrial hyperplasia, which may produce the abnormal bleeding pattern.

2. **Pain.** Uncomplicated uterine leiomyomas generally do not produce pain. Acute pain associated with fibroids is usually due to either torsion of a pedunculated myoma or infarction progressing to carneous degeneration within a myoma. Pain is often crampy in nature when a submucous myoma within the endometrial cavity acts as a foreign body. Some patients with intramural myomas experience the reappearance of dysmenorrhea after many years of pain-free menses.

3. Pressure. As myomas enlarge, they may cause a feeling of pelvic heaviness or produce pressure symptoms on the surrounding structures.
   a. Urinary frequency is a common symptom when a growing myoma exerts pressure on the bladder.
   b. Urinary retention can result when myomatous growth creates a fixed retroverted uterus that pushes the cervix anteriorly under the symphysis pubis in the area of the posterior urethrovesicular angle.
   c. Asymptomatic pressure effects of myomas are generally caused by lateral extension or intraligamentous myomas, which produce unilateral ureteral obstruction and hydronephrosis.
   d. Constipation and **difficult defecation** can be caused by large posterior myomas.

4. Reproductive disorders. Infertility may result when myomas interfere with normal tubal transport or implantation of the fertilized ovum.
   a. Large intramural myomas located in the cornual regions may effectively close the interstitial portion of the tube.
   b. Continuous bleeding in patients with submucous myomas may impede implantation; the endometrium overlying the myoma may be out of phase with the normal endometrium and thus provide a poor surface for implantation.
   c. There is an increased incidence of abortion or premature labor in patients with submucous or intramural myomas.

B. Signs

1. Abdominal examination. Uterine leiomyomas may be palpated as irregular, nodular tumors protruding against or through the anterior abdominal wall. Leiomyomas are usually firm upon palpation; softness or tenderness suggests the presence of edema, sarcoma, pregnancy, or degenerative changes.

2. Pelvic examination. The most common finding is uterine enlargement; the shape of the uterus is usually asymmetric and irregular in outline. The uterus is usually freely movable unless residuals of an old inflammatory disease persist.
   a. In the case of submucous myomas, the uterine enlargement is usually symmetric.
   b. Some subserous myomas may be very distinct from the main body of the uterus and may move freely, which often suggests the presence of adnexal or extrapelvic tumors.
   c. The diagnosis of cervical myomas or pedunculated submucous myomas may be made by tumor extension into and effacement of the cervical canal; occasionally a submucous myoma may be visible at the cervical os or the introitus.

IV. TREATMENT. The treatment of myomas must be adapted to each patient. If the tumor is not excessively large and there are no symptoms, treatment may not be necessary.

A. Observation. In the absence of pain, abnormal bleeding, pressure symptoms, or large myomas, periodic examinations are sufficient management. This is especially true if the patient is nearing the menopause at which time the myomas will atrophy as estrogen levels fall.

   1. Bimanual examinations should be made every 3–6 months to determine uterine size.

   2. Palpation of the uterosacral ligaments for evidence of endometriosis is important since this lesion often coexists with leiomyomas.

   3. Because of the increased bleeding with myomas, patients should have regular blood counts; iron deficiency anemia is common with hypermenorrhea, and oral iron may be required to keep pace with the uterine bleeding.

   4. Pelvic ultrasound may be helpful in documenting growth of myomas and ovarian enlargement when clinical evaluation of the pelvis is difficult because the enlarged uterus fills the pelvis; ultrasound can also demonstrate hydroureter and hydronephrosis secondary to compression by the myomatous uterus.

B. Gonadotropin-releasing hormone (GnRH) agonists. Long-acting GnRH agonists, which suppress gonadotropin secretion and create a pseudomenopause, may be given subcutaneously on a monthly basis for 6 months.

   1. A 55% reduction in the size of the myomas has been noted with this regimen.

   2. The myomas usually regrow after the GnRH therapy is discontinued.

C. Indications for surgery

1. **Bleeding** produced by myomas is a primary indication for surgery; the hypermenorrhea is associated with submucous or intramural myomas, which no longer can be observed, especially when the bleeding leads to anemia.

2. **Pain** in association with myomas suggests degeneration within the myoma or torsion of a pedunculated myoma.

3. **The size** of a myomatous uterus is important. Surgery is indicated when the conglomerate size of the myomas exceeds that of a 12-week gestation because a uterus of that size fills the entire true pelvis and makes examination of the adnexa very difficult. Adnexal examination is important in women over 40 years of age because of the increased risk of ovarian neoplasm. Rapid growth in a myomatous uterus at any age warrants exploration since malignant change must be ruled out.

4. **The signs and symptoms of pressure** on the bladder, bowel, or ureters may be indications for surgical intervention. **Hydronephrosis**, demonstrated by sonography or intravenous pyelography, is a clear indication for surgery.

5. **When the reproductive process is complicated by myomas** by repetitive pregnancy loss, surgery is indicated.

D. **Surgical procedures**. The type of surgery to be performed depends on the age of the patient, the nature of the symptoms, and the patient's desires regarding future fertility.

1. **Myomectomy** involves the removal of single or multiple myomas while preserving the uterus; this procedure is usually reserved for women who desire pregnancy and in whom pregnancy is not contraindicated.
   a. It may be necessary to open the uterine cavity to remove submucous myomas; this usually means that a cesarean section is necessary with the successful completion of a pregnancy.
   b. Major complications of the procedure are intraoperative and postoperative hemorrhage and early or late intestinal obstruction.
   c. The recurrence of myomas following myomectomy depends on the race (higher in blacks) and age of the patient as well as the completeness of the original myomectomy; a 30% recurrence rate within 10 years has been reported.
   d. The incidence of pregnancy following myomectomy has been estimated to be 40%.

2. **Hysterectomy**. If the indications for surgery are present and if the patient's childbearing is complete, total removal of the uterus is the procedure of choice.
   a. Hysterectomy should not be performed on the assumption that the bleeding is due to the myomas. Curettage of the endometrial cavity is essential prior to hysterectomy to rule out pathology, especially endometrial neoplasia.
   b. With hysterectomy, both the leiomyomas and any associated disease are removed permanently, and there is no risk of recurrence.
   c. Ovaries should be retained in women less than 40–45 years of age. Patients must play an important part in the decision concerning oophorectomy at any age, keeping in mind that there is little evidence to support the contention that the residual ovary after a hysterectomy is at greater risk for developing ovarian cancer.

STUDY QUESTIONS

Directions: Each question below contains five suggested answers. Choose the **one best** response to each question.

1. Submuous myomas may be associated with all of the following signs and symptoms EXCEPT

(A) abnormal bleeding
(B) reproductive failure
(C) anemia
(D) parasitic myomas
(E) pedunculated myomas

2. Typical symptoms associated with an abnormally enlarged 6- to 8-week myomatous uterus are

(A) acute crampy pain
(B) urinary frequency
(C) constipation
(D) urinary retention
(E) none of the above

3. Abnormal uterine bleeding associated with myomata uteri is characterized by all of the following EXCEPT

(A) a gradual increase in the bleeding
(B) excessively long menstrual bleeding
(C) excessive bleeding during a menses of normal length
(D) the development of anemia
(E) irregular cycles with hypermenorrhea

4. Gross and microscopic features of myomas include all of the following EXCEPT

(A) a whorl-like appearance
(B) bundles of smooth muscle fibers
(C) a well-defined capsule of fibrous tissue
(D) central degeneration
(E) peripheral vascularity

Directions: Each question below contains four suggested answers of which **one or more** is correct. Choose the answer

A   if **1, 2, and 3** are correct
B   if **1 and 3** are correct
C   if **2 and 4** are correct
D   if **4** is correct
E   if **1, 2, 3, and 4** are correct

5. Large subserous myomas are associated with which of the following conditions?

(1) Anemia
(2) Hydronephrosis
(3) Reproductive loss
(4) Constipation

6. Reproductive problems associated with myomas include

(1) recurrent abortion
(2) poor implantation
(3) blocked tubes
(4) luteal phase defect

Directions: The group of questions below consists of lettered choices followed by several numbered items. For each numbered item select the **one** lettered choice with which it is **most** closely associated. Each lettered choice may be used once, more than once, or not at all.

Questions 7–9

For each of the following clinical situations involving a myomatous uterus, select the therapy that is most appropriate.

(A) Oral iron therapy
(B) Hormone suppression
(C) Dilatation and curettage
(D) Myomectomy
(E) Hysterectomy

7. A 50-year-old woman with a known myomatous uterus presents with the complaint of irregular bleeding. She states that her menses are heavy and occur every 5–6 weeks. She also mentions that she has had 5–7 days of intermenstrual spotting over the past three cycles.

8. A 32-year-old black woman with known myomas returns to the office after 3 years, complaining of mild left lower quadrant pain. Three years ago she had a tubal ligation. Physical examination reveals a 14-week, irregular uterus with an apparent 4-cm left fundal myoma.

9. A 28-year-old primipara presents with a 14-week uterine mass, pain, and hypermenorrhea. On physical examination, she has a prominent posterior fundal mass, which seems to make up the bulk of the uterine mass.

ANSWERS AND EXPLANATIONS

1. The answer is D. (*II A 2, 3*) Submucous myomas are the type most commonly associated with abnormal bleeding because of changes in the overlying endometrium that result in a disturbed bleeding pattern. This then can lead to anemia and reproductive failure through poor implantation of the embryo in the abnormal endometrium overlying the myoma. These same myomas can grow within the uterine cavity, remain connected to the endometrium via pedicles, and become pedunculated with actual prolapse through the cervical os. These myomas, however, cannot become parasitic myomas, as do some subserous myomas, because there is nothing to which they can attach and establish a secondary blood supply as may happen within the abdominal cavity.

2. The answer is C. (*II B 1, 2*) Myomas are made up of bundles of smooth muscle fibers that have a whorl-like appearance when cut on cross section. Degenerative changes within the myoma are common and may be due to alterations in circulation, infection, or malignant transformation. The vascularity is on the periphery of the myoma, making the central part susceptible to degenerative changes. Myomas are encapsulated in the sense that they do not invade adjacent tissue, although no real capsule exists. The pseudocapsule is composed of fibrous and muscle tissue that has been flattened by the myoma and has the appearance of a capsule.

3. The answer is E. (*III A 1*) Abnormal menstrual bleeding is the most common characteristic associated with myomata uteri. Hypermenorrhea is common with excessive bleeding at the time of the menses either in length or amount. The bleeding usually increases gradually and may eventually result in a significant anemia. Myomas are discrete objects and are not related to the hormonal aspects of the cycle. Therefore, irregular cycles are not characteristic because the length and regularity of the menstrual cycle is hormonally controlled.

4. The answer is E. (*III A 2, 3*) A 6- to 8-week myomatous uterus is not very big and should not cause the pressure symptoms of constipation, urinary frequency, or urinary retention as would a grossly enlarged uterus that fills the pelvis. In addition, small, uncomplicated myomas, as is the case in this uterus, without any pedunculated myomas, generally do not produce pain. Acute pain is usually associated with torsion of a pedunculated myoma.

5. The answer is C (2, 4). (*II A 1–3*) Myomas can be of three different types, depending on their location on or within the uterus. The clinical conditions associated with myomas in part depend on the location of the myomas. The submucous myomas, because of their strategic location within the uterine cavity, can lead to excessive blood loss and anemia along with reproductive problems, such as infertility and pregnancy wastage. The large subserous myomas, especially those on the posterior aspect of the uterus, are on the surface of the uterus and can put pressure on nearby structures, such as the ureters and rectum, resulting in hydronephrosis and constipation.

6. The answer is A (1, 2, 3). (*III A 4 a–c*) Because of the thinned, sometimes poorly vascularized endometrium that can overlie a submucous myoma, there is the likelihood of poor implantation of an embryo with the possibility of recurrent spontaneous abortion early in the first trimester. Myomas growing at or near the cornual regions of the uterus can put pressure on the interstitial portions of the tubes and block them. A luteal phase defect is a hormonal problem and is not caused by the mechanical problems associated with intramural and submucous myomas.

7–9. The answers are: 7-C, 8-E, 9-D. (*IV C 3, D 1, 2 a*) One cannot assume that abnormal bleeding in a 50-year-old woman is caused by the myomas simply because she has a myomatous uterus. At this age, the risk of endometrial pathology, such as polyps, hyperplasia, or carcinoma, is significant and must be ruled out. Therefore a dilatation and curettage is indicated before considering any other therapy.

Hysterectomy is indicated in the 32-year-old black woman who has had a tubal ligation as reproduction is no longer a consideration. She has 15–20 years of ovarian activity remaining, and estrogen secretion over that time will only stimulate the growth of the myomas. The size of this uterus is greater than a 12-week gestation and has an apparent left fundal myoma. Both the size and the configuration of this uterus preclude a good adnexal examination to determine if she has an ovarian mass on the left. Because she no longer has need of her uterus and because of its size, this patient should have a hysterectomy.

This patient is a young woman of low parity who is probably not finished with her childbearing. She has many years of estrogen stimulation ahead of her, which will only cause the uterus to enlarge further. Physical examination suggests a single, large myoma in the uterus. The size of the uterine mass has already exceeded that recommended for observation alone. To preserve fertility in a young woman with a myomatous uterus, which will increase in size over time, a myomectomy is the treatment of choice.

32
Stress Urinary Incontinence
John M. Riva

I. INTRODUCTION. Voluntary control of micturation is learned at an early age. In women, this control is relative. Studies have indicated that more than 50% of young nulliparous women admit to an involuntary loss of urine when the bladder is full. When the involuntary loss of urine occurs as a result of an incompetent urethral closure mechanism during an increase in intra-abdominal pressure, such as occurs with coughing or sneezing, it is known as stress urinary incontinence (SUI).

A. Epidemiology of SUI

  1. It occurs most often in white parous women.

  2. It is rare in nulliparous women.

  3. It is infrequent in black and Oriental women.

  4. It is unknown in men.

B. Pathophysiology of SUI. SUI is strictly an anatomic problem. In the normal continent woman, the bladder neck and the proximal urethra are intra-abdominal or above the pelvic floor in the standing position. Consequently, the urethral pressure equals or exceeds the intravesical pressure. In SUI:

  1. Distortion of the normal anatomic urethrovesical relationship can result from increases in intra-abdominal pressure, leading to increases in intravesical pressure, which exceeds urethral pressure, resulting in incontinence. Examples of this distortion include:
  a. Funneling and descent of the vesical neck
  b. Abnormal downward and backward rotation of the urethral axis
  c. Loss of the posterior urethrovesical angle

  2. Alterations in the circular muscular arrangement lead to a reduction in urethral resting tone and closing pressure.

II. DIAGNOSIS OF SUI

A. History. Incontinence of urine is not always purely of anatomic origin. A detailed history is mandatory to differentiate pure anatomic SUI from other causes of involuntary loss of urine. The history should include a characterization of the:

  1. Voiding patterns

  2. Stresses that evoke a loss of urine

  3. Temporal relationship between the stress and the loss of urine

  4. Use of medications

  5. History of:
  a. Urinary tract infections
  b. Urologic surgery
  c. Obstetric trauma
  d. Central nervous system or spinal cord disorders

B. Physical examination may detect:

  1. Exacerbating conditions, such as chronic obstructive pulmonary disease, obesity, or intra-abdominal masses

2. Genitourinary descensus

3. Neurologic abnormalities

C. Diagnostic tests

1. Midstream urine specimen is collected for culture and sensitivity. Chronic infection may aggravate SUI.

2. Residual urine volume should be measured.

3. Cystoscopy is performed to evaluate the bladder mucosa for intrinsic lesions (e.g., infection, calculi, neoplasms, fistulae, or cicatrix) and to identify the ureteral orifices.

4. Cystometry evaluates bladder capacity, tone, and dynamics. The urethra and intravesical pressures are measured, using either fluids (balanced salt) or air (carbon dioxide). The bladder is filled in the supine position.

    a. If the bladder pressure after filling rises more than 10 cm of water on standing, detrusor instability is suspected.

    b. Bladder capacity may be reduced (less than 250 ml), suggesting urge incontinence and psychogenic or interstitial cystitis as possible etiologies.

    c. Bladder capacity may be increased (greater than 600 ml), which almost always indicates neurologic disease.

5. Bladder neck elevation test (Marchetti test). In this test, the physician places a finger on each side of the urethra as the patient strains; if this relieves incontinence, then bladder neck elevation may offer hope of therapeutic success.

6. Q-tip or straight catheter test is an indirect measure of the urethral axis (angle of inclination). A Q-tip or catheter is inserted with the patient in the lithotomy position. If it points downward from the horizontal, the axis is normal; if it points upward, the urethra is rotated posteriorly.

7. Metallic bead chain urethrocystogram (cystourethrography) displays the bladder and urethra radiographically. It does not distort the urethra and allows urethral mobility. A metallic bead chain is placed inside the urethra and bladder with radiopaque dye.

    a. First, anterior–posterior and lateral films are taken with the patient standing with her feet 14–16 inches apart, nonstraining, to allow complete freedom of movement of the bladder base, neck, and urethra.

    b. Anterior–posterior and lateral films are taken while the patient is straining. The spatial relationship of the urethra and bladder is noted.

    c. The metallic bead chain technique demonstrates two important anatomic abnormalities:

        (1) Type I SUI is indicated by a loss of the posterior urethrovesical angle, which is normally 90–100 degrees (Fig. 32-1), with retention of the angle of inclination (the urethral axis in relation to the vertical axis of the symphysis pubis), which is normally less than 45 degrees.

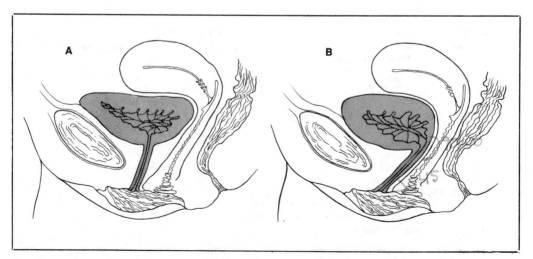

Figure 32-1. Abnormalities demonstrated by metallic bead chain urethrocystogram. *A*, Normal vesical neck–proximal urethra angle posteriorly (90°). *B*, Loss of the posterior urethrovesical angle.

(2) Type II SUI is indicated by a loss of both the posterior urethrovesical angle and the angle of inclination. Type II reflects profound weakness of the supporting tissues. Symptoms are severe, and cure is difficult.

D. Differential diagnosis

1. **Detrusor instability (dyssynergia)**, as a result of involuntary contractions of the detrusor muscle, which elevate intravesical pressure and lead to incontinence

2. **Urine retention with overflow**, as a result of neurologic disease, drugs, and pelvic surgery

3. **Congenital anomalies** (ectopic ureter and epispadias)

4. **Functional** (no organic cause can be found)

5. **Chronic infection**, **neoplasms**, **calculi**, **cicatrix** (postirradiation and surgery), **and fistulae**

III. MANAGEMENT OF SUI.
Patients with SUI are often suffering from more than one disorder. Some abnormalities may be functional and others due to anatomic etiologies. Nonsurgical treatment should be instituted first, and if symptoms persist, surgery can be performed. When patients fail to respond to therapy, or no organic cause can be found for the incontinence, psychiatric consultation should be obtained. Emotional stress, anxiety, and depression can manifest as SUI. An error in diagnosis can lead to erroneous, unnecessary, and unsuccessful therapy.

A. Nonsurgical treatment

1. **Pelvic exercises** strengthen the pelvic floor and perineal muscles.

2. **Weight reduction** in obese patients alleviates some of the symptoms.

3. **Chronic cough** should be evaluated and treated. Smoking should be stopped.

4. **Infection** should be treated.

5. **Faradism** is the therapeutic use of an interrupted current to stimulate muscles and nerves. Success obtained has not yet been determined.

6. **Drug therapy**
   a. **Anticholinergics** (e.g., propantheline and imipramine) reduce bladder motility and capacity increases. These drugs are particularly beneficial in detrusor instability.
   b. **Sympathomimetics** may elevate urethral pressure.
   c. **Hormones**, especially estrogen, are beneficial in postmenopausal patients. They cause a proliferation of the lining of the urethrovesical mucosa.
   d. **Muscle relaxants** (central acting), such as diazepam, tend to improve symptoms of frequency, urgency, and urge incontinence.
   e. **Cholinergic and anticholinesterase drugs** promote emptying of the bladder in cases of retention overflow.

7. **Mechanical devices**, such as catheters (indwelling and intermittent use), collecting devices, pads, and vaginal pessaries have palliative effects.

B. Surgical treatment.
Many procedures have proved quite successful in elevating the bladder neck and proximal urethra to the normal anatomic position, thus restoring the normal urethrovesical pressure differential. There are three basic surgical approaches.

1. **Vaginal cystourethropexy** is plication of the paraurethral and bladder neck tissues. This is the oldest, most commonly employed, and simplest procedure for the treatment of SUI. The anterior vaginal wall is dissected to expose the bladder neck and proximal urethra. The bladder is displaced upward and plicated by the Kelly technique. A vaginal hysterectomy and posterior colporrhaphy are also performed to strengthen the pelvic diaphragm and prevent future pelvic relaxation, which could result in descent of the bladder neck and proximal urethra. This procedure is employed for type I bladders with a cure rate of 75%–90%.

2. **Retropubic urethropexy** elevates the urethra and bladder neck by fixation to paraurethral and paravesical structures. A disadvantage of retropubic procedures is the delayed postoperative complication of **osteitis pubis**, which is an inflammation of the periosteum of bone, in this case, the pubis.
   a. **The Marshall-Marchetti-Krantz procedure** fixes the bladder neck and proximal urethra to the periosteum of the symphysis pubis. Long-term results are excellent with a cure rate of 85%–100%.
   b. **The Everard Williams procedure** fixes the bladder wall rather than paraurethral tissues to the periosteum of the symphysis pubis.

    c. The Burch procedure is fixation of the paraurethral and paravesical tissues to the ileopectineal ligament (Cooper's).

    d. The Peyrera procedure suspends the paraurethral and paravesical tissues on either side of the rectus sheet.

3. Sling procedures are rarely used as primary procedures, but the cure rate is good (90%). Because these procedures are very complicated and require additional materials, which can lead to infection and ulceration, they are often reserved for failed vaginal and retropubic procedures. Overcorrection with any of the procedures can lead to urinary retention. Three sling procedures are described below.

    a. The Aldridge sling procedure uses strips of the anterior abdominal oblique aponeurosis to elevate the bladder neck.

    b. The Goebell-Stoeckel-Frangenheim procedure uses the autogenous fascia lata strap as the sling.

    c. The Chassar moir sling uses mersilene tape.

STUDY QUESTIONS

Directions: Each question below contains five suggested answers. Choose the **one best** response to each question.

1. The most important etiologic abnormality in the anatomy of the urethra and bladder that leads to stress urinary incontinence is

(A) loss of estrogen in the postmenopausal period
(B) loss of normal urethral length
(C) loss of normal urethral position when supine
(D) loss of posterior urethrovesical angle
(E) rapid weight gain

2. Cystoscopy and cystometry are important in the evaluation of stress urinary incontinence because

(A) most causes other than bladder neck descent can be eliminated
(B) the posterior urethrovesical angle can be measured directly
(C) the angle of inclination can be estimated
(D) there is no risk of infection
(E) urethral length can be measured

3. Detrusor instability, an intrinsic bladder abnormality that can cause stress urinary incontinence, should be managed primarily by

(A) drug therapy
(B) electrical therapy
(C) operative therapy
(D) psychiatric therapy
(E) no therapy

Directions: Each question below contains four suggested answers of which **one or more** is correct. Choose the answer

    A   if **1, 2, and 3** are correct
    B   if **1 and 3** are correct
    C   if **2 and 4** are correct
    D   if **4** is correct
    E   if **1, 2, 3, and 4** are correct

4. The correct technique of the metallic bead chain cystourethrography includes which of the following steps?

(1) It requires the manual elevation of paraurethral tissues during the Valsalva maneuver
(2) The patient must stand with the feet spread apart to allow full mobility of the urethra
(3) The patient must stand because the symphysis pubis is not visible on x-ray in the sitting position
(4) Nonstraining films should always be taken first

Directions: The group of questions below consists of lettered choices followed by several numbered items. For each numbered item select the **one** lettered choice with which it is **most** closely associated. Each lettered choice may be used once, more than once, or not at all.

Questions 5–7

For each result described below, select the procedure most likely to be associated with it.

(A) Marshall-Marchetti-Krantz procedure
(B) Burch procedure
(C) Goebell-Stoeckel-Frangenheim procedure
(D) Peyrera procedure
(E) Kelly plication procedure

5. Associated with the complications of infection and ulceration

6. Suspends the urethra and vagina to the ileopectineal ligament

7. Associated with an excellent cure rate (85%–100%) but may be complicated by delayed postoperative osteitis pubis

ANSWERS AND EXPLANATIONS

1. The answer is D. (*I B 1; II C 7 c; Figure 32-1*) The normal posterior urethrovesical angle is 90–100 degrees. When standing, this implies that the bladder neck and proximal urethra are above the pelvic floor. When this relationship is lost, the normal pressure differential is also lost and incontinence results.

2. The answer is A. (*II C 3, 4*) Cystoscopy permits internal visualization of the bladder to detect neoplasms, infections, stones, fistulae, and the ureteral orifices. Cystometry allows assessment of bladder tone and dynamics, which completes the gamut of most causes of stress urinary incontinence. Only cystourethrography (metallic bead chain urethrocystogram) permits assessment of the anatomy of the bladder neck and proximal urethra.

3. The answer is A. (*II D 1; III A 6 a*) Chronic involuntary contractions of the detrusor muscle result in stress urinary incontinence (SUI) and should be treated with anticholinergic drugs to maintain stability of the muscle. If detrusor instability is found in combination with an anatomic alteration, surgery should be performed if relief is not satisfactory from drug therapy alone. When SUI does not respond to any therapy or no etiology is found, psychiatric evaluation is indicated.

4. The answer is C (2, 4). (*II C 5, 7*) It is of utmost importance that the correct technique of cystourethrography be followed to assess accurately the bladder neck–urethral spatial relationships. The patient must be erect with feet spread apart to allow full mobility (descent) of the bladder neck and proximal urethra. Nonstraining films must be taken first. The reverse may not allow time for the urethra to come to rest before obtaining the baseline film. The manual elevation of the paraurethral tissues is known as the Marchetti test. This simple test can be an aid in judging the potential success with surgery for stress incontinence.

5–7. The answers are: 5-C, 6-B, 7-A. (*III B 2 a, c, 3 b*) Infection and ulceration are a problem with sling procedures (e.g., Goebell-Stoeckel-Frangenheim procedure) because of the introduction of materials beneath the bladder neck in the retropubic space.

The Burch procedure, a retropubic urethropexy, fixes the paraurethral and paravesical tissues to the ileopectineal ligament, which corrects symptoms of prolapse, something that is not routinely possible with other procedures.

All retropubic procedures have excellent cure rates, but when the adjacent bone periosteum is used as in the Marshall-Marchetti-Krantz and Everard Williams procedures, a reaction may ensue (osteitis pubis) that proves to be a bothersome delayed complication in some cases.

The simplest and least complicated procedure is still the Kelly plication procedure, which is accompanied by an acceptable success rate of 75%–90%.

33
The Infertile Couple
Edward E. Wallach

I. INTRODUCTION

A. Definition. Conception is a complex process accomplished through a series of intricate steps. Thus, even couples with normal reproductive function may require several cycles to conceive. Infertility implies the inability to conceive. The **American Fertility Society** considers couples infertile when pregnancy has not occurred after 1 year of coitus without contraception. A "normal" cumulative fecundity curve has been proposed in which 95% of couples attempting pregnancy should conceive within 13 months.

1. **Primary infertility** refers to couples who have never established a pregnancy.

2. **Secondary infertility** refers to couples who have conceived previously but are currently unable to establish a subsequent pregnancy.

B. Incidence

1. Approximately 10% of couples are infertile, using the criteria of at least 1 year of unprotected coitus.

2. Approximately 15% of infertile couples have no identifiable cause of infertility.

II. PHYSIOLOGY OF CONCEPTION

A. Basic requirements for successful completion of the reproductive process

1. Release of ova from the ovaries (ovulation) on a regular cyclic basis

2. Production of an ejaculate containing an ample number of motile spermatozoa

3. Deposition of spermatozoa in the female reproductive tract, usually at or near the cervical os

4. Migration of the spermatozoa through the female reproductive tract to the fallopian tubes

5. Arrival of the recently ovulated ovum capable of being fertilized in the fallopian tube

6. Patency of the fallopian tube

7. Normal intrauterine environment from the cervix to fallopian tube lumen to enable active movement of spermatozoa capable of fertilizing an ovum

8. Conditions appropriate for fusion of gametes (ovum and spermatozoa) within the fallopian tube

B. Factors involved in fertility

1. Spermatogenesis (the male factor)

2. Ovulation (the ovarian factor)

3. Mucus and sperm interactions (the cervical factor)

4. Endometrial integrity and cavity size and shape (the uterine factor)

5. Oviductal patency and anatomic relationships to the ovary (the tubal factor)

6. Insemination (the coital factor)

III. INFERTILITY EVALUATION

A. **Male factor.** The male gamete can be examined in its own environment, seminal fluid, as well as in its new environment, cervical mucus. The following tests are used to evaluate the male factor.

1. **Semen analysis.** The customary standards for normalcy include the following ranges:
   a. Volume: 2.5–6.0 ml
   b. Count: more than 20×10^6/ml
   c. Motility: more than 75%
   d. Quality of motion: 3– or above when graded 1–4 (with + / –) going from poor to excellent (quality worsens with increasingly wobbly motion of spermatozoa)
   e. Morphology: more than 70% normal

2. **Postcoital test.** Mucus is examined microscopically between 2 and 12 hours after coitus at midcycle for total number of sperm seen per high-powered field and percentage and quality of motility. A satisfactory test is one in which many (more than 10) motile spermatozoa are seen per high-powered field. The results of the test are unsatisfactory if:
   a. No spermatozoa are seen.
   b. The majority of spermatozoa are immotile.
   c. Very few spermatozoa are present.
   d. Motility is characterized by a "shaking" movement rather than forward motility.
   e. Hostile cervical mucus is present.

3. **Sperm antibodies.** Occasionally antibodies to sperm may be present in the male or female and are responsible for fertility impairment. Sperm antibodies may be measured in:
   a. Seminal plasma
   b. Male serum
   c. Female reproductive tract fluids
   d. Female serum

4. **Tests of fertilizing capacity of spermatozoa** have been devised to assess the ability of sperm to fertilize an ovum.
   a. **Measurement of sperm acrosin,** an enzyme in the sperm head that is responsible for preliminary changes in the sperm, can determine fertilizing capacity.
   b. **Zona-free hamster ovum penetration test** measures the ability of spermatozoa to enter the ooplasm of the hamster egg when compared with control spermatozoa (such as donor sperm).
   c. **Human ovum fertilization test** is rarely performed except at the time of in vitro fertilization. This procedure evaluates the ability of sperm not only to penetrate the zona pellucida of a human egg but also to initiate cell cleavage.

B. **Coital factor.** Details of coital frequency and technique can help to determine if coital dysfunction is a cause of infertility. Coital dysfunction can be studied by:

1. Taking a history of coital frequency, patterns, technique, satisfaction, and use of adjuvants (creams, jellies, or douches)

2. Anatomic evaluation of the position of the cervix with relationship to the vagina

3. Postcoital testing

C. **Cervical factor.** The cervix is the first major barrier encountered by sperm after arrival in the female reproductive tract. Spermatozoa migrate rapidly through the endocervical canal and have been demonstrated in the fallopian tube as early as 5 minutes after deposition at the cervix.

1. **Abnormalities in the cervix or the cervical mucus** that interfere with sperm migration include:
   a. Abnormal position of the cervix (prolapse or uterine retroversion)
   b. Chronic infection, which may produce an unfavorable mucus (e.g., *Streptococcus, Staphylococcus,* and *Gardnerella*)
   c. Colonization with organisms that are cytotoxic to sperm (e.g., *Ureaplasma*)
   d. Previous cervical surgery (e.g., conization), which may lead to mucus depletion
   e. Previous electrocautery
   f. The presence of antisperm antibodies in the cervical mucus

2. **Mucus quality** can be assessed by physical, biochemical, and physiologic parameters including:
   a. pH, using Tes-Tape [an alkaline pH is optimum (pH 8.0)]
   b. Bacteriologic culture for microorganisms

    c. Crystallization (ferning) and spinnbarkeit (thread formation) of midcycle mucus
    d. Serologic tests for antibodies
    e. Postcoital testing
    f. Tests of sperm behavior in mucus
        (1) Examination of mucus after artificial placement of the partner's specimen
        (2) In vitro microscopic study of penetration of sperm through cervical mucus
        (3) In vitro cross-testing whereby the behavior of sperm in donor mucus is compared to the behavior of sperm in the patient's mucus, and the behavior of the partner's sperm is compared to the behavior of the donor sperm in the patient's mucus

D. Uterine factor. The uterus supports the journey of spermatozoa from the cervix to fallopian tube and performs many significant roles in reproduction.

    1. The roles of the uterus in reproduction include:
      a. Retention of the zygote after arrival from the fallopian tube for several days before implantation
      b. Provision of a suitable environment for implantation
      c. Protection of embryo/fetus from the external environment

    2. Evaluation of the uterine factor by:
      a. Endometrial sampling for histology by biopsy to determine:
        (1) The occurrence of ovulation when evidence of progesterone secretion (i.e., secretory endometrium) is found on biopsy
        (2) The duration of hormonal influence and defects in corpus luteum secretion of progesterone
        (3) The presence of infection (e.g., endometritis)
      b. Endometrial culture to identify bacterial organisms in the presence of endometritis
      c. Hysterography to visualize the contour of the uterine cavity, using a radiopaque contrast medium and fluoroscopy/radiography
      d. Hysteroscopy to visualize the uterine cavity to detect anomalous development, polyps, tumors, or adhesions (synechiae)
      e. Laparoscopy to detect and delineate anomalous uterine development or myomata. This procedure requires anesthesia and can be done at the time of hysteroscopy.

E. Tubal factor. The fallopian tube is responsible for efficient transfer of gametes and for fostering their approximation.

    1. Functions of the fallopian tube are twofold.
      a. Mechanical functions act to:
        (1) Convey recently ovulated ova into the fallopian tube
        (2) Permit spermatozoa to enter the oviduct
        (3) Effect transfer of the blastocyst into the uterine cavity
      b. Environmental functions provide for:
        (1) Fertilization of the ovum
        (2) Capacitation of spermatozoa
        (3) Early development and segmentation of the fertilized ovum

    2. Tests used to evaluate the function of the fallopian tube evaluate patency, location with respect to the ovary, and, to a lesser extent, function.
      a. Hysterosalpingography enables visualization of the lumen and patency of the fallopian tube using a radiopaque contrast medium.
      b. Laparoscopy allows direct visualization of the fallopian tube in order to identify abnormalities in structure or location and detect peritubal adhesions. This procedure is usually carried out in conjunction with transcervical lavage with a dye (usually indigo carmine) as a test of tubal patency.
      c. Tubal insufflation with carbon dioxide and manometric measurements of pressure is rarely performed today.
      d. Other rarely performed procedures
        (1) Pneumosalpingography (hysterosalpingography combined with pneumoperitoneum)
        (2) Phenolsulfonphthalein (PSP) testing in which the dye is placed in the uterine cavity and found excreted in the urine, suggesting transperitoneal absorption
        (3) Methylene blue lavage of the uterus with methylene blue dye and recovery of dye from the pouch of Douglas

F. Ovarian factor. The ovarian factor refers to the ability of the ovaries to release ova on a cyclic basis.

1. **Ovarian functions**
   a. The ovaries serve as a repository for oocytes and release matured oocytes at regular intervals throughout reproductive life.
   b. The ovaries secrete steroid hormones that influence the structure and function of tissues in the reproductive tract, promoting fertility.

2. **Documentation of ovulation**
   a. **Direct means** (impractical)
      (1) Observation of ovulation at laparoscopy or laparotomy
      (2) Recovery of an ovum from the fallopian tube or uterus
      (3) Establishment of pregnancy
   b. **Indirect means** (practical)
      (1) Basal body temperature records demonstrate a 14-day elevation of basal temperature beginning at or after ovulation, as a result of progesterone secretion, which has a thermogenic effect.
      (2) Elevated blood progesterone levels, exceeding 3 ng/ml, are usually found after ovulation and corpus luteum formation.
      (3) Endometrial biopsy demonstrates the characteristic histologic changes of the endometrium achieved by circulating progesterone levels, namely, a secretory endometrial pattern.

3. **Corpus luteum production of progesterone** must be sufficient to prepare the endometrium for implantation and maintenance of the pregnancy. Defects in luteal function can be reflected by:
   a. Short life span of the corpus luteum with a thermal shift of less than 12 days.
   b. Reduced progesterone production during the luteal phase.

4. **Reasons for ovulatory defects**
   a. Hypothalamic–pituitary insufficiency
      (1) Tumors or destructive lesions
      (2) Drugs that interfere with normal hypothalamic function
      (3) Hyperprolactinemia due to a pituitary adenoma
   b. Thyroid disease
      (1) Hypothyroidism
      (2) Hyperthyroidism
   c. Adrenal disorders
      (1) Adrenal insufficiency
      (2) Hyperadrenalism
         (a) Cortisol excess
         (b) Androgen excess
   d. Emotional disturbances
   e. Metabolic and nutritional disorders
      (1) Obesity
      (2) Malnutrition
   f. Excessive exercise (e.g., running and dancing)

IV. **THERAPY.** Treatment is based upon documentation of the abnormality or abnormalities leading to infertility and can include surgical or medical means.

A. **Correction of male factor**

1. **Medical**
   a. Correction of underlying deficiencies (e.g., thyroid disorders, prolactin excess, and dietary disturbances)
   b. Artificial donor insemination

2. **Surgical**
   a. Reversal of sterilization
   b. Varicocele surgery

B. **Correction of coital factor**

1. Psychotherapy

2. Sexual therapy

3. Artificial insemination, using partner's sperm

C. Correction of cervical factor

  1. Low-dose estrogen therapy

  2. Antibiotics

  3. Either cervical or intrauterine artificial insemination

  4. Corticosteroids for antisperm antibodies

  5. Human gonadotropins

  6. In vitro fertilization and embryo transfer

D. Correction of uterine factor

  1. Medical
    a. Antibiotic therapy for endometritis
    b. High-dose estrogen/estrogen–progestogen therapy for endometritis, following removal of intrauterine adhesions

  2. Surgical
    a. Myomectomy for myomata
    b. Metroplasty in certain anomalies
    c. Removal of intrauterine synechiae

E. Correction of tubal factor

  1. Tubal anastomosis for reversal of sterilization

  2. Salpingoplasty for occluded fallopian tubes, distal or proximal

  3. Lysis of peritubal adhesions

  4. In vitro fertilization and embryo transfer when fallopian tubes are absent or irreparable

F. Correction of ovarian factor

  1. Induction of ovulation
    a. Correction of underlying endocrine disorders, such as thyroid disease
    b. Clomiphene citrate to correct hypothalamic dysfunction
    c. Human gonadotropins for pituitary insufficiency or when clomiphene citrate fails
    d. Bromocryptine for anovulation due to prolactin excess
    e. Glucocorticoids for androgen excess due to adrenal hyperplasia

  2. Correction of luteal phase defects
    a. Clomiphene citrate
    b. Human chorionic gonadotropin
    c. Postovulatory progesterone supplementation
    d. Human gonadotropins [follicle-stimulating hormone and luteinizing hormone (Pergonal)]

G. Unexplained infertility

  1. With in vitro fertilization and embryo transfer (IVF/ET), the ovum is fertilized in a culture dish after cell division (8–16 cell stage). The embryo is then placed back into the uterus.

  2. In gamete intrafallopian transfer (GIFT), the ovum and the spermatozoa are mixed and together are placed in the fallopian tube via the laparoscope; fertilization occurs in the fallopian tube.

STUDY QUESTIONS

Directions: Each question below contains five suggested answers. Choose the **one best** response to each question.

1. Abnormalities in the cervical mucus may result from all of the following conditions EXCEPT

(A) colonization of the cervix with cytotoxic organisms
(B) uterine retroversion
(C) chronic infection of the cervix
(D) previous electrocauterization of the cervix
(E) antisperm antibodies

2. Defects in corpus luteum function may be demonstrated by all the following procedures EXCEPT

(A) basal body temperature
(B) endometrial biopsy and histologic dating
(C) measurement of serum progesterone levels
(D) determination of the length of the luteal phase
(E) measurement of serum estrogen levels

3. All of the following procedures are appropriate for evaluation of the endometrial cavity EXCEPT

(A) laparoscopy
(B) endometrial biopsy
(C) hysteroscopy
(D) endometrial culture
(E) hysterography

4. Therapy for the correction of a cervical factor in infertility includes all of the following EXCEPT

(A) intrauterine insemination
(B) low-dose estrogen
(C) antibiotics
(D) human chorionic gonadotropin injection
(E) in vitro fertilization and embryo transfer

5. All of the following factors are evidence that ovulation has occurred EXCEPT

(A) rise in the basal body temperature
(B) pregnancy
(C) progesterone level above 3 ng/ml
(D) secretory endometrium
(E) the occurrence of menses

Directions: Each question below contains four suggested answers of which **one or more** is correct. Choose the answer

A   if **1, 2, and 3** are correct
B   if **1 and 3** are correct
C   if **2 and 4** are correct
D   if **4** is correct
E   if **1, 2, 3, and 4** are correct

6. The postcoital test examines cervical mucus at some point following intercourse. Correct statements about this procedure include which of the following?

(1) It is performed 2–12 hours after coitus
(2) It tests sperm and mucus interaction
(3) It is satisfactory when more than 10 motile sperm per high-powered field are seen
(4) It is performed early in the luteal phase

7. Important functions of the ovary include

(1) secretion of human chorionic gonadotropin
(2) release of mature oocytes
(3) regulation of cervical mucus
(4) secretion of steroid hormones

8. Indications for in vitro fertilization include which of the following?

(1) Poor coital technique (impotence)
(2) Absent cervical mucus
(3) Endometritis
(4) Tubal disease

9. Clomiphene citrate is used to correct which of the following clinical problems?

(1) Infrequent ovulation
(2) High prolactin levels
(3) A corpus luteum defect
(4) Cervical mucus of poor quality

ANSWERS AND EXPLANATIONS

1. The answer is B. (*III C 1 a–f*) Both conization and electrocauterization of the cervix destroy cervical endothelium and thus reduce or eliminate epithelium capable of producing mucus. Infection produces a viscous, hostile mucus with respect to spermatozoa. Antisperm antibodies also create a hostile mucus that inhibits sperm motility. Uterine retroversion has nothing to do with the cervical mucus. Because of the consequent anterior cervix in a retroverted uterus, there can be an insemination problem.

2. The answer is E. [*III D 2 a, F 2 b (1)–(3), 3*] Measurement of serum estrogen levels is not useful when assessing a suspected inadequate luteal phase because progesterone is the hormone responsible for the luteal phase. The basal body temperature may show a slow rise and a short span of 10 days or less. Measurement of serum progesterone levels is helpful as it will be lower than the norm. Endometrial biopsy will show a lag of at least 48 hours between the histologic dating and the cycle day of the biopsy.

3. The answer is A. (*III D 2 a–e*) Various clinical problems can occur within the endometrial cavity that contribute to infertility, such as, chronic infection, inadequate hormonal preparation of the endometrium, submucous myomas, polyps, or adhesions. Tests, such as endometrial culture and biopsy, hysteroscopy for direct visualization of the cavity, and hysterography for the radiographic outline of the cavity are helpful in defining these problems. Laparoscopy is not helpful because the laparoscope cannot see into the uterine cavity; it merely reveals the external surface and is used to define anomalous uterine development.

4. The answer is D (*IV C 1–6*) Poor cervical mucus that is hostile to the penetration of spermatozoa can be a major factor in infertility. The poor cervical mucus may be due to inadequate estrogen preparation of the mucus or infection. Therefore, low-dose estrogen or antibiotics could be used. With persistently poor cervical mucus despite therapy, the cervix may have to be bypassed with either intrauterine insemination or in vitro fertilization with implantation of the embryo. Human chorionic gonadotropin is not useful because it has no way of stimulating estrogen production. It could, however, be used at ovulation to help stimulate the secretion of progesterone from the corpus luteum.

5. The answer is E. (*III F 2 a, b*) Pregnancy is the best possible way to document ovulation. The other methods listed in the question depend on the secretion of progesterone from the corpus luteum, and the corpus luteum does not exist in the absence of ovulation. The secretory endometrium and the rise in the basal body temperature are reflective of progesterone secretion and, thus, ovulation. The menses can occur in the absence of ovulation as happens in dysfunctional uterine bleeding.

6. The answer is A (1, 2, 3). (*III A 2*) The postcoital test is timed to coincide with ovulation when cervical mucus is the most receptive to spermatozoa. Performing the test in the luteal phase would be too late because the mucus would not be favorable as ovulation would have already occurred. The test is performed 2–12 hours after coitus and is a good in vivo test of sperm and mucus interaction. A good test reveals at least 10 motile sperm per high-powered field.

7. The answer is C (2, 4). (*III F 1 a, b*) The ovary has two main functions: the regular release of mature oocytes and the secretion of steroid hormones that influence the structure and function of tissues in the reproductive tract. Trophoblastic or placental tissue secretes human chorionic gonadotropin. The regulation of the cervical mucus is controlled by estrogen, which is secreted by the ovary. However, estrogen has many other functions, and the ovary would secrete estrogen whether or not there was any possibility of cervical mucus production.

8. The answer is C (2, 4). (*IV C 6, E 4*) Poor coital technique, due to impotence, is solved by psychotherapy or partner insemination. Endometritis is treated with antibiotics. In vitro fertilization and embryo transfer are used with infertility patients when the sperm cannot get to the ovum because of tubal disease, which prevents the ovum from entering the tube, or absent cervical mucus, in which case the sperm cannot get into the reproductive tract to migrate to the tube.

9. The answer is B (1, 3). (*IV F 1 b, 2 a*) The primary use for clomiphene citrate is the induction of ovulation. Infrequent ovulations suggest the use of clomiphene to increase the likelihood of conception. By improving the quality of the cycle, clomiphene corrects a defect in the corpus luteum. Bromocryptine reduces the level of prolactin, and low-dose estrogen can be used to correct the poor quality of the cervical mucus.

I. INTRODUCTION

A. Amenorrhea is the absence of menses, which may be eugonadotropic, hypergonadotropic, or hypogonadotropic. It is important to realize that amenorrhea is not a diagnosis in and of itself, but is a symptom, indicating an anatomic, genetic, biochemical, physiologic, or emotional abnormality. The pathophysiology of amenorrhea must be understood in terms of the physiology of menstruation.

1. Physiologic amenorrhea, the absence of menses prior to or directly after menarche, during pregnancy and lactation, and after the menopause, is not a manifestation of disease and need not be evaluated.

a. A significant number of teenage girls have intervals of amenorrhea lasting 2–12 months during the first 2 years after menarche.

b. Spontaneous menopause may occur in women in their mid-thirties.

2. Pathologic amenorrhea is suspected in the following situations:

a. At 14 years of age in the absence of both menstruation and secondary sexual characteristics

b. At 16 years of age regardless of whether or not there are secondary sexual characteristics

c. At any age in which there has been a cessation of menses in a woman who previously had normal menstrual function

B. Menstruation depends on the following interrelated factors that culminate in the visible discharge of menstrual blood. An interruption of any of these can result in amenorrhea.

1. An intact outflow tract, which assumes patency and continuity of the vaginal orifice, the vaginal canal, and the uterine cavity

2. An endometrium that is responsive to hormonal stimulation

3. An intact hypothalamic–pituitary–ovarian axis, allowing the sequential elaboration of steroid hormones from the ovary. The cascade begins in the hypothalamus with the secretion of gonadotropin-releasing hormone (GnRH), which stimulates the pituitary to release the gonadotropins: follicle-stimulating hormone (FSH) and luteinizing hormone (LH).

4. Secretion of estrogen from the ovary, resulting ultimately in ovulation with the secretion of progesterone as a result of FSH and LH stimulation.

II. EUGONADOTROPIC AMENORRHEA.

The eugonadotropic causes of amenorrhea involve congenital and acquired anomalies of the uterus and the outflow tract as well as some forms of androgen excess. The ovaries are functional, producing normal levels of estrogen and progesterone, and the usual feedback to the pituitary results in normal gonadotropin levels.

A. Congenital anomalies

1. The Rokitansky-Küster-Hauser syndrome, the most common congenital anomaly of the uterus, is characterized by:

a. Failure of fusion of the two müllerian ducts, vaginal agenesis, normal ovaries, and kidney abnormalities

b. Delayed menarche and the presence of a vaginal pouch

2. Imperforate hymen and transverse vaginal septum, also causes for delayed menarche, are characterized by:

a. Normal sexual development, pelvic pain, urinary frequency, and a perineal bulge (in patients with an imperforate hymen)

    b. Continued reflux of menstrual debris, which can lead to endometriosis and impaired future fertility, making these diagnoses relative emergencies

B. Acquired anomalies

    1. Asherman's syndrome is an acquired form of uterine dysfunction. The amenorrhea associated with this syndrome is caused by intrauterine adhesions that partially or completely obliterate the uterine cavity. The cause of these adhesions is traumatization of the endometrium and myometrium as a result of a vigorous curettage of the postabortal or postpartum uterus (because of bleeding) upon which is superimposed an endometritis.

    2. Tuberculosis can lead to scarring of the endometrial cavity, causing amenorrhea, but this etiology is now rare in the United States.

C. Androgen excess from either the adrenal gland or the ovary can cause amenorrhea.

    1. Androgen excess from the adrenal gland may be secondary to a virilizing tumor or congenital adrenal hyperplasia.

    2. Androgen excess from the ovary may be due to a rare virilizing ovarian tumor or the more common polycystic ovarian syndrome. The latter results in an hirsute patient who is well estrogenized due to the conversion of excess amounts of the weak androgen, androstenedione, to testosterone and estrone.

III. HYPERGONADOTROPIC AMENORRHEA, or primary amenorrhea, involves gonadal, chromosomal, or genetic defects that inhibit the normal hormonal feedback mechanisms to suppress the secretion of gonadotropin.

A. Chromosomal abnormalities. Patients with sex chromosomal abnormalities (45,XO or mosaicism) and absent or limited ovarian function are categorized as having **gonadal dysgenesis**. They usually express phenotypic differences, such as short stature. Identification of Y chromosomal material in these patients is essential because of the malignant potential of such a gonad.

B. Normal chromosomes

    1. Pure gonadal dysgenesis encompasses that group of women with ovarian failure who are phenotypically normal and who have 46,XX or 46,XY karyotypes. Receptor problems are evident in both karyotypes.

    2. Resistant ovary syndrome encompasses women with 46,XX karyotypes who present with amenorrhea and who have an ovarian membrane receptor defect. Gonadotropin levels are elevated because the ovaries do not:
      a. Respond to gonadotropin
      b. Secrete hormones
      c. Suppress the pituitary

    3. Androgen insensitivity syndrome, or testicular feminization syndrome, is characterized by patients who are gonadal males (46,XY) but phenotypic females. Other characteristics include the following:
      a. The cytosol receptors for testosterone are defective.
      b. The testosterone level is in the male range, but there is no biologic evidence of circulating testosterone, such as pubic and axillary hair.
      c. Patients have a vaginal pouch with no uterine remnants due to the active presence of testicular müllerian-inhibiting factor.
      d. These patients should not have their gonads removed until after full sexual development as the risk of dysgerminoma or other gonadal neoplasms is minimal until the patient is over 20 years of age.
      e. Pubescence occurs normally in the presence of the patient's own endogenous hormones.

IV. HYPOGONADOTROPIC AMENORRHEA, or secondary amenorrhea, occurs after a menstrual pattern has been established. Most hypogonadotropic amenorrheas are acquired, resulting from a number of different causes: emotional stress, drugs, diseases of the pituitary, nutritional deficiencies, excessive exercise, and abnormalities of the adrenal and thyroid glands. These amenorrheas are both hypogonadotropic and hypoestrogenic.

A. Kallmann's syndrome. This is the most common congenital form of hypogonadotropic amenorrhea. There is both an irreversible defect in gonadotropin synthesis and an olfactory sensory defect.

B. Emotional stress. The most common forms of acquired hypogonadotropic amenorrhea are psychogenic in nature, occurring in association with either acute or chronic emotional stress.

C. Nutritional deficiency. Hypothalamic suppression in patients with classic anorexia nervosa is often manifested by secondary amenorrhea.

D. Excessive exercise. Women who are able to maintain a borderline body weight but who undergo strenuous physical activity, such as marathon running, swimming, gymnastics, or ballet, may all present with secondary amenorrhea.

E. Drugs. Drug-induced amenorrheas include those associated with birth control pills, phenothiazine derivatives, reserpine, and ganglion-blocking agents.

    1. Less than 1% of women on birth control pills experience amenorrhea on discontinuation, and many of these had menstrual irregularities prior to using the pills.

    2. The other drugs listed affect the hypothalamus, probably the dopamine/norepinephrine balance, and are sometimes associated with galactorrhea.

F. Diseases of the pituitary. Pituitary tumors and ischemia and necrosis of the pituitary can lead to amenorrhea.

    1. The pituitary tumors include craniopharyngiomas (in the younger age group), chromophobe adenomas, and prolactin-producing adenomas. These tumors may be accompanied by neurologic symptoms (blindness), galactorrhea, and signs of other tropic hormone deficiencies, including hypothyroidism, amenorrhea, and Addison's disease.

    2. Ischemia and necrosis of the pituitary gland secondary to obstetric shock (blood loss) are associated with varying degrees of insufficiency of all the pituitary tropic hormones.

G. Other hormonal etiologies. Amenorrhea is also seen secondary to thryoid or adrenal hyper- or hypofunction; the thyroid component of amenorrhea is the more common of the two.

V. EVALUATION OF AMENORRHEA

A. History. The first step in the workup of a patient with amenorrhea is a detailed history, which should include:

    1. The age of the patient, the presence or absence of secondary sexual characteristics, and the time of the onset of the amenorrhea.

    2. A history of emotional stress, weight gain or loss, eating habits, exercise program, use of medication, recent pregnancy, body hair growth, symptoms suggestive of thyroid or adrenal disease, or galactorrhea.

    3. A history of sexual exposure to rule out the possibility of pregnancy. (Discretion is necessary when eliciting sexual histories from young patients.)

B. Physical examination. The physical examination can be instructive by either the presence or absence of findings.

    1. In the case of delayed menarche, it is important to evaluate the status of the secondary sexual characteristics, the presence or absence of a functional vagina, and a palpable mass on rectal examination.

    2. Evidence of defeminization, masculinization, thyroid or adrenal dysfunction, and somatic abnormalities can help to formulate a differential diagnosis.

C. Laboratory studies. The appropriate tests depend on whether or not a patient has ever had a menstrual flow and on her pelvic examination. If there has been previous menstrual function, the physician can assume that the ovaries have functioned and that there is a patent outflow tract.

    1. Previous menstrual function
        a. Measurement of serum human chorionic gonadotropin (HCG) levels to rule out the possibility of pregnancy
        b. A progesterone challenge [medroxyprogesterone (Provera), 10 mg per day for 5 days] to determine the status of the hypothalamic–pituitary–ovarian axis
           (1) There will be no progesterone withdrawal flow in the absence of estrogen priming of the endometrium or in the presence of a nonfunctional endometrium.

(2) Progesterone withdrawal in the presence of amenorrhea indicates anovulation with estrogen secretion.

c. **Evaluation of endometrial potential**

(1) The evaluation is accomplished by the sequential use of estrogen and progesterone (a conjugated estrogen, 2.5 mg daily for 21 days, with medroxyprogesterone, 20 mg daily for the last 5 days of the estrogen therapy).

(2) Subsequent bleeding suggests one of the hypo- or hypergonadotropic amenorrheas.

(3) Absence of bleeding suggests either an abnormal outflow tract or a nonfunctional endometrium (as in Asherman's syndrome).

(4) The existence of a nonfunctional endometrium can be confirmed by hysterosalpingography or hysteroscopy.

d. **Measurement of prolactin levels**

(1) A normal level in the presence of a progesterone withdrawal flow and the absence of galactorrhea essentially eliminates the possibility of a pituitary tumor.

(2) An elevated level demands a workup of the pituitary gland.

(a) An abnormal coned-down view (x-ray) of the pituitary requires a CAT scan.

(b) A normal coned-down view requires polytomography of the pituitary to evaluate the abnormal prolactin level.

(c) Abnormal polytomography requires a CAT scan.

(d) Thyroid-stimulating hormone (TSH) is the most sensitive evaluation of hypothyroidism. Elevated TSH in hypothyroidism stimulates the pituitary lactotropes to give the elevated prolactin levels.

e. **Measurement of plasma testosterone and dehydroepiandrosterone sulfate** (DHEASO$_4$), which may be elevated in diseases of the ovary and the adrenal gland

f. **Thyroid indices** (T$_3$ and T$_4$), A.M. and P.M. cortisol, and a glucose tolerance test to diagnose the cause of the amenorrhea

2. **No previous menstrual function**

a. **Measurement of serum gonadotropin levels**

(1) High levels of FSH (over 40 mIU/ml) indicate gonadal failure as the cause of the amenorrhea.

(2) High levels of FSH dictate that a karyotype be done to determine the sex chromosomes and to rule out the presence of a Y chromosome.

(3) Low levels of FSH indicate pituitary failure or inactivity, the latter probably due to hypothalamic dysfunction.

b. **Intravenous pyelogram.** This should be obtained on all patients with any degree of müllerian dysgenesis because of the renal abnormalities that are associated with the developmental abnormalities of the müllerian system.

c. **Laparoscopy.** Visual examination of the pelvis may be necessary to delineate the extent of müllerian dysgenesis or to ascertain the nature of the dysgenetic gonad (i.e., the streak ovary).

VI. TREATMENT OF AMENORRHEA

A. **Eugonadotropic amenorrhea**

1. **Congenital anomalies**

a. Incision of an imperforate hymen or a transverse vaginal septum to establish outlet patency and to release accumulated menstrual blood

b. Creation of an artificial vagina to correct the vaginal agenesis seen in some forms of müllerian dysgenesis

2. **Acquired anomalies. Asherman's syndrome** should be treated in the following ways:

a. Dilatation and curettage with or without hysteroscopy

b. Insertion of a pediatric Foley catheter or an intrauterine device to keep the uterine cavity open

c. Sequential hormonal therapy with high-dose estrogen (10 mg of conjugated estrogen daily for 21 days with medroxyprogesterone, 10 mg daily during the last week) for 6 months to help reestablish the endometrium

d. Antibiotics for 10 days

B. **Hypergonadotropic amenorrhea.** There is no curative therapy for these amenorrheas.

1. Estrogen replacement is administered to dysgenetic patients for the development of secondary sexual characteristics (2.5 mg of conjugated estrogen for 21 days with medroxyprogesterone, 10 mg daily for the last 7 days).

   2. Sequential hormonal therapy is given as above to maintain secondary sexual characteristics whenever a deficiency develops.

   3. Surgical excision of gonads containing Y chromosomal material should be undertaken:
      a. Prior to puberty or at the time of discovery in dysgenetic patients with abnormal chromosomes
      b. Following puberty in dysgenetic patients with normal chromosomes, such as with the androgen insensitivity syndrome

C. Hypogonadotropic amenorrhea. Therapy depends on the patient's desires regarding pregnancy or the presence or absence of regular menses, unless the situation is potentially life-threatening as with a pituitary tumor.

   1. Periodic progestin is administered to anovulatory patients who do not desire pregnancy (medroxyprogesterone, 10 mg daily for 5 days every 8 weeks).

   2. Ovulation is induced with clomiphene or gonadotropins in women who desire a pregnancy.

   3. Bromocryptine is recommended for patients with hyperprolactinemia and a normal pituitary or microadenomas.

   4. Surgery is recommended for central nervous system tumors.

   5. Thyroid or adrenal medication is given as indicated.

STUDY QUESTIONS

Directions: Each question below contains five suggested answers. Choose the **one best** response to each question.

1. The occurrence of menstruation is dependent upon all of the following factors EXCEPT

(A) hypothalamic-releasing hormone
(B) an endometrium responsive to sex steroids
(C) gonadotropins
(D) patent fallopian tubes
(E) ovarian steroidal hormones

2. Which of the following statements regarding the testicular feminization syndrome is correct?

(A) The testosterone level is in the male range, resulting in pubic and axillary hair
(B) The gonads should not be removed until after full sexual development
(C) The risk of dysgerminoma or other gonadal neoplasms is great until 20 years of age
(D) Pubescence is delayed because of the absence of endogenous hormones
(E) None of the above statements is true

3. All of the following conditions can be found in a patient with a pituitary chromophobe adenoma EXCEPT

(A) amenorrhea
(B) hypothyroidism
(C) galactorrhea
(D) blindness
(E) Cushing's syndrome

Directions: Each question below contains four suggested answers of which **one or more** is correct. Choose the answer

    A if **1, 2, and 3** are correct
    B if **1 and 3** are correct
    C if **2 and 4** are correct
    D if **4** is correct
    E if **1, 2, 3, and 4** are correct

4. Elevated gonadotropins are expected with which of the following conditions associated with amenorrhea?

(1) Rokitansky-Küster-Hauser syndrome
(2) Kallmann's syndrome
(3) Anorexia nervosa
(4) Gonadal dysgenesis

5. The development of adhesions seen in Asherman's syndrome is commonly preceded by which of the following events?

(1) Delivery
(2) Endometritis
(3) Dilatation and curettage
(4) Postabortal hemorrhage

6. Clinical conditions that are suitable for clomiphene stimulation of ovulation include

(1) gonadal dysgenesis
(2) Asherman's syndrome
(3) resistant ovary syndrome
(4) psychogenic amenorrhea

Directions: The group of questions below consists of lettered choices followed by several numbered items. For each numbered item select the **one** lettered choice with which it is **most** closely associated. Each lettered choice may be used once, more than once, or not at all.

Questions 7–9

For each of the following clinical situations, select the laboratory study that would be most appropriate.

(A) Gonadotropin levels
(B) Serum prolactin levels
(C) Progesterone challenge
(D) Thyroid-stimulating hormone levels
(E) Serum testosterone levels

7.   A 24-year-old nulligravida stopped taking birth control pills in order to conceive. After the last pill withdrawal flow, she was amenorrheic for 6 months.

8.   A 24-year-old primipara returns 6 months postpartum, complaining of amenorrhea. Her pregnancy terminated with a cesarean section because of abruptio placentae and fetal distress with an estimated blood loss of 2000 ml due to a transient coagulation problem.

9.   A 24-year-old woman with previously normal menstrual cycles develops irregular cycles and anovulation. Serum prolactin levels are elevated.

ANSWERS AND EXPLANATIONS

1. The answer is D. (*I B 1–4*) Menstruation depends on a series of interrelated events that culminate in the visible discharge of menstrual blood. It is a cascade phenomenon that involves the stimulation of the pituitary by hypothalamic-releasing hormone with secretion of gonadotropins. These gonadotropins stimulate the ovary to release steroidal hormones (estrogen and progesterone), which produce changes in a responsive endometrium. This whole process takes place with or without patent fallopian tubes as the tubes are not involved in menstruation.

2. The answer is B. (*III A, B 3 a–e*) One of the entities with normal chromosomes in the group of diseases characterized by gonadal dysgenesis is the XY gonad found in the testicular feminization syndrome. That gonad has a much lower malignant potential than the dysgenetic gonad with Y material and abnormal chromosomes. Pubescence occurs normally in these patients so they should not have their gonads removed until after sexual development has occurred.

3. The answer is E. (*IV F 1, 2*) The pituitary tumors can produce galactorrhea, neurologic signs (blindness) because of the close proximity of the optic nerve, and signs of other tropic hormone deficiencies, such as hypothyroidism, amenorrhea, and Addison's disease. Cushing's syndrome would not be found in these patients because it is a disease of cortisol excess, and the opposite would be expected with an adrenocorticotropic hormone deficiency.

4. The answer is D (4). (*II A 1; III B 1; IV A, C*) Even though the Rokitansky-Küster-Hauser syndrome is characterized by müllerian deficiencies, the ovaries are normal and so are the gonadotropin levels. Because of hypothalamic suppression, the gonadotropins are low in the nutritional deficiency that characterizes anorexia nervosa. Gonadotropin levels are low in Kallmann's syndrome because there is a congenital defect in gonadotropin synthesis. Gonadal dysgenesis is characterized by sex chromosomal abnormalities and absent or limited ovarian function. Because the ovaries do not secrete estrogen, there is no negative feedback on the pituitary, and thus, the gonadotropin levels remain high.

5. The answer is E (all). (*II B 1*) Asherman's syndrome, characterized by intrauterine adhesions, is an acquired form of uterine dysfunction. A common history preceding the establishment of the adhesions, which partially or completely obliterate the uterine cavity, involves the curettage of a postpartum or a postabortal uterus upon which is superimposed an endometritis. Postabortal hemorrhage may be a component in the pathophysiology of Asherman's syndrome, in that it may have been the reason for the curettage.

6. The answer is D (4). (*II B 1; III B 1–3; IV B; VI C 2*) Clomiphene citrate is an ovulation-inducing drug, which stimulates the pituitary gland to secrete the gonadotropins necessary to induce the ovaries to ovulate. Therefore, clomiphene would not be useful in clinical conditions in which the gonadotropin levels are already high, such as gonadal dysgenesis or resistant ovary syndrome. The amenorrhea of Asherman's syndrome is due to intrauterine adhesions, not low gonadotropin levels. The women with amenorrheas associated with low gonadotropin levels are candidates for clomiphene therapy if they desire pregnancy; these include women with the psychogenic (emotional stress) amenorrheas.

7–9. The answers are: 7-B, 8-A, 9-D. [*IV E 1, F 2; V C 1 d (1), (2) (d), 2 a (3)*] The most important diagnosis to make in an amenorrheic woman coming off birth control pills is a pituitary adenoma. She could be amenorrheic because of the pills, but it is essential not to miss a pituitary lesion. Thus, measurement of serum prolactin should be the first test ordered.

From the clinical history of the 24-year-old primipara, the physician can assume that the patient was in shock and suffered ischemia or necrosis of the pituitary gland. In this situation, there may be deficiencies of all the pituitary tropic hormones. Amenorrhea is the most obvious sign, so measurement of gonadotropin levels would be the appropriate test in this patient.

One cause of hyperprolactinemia is an elevated thyroid-stimulating hormone (TSH) level with stimulation of the lactotropes found in hypothyroidism. Thus, measurement of TSH levels would be indicated to rule out hypothyroidism as the cause of the hyperprolactinemia.

35
Hirsutism
William W. Beck, Jr.

I. INTRODUCTION. Increased hair growth in a woman may be associated with normal or increased levels of circulating androgens. It is important to view hirsutism as a potential endocrine abnormality as well as a psychological and cosmetic problem.

A. Definitions

1. **Hypertrichosis** involves excessive growth of nonsexual hair, including eyebrows, eyelashes, and hair on the forearms and lower legs.

2. **Hirsutism** involves increased growth of male-like, pigmented, terminal hairs on midline portions of the body, including the face, chest, abdomen, and inner thigh. It may be accompanied by anovulatory amenorrhea, dysfunctional uterine bleeding, or infertility.

3. **Virilization** involves hirsutism accompanied by increased muscle mass, clitorimegaly, temporal balding, voice deepening, and increased libido. There may also be signs of defeminization, such as decreased breast size and loss of vaginal lubrication.

B. Etiology. Cosmetically disturbing hirsutism is the result of:

1. The number of hair follicles present; for example, hirsutism is rarely seen in Asian women who have low concentrations of hair follicles.

2. The degree to which androgens are actively available to convert vellus hairs, which are finely textured and relatively unpigmented, to terminal hairs, which are coarse, thick, and pigmented, in the male sexual hair areas

3. The ratio of growth to resting phases in affected hair follicles

4. The thickness and degree to which individual hairs are pigmented

II. ANDROGENS. Androgens are steroids that promote the development of masculine secondary sexual characteristics and that cause nitrogen retention. In women, androgens are thought to be derived from three major sources—the adrenal gland, the ovary, and the peripheral transformation of preandrogens, such as dehydroepiandrosterone (DHEA), DHEA sulfate, and androstenedione, to testosterone. This transformation is thought to occur in the liver with extrahepatic conversion in tissues, such as skin, particularly in patients that manifest hirsutism. The most important androgen is **testosterone.**

A. Total testosterone. Blood testosterone levels are a function of blood production rates and metabolic clearance rates; thus, blood levels may not represent the actual state of androgenicity.

1. Total testosterone levels are as follows:
   a. **Normal women:** 30 ng/100 ml
   b. **Hirsute women:** 120 ng/100 ml
      (1) As a group, hirsute women have elevated total testosterone levels, but tests are not specific enough to answer questions about excess androgen production unless it is in the male range, which suggests a tumor.
      (2) For clinical purposes, every woman with hirsutism has an increased production rate of testosterone. However, mild elevations do not localize the cause of the elevated level.
   c. **Men:** 600 ng/100 ml

2. Circulating testosterone in women is derived from the following sources:
   a. **Ovarian origin** (probably the stroma): 5%–20%
   b. **Adrenal origin:** 0%–30%

    c. Peripheral transformation: 50%–70%

B. Free testosterone

    1. Most testosterone in the blood circulates bound either to albumin or to a binding globulin; only a small portion exists in the free form.
      a. Normal women: 1.6%
      b. Hirsute women: 2.6%
      c. Men: 2.85%

    2. Free testosterone seems to correlate well with the state of excess androgenicity and with testosterone production rates.
      a. Normal women: 250 μg/day
      b. Hirsute women: 600 μg/day
      c. Men: 7000 μg/day

C. Sex hormone binding globulin (SHBG)

    1. Most circulating testosterone is tightly bound and not biologically active.

    2. As SHBG decreases, the percentage of free testosterone increases; when SHBG increases, the percentage of free testosterone decreases.
      a. There is a decrease in plasma SHBG in:
        (1) Obesity
        (2) Increased androgen production
        (3) Corticosteroid therapy
        (4) Hypothyroidism
        (5) Acromegaly
      b. There is an increase in plasma SHBG with:
        (1) Estrogen therapy
        (2) Pregnancy
        (3) Hyperthyroidism

    3. Hirsute women in general have reduced serum concentrations of SHBG.

D. 5α-Reductase enzyme

    1. 5α-Reductase converts testosterone to dihydrotestosterone (DHT) in androgen-sensitive tissues, such as hair follicles and skin.

    2. It is significantly elevated in the skin of hirsute women as compared to controls.

    3. DHT is thought to be responsible for stimulating hair growth and is two to three times as potent as testosterone.

E. Pathophysiology of hirsutism involves a combination of the following:

    1. Increased concentration of serum androgens, especially free testosterone

    2. Decreased levels of SHBG, resulting in an increase in percentage of free or bioavailable androgen

    3. Increased activity of 5α-reductase, which converts testosterone to DHT in the skin and hair follicles

III. CLASSIFICATION OF HIRSUTISM

A. Patients with regular menstrual cycles

    1. Intrinsic factors
      a. Genetic: racial, familial, and individual differences
      b. Physiologic: premature pubarche, precocious puberty, puberty, pregnancy, and menopause
      c. Idiopathic

    2. Extrinsic factors
      a. Local trauma
      b. Drug-related
        (1) Without virilization
          (a) Phenytoin
          (b) Diazoxide

            (c) Hexachlorobenzene
            (d) Adrenocorticotropic hormone
            (e) Corticosteroids
        (2) With potential virilization
            (a) Progestogens
            (b) Anabolic agents
            (c) Androgen therapy

    3. Hamartomas or nevi
       a. Pigmented nevi with hair
       b. Nevus pilosus
       c. Pigmented hairy epidermal nevus

  B. Patients with irregular menstrual cycles

    1. Disorders of adrenal origin
       a. Congenital or adult onset adrenal hyperplasia
       b. Androgen-producing tumors

    2. Disorders of ovarian origin
       a. Polycystic ovary disease (Stein-Leventhal syndrome)
       b. Androgen-producing tumors
         (1) Arrhenoblastoma
         (2) Granulosa–theca cell tumor
         (3) Luteoma of pregnancy
       c. Hyperthecosis
       d. Chronic anovulation associated with:
         (1) Hypothalamic amenorrhea
         (2) Emotional disorders
         (3) Thyroid disease

    3. Disorders of pituitary origin
       a. Cushing's syndrome
       b. Acromegaly

    4. Intersex problems
       a. Male pseudohermaphroditism
       b. Gonadal dysgenesis (Turner's syndrome) with androgenic manifestations

IV. DIAGNOSTIC WORKUP OF HIRSUTISM

  A. History. Important factors to note while taking a history include:

    1. The onset of hirsutism
       a. Gradual. A gradual onset of hirsutism is often accompanied by acne, weight gain, and increasing irregularity of the menstrual cycles as seen with polycystic ovary disease.
       b. Abrupt. An abrupt onset of hirsutism is often accompanied by signs of virilization as seen with androgen-producing tumors.

    2. The presence or absence of other virilizing signs

    3. Drug ingestion

    4. The presence or absence of regular menstrual cycles. Patients with regular menstrual cycles almost always represent idiopathic, ethnic, or familial hirsutism; workup of these patients is unnecessary.

  B. Blood studies

    1. Serum testosterone
       a. Total testosterone of less than 200 μg/100 ml, which declines with birth control pills or prednisone administration, is usually present in polycystic ovary disease.
       b. Total testosterone of more than 200 μg/100 ml suggests a tumor.
         (1) A CAT scan is indicated to define the location of the tumor.
         (2) Laparoscopy can be helpful in ruling out an ovarian neoplasm.

    2. Serum DHEA sulfate is usually a marker for adrenal secretory activity.
       a. A level above 700 μg/100 ml, which is suppressed with dexamethasone, suggests adrenal hyperplasia.
       b. Elevated DHEA sulfate levels that cannot be suppressed suggests an adrenal tumor.

3. Serum androstenedione. Elevated levels of androstenedione suggest ovarian disease.

4. Serum 17-hydroxyprogesterone

   a. 17-Hydroxyprogesterone is an intermediate metabolite in the steroidogenesis process in the adrenal.

   b. As an intermediate metabolite, it is elevated in the various enzyme deficiencies (i.e., 21-hydroxylase and 11β-hydroxylase) seen in congenital adrenal hyperplasia.

5. Cortisol. Elevated serum levels suggest Cushing's syndrome.

6. Gonadotropins. Relatively elevated luteinizing hormone over follicle-stimulating hormone suggests polycystic ovary disease.

↑LH/FSH

V. TREATMENT OF HIRSUTISM

A. Goals

1. Patients should be told that the goal of therapy, due to the pathophysiology of hirsutism, is the arrest of the virilizing process, not the removal of hair.

2. Once terminal hair has been established in the area of sexual hair, withdrawal of the androgen will not affect the established hair pattern.

3. Amelioration of a specific disease state will not rid one totally of the excess hair growth, but it will help to slow the rate of growth.

B. Elimination of specific causes

1. Removal of ovarian or adrenal tumors

2. Elimination of drugs suspected to contribute to the abnormal hair growth

3. Suppression with prednisone or dexamethasone of the adrenal contribution to the androgen pool

4. Treatment for Cushing's syndrome, hypothyroidism, or acromegaly

5. Clomiphene induction for ovulatory cycles in patients with polycystic ovary disease and possible bilateral ovarian wedge resection for patients with ongoing hirsutism and anovulation who are resistant to clomiphene

C. Reduction of gonadotropins

1. In most idiopathic or ovarian-related hirsutism, suppression of ovarian steroidogenesis is the goal.

2. The combination oral contraceptives have both a potent negative feedback effect on the pituitary and other effects that ameliorate peripheral androgen stimulation.

   a. Both estrogen and progestogen cause a decrease in gonadotropin secretion with a consequent decrease of ovarian steroidogenesis.

   b. Estrogen causes an increased binding of testosterone by stimulating the increase of steroid-binding globulin.

   c. Progestogen can displace active androgens at the hair follicle level in the skin.

   d. Blood testosterone levels are effectively suppressed within 1–3 months of suppression therapy; this reduction has been associated with a clinical improvement in the progression of hirsutism.

3. Medroxyprogesterone (Depo-Provera), 150 mg intramuscularly every 3 months, is effective in suppressing gonadotropin secretion in patients for whom oral contraceptives are contraindicated.

   a. There is a decreased production of androgens as is seen with the oral contraceptives.

   b. There is an increased clearance of testosterone from the circulation.

D. Androgen antagonists

1. Spironolactone may act at the cellular level by inhibiting 5α-reductase, thereby lowering the conversion of testosterone to DHT.

2. Cyproterone acetate is a progestogen that acts by blockage of androgen receptors at the cellular level.

3. Cimetidine is a histamine receptor antagonist that blocks androgen action at the receptor level.

E. Additional measures

1. Supportive therapy is very important for the hirsute female.
   a. Realistic goals should be set, and the patient should understand that the therapy is a long-term process.
   b. Treatment with the oral contraceptives may be necessary for 6–12 months before an observable diminution of hair growth occurs.

2. Although shaving is often undertaken by hirsute women, they should be told that this eventually results in the need for daily shaving.

3. Chemical depilatories often produce skin rashes and may also have to be used daily.

4. Wax depilatories offer better long-term results than shaving and chemical depilatories.

5. Bleaching is often effective with mild cases and can be used early in the treatment.

6. Plucking of terminal hairs should be avoided, as it often causes pustule formation and scarring.

7. Electrolysis, which involves the destruction of hair follicles, is the main supportive measure; however, it is expensive, time-consuming, and uncomfortable.

8. A combination of hormonal suppression and supportive measures offers the best long-term results for hirsute patients.

STUDY QUESTIONS

Directions: Each question below contains five suggested answers. Choose the **one best** response to each question.

1. The least amount of hirsutism would be expected in women of which of the following nationalities?

(A) Italian
(B) Greek
(C) Chinese
(D) Irish
(E) French

2. Measurement of which of the following substances best demonstrates the ovary as the source of excess androgen?

(A) Androstenedione
(B) Dehydroepiandrosterone
(C) Dehydroepiandrosterone sulfate
(D) 17-Hydroxyprogesterone
(E) Total testosterone

3. Decreased levels of sex hormone binding globulin are found in all of the following clinical conditions or situations EXCEPT

(A) corticosteroid therapy
(B) increased androgen productivity
(C) hyperthyroidism
(D) obesity
(E) acromegaly

4. The most effective therapy for hirsutism in a young woman with irregular menstrual cycles includes

(A) chemical depilatories
(B) plucking
(C) electrolysis
(D) birth control pills
(E) bleaching

Directions: Each question below contains four suggested answers of which **one or more** is correct. Choose the answer

A if **1, 2, and 3** are correct
B if **1 and 3** are correct
C if **2 and 4** are correct
D if **4** is correct
E if **1, 2, 3, and 4** are correct

5. Most circulating testosterone in women is derived from the

(1) liver
(2) ovary
(3) skin
(4) adrenal gland

6. Androgen activity is blocked at the receptor level by

(1) cyproterone acetate
(2) spironolactone
(3) cimetidine
(4) prednisone

7. The estrogen/progestogen combination in oral contraceptive pills is effective in ameliorating hirsutism by

(1) decreasing ovarian steroidogenesis
(2) displacing androgens at the skin level
(3) increasing steroid-binding globulin
(4) decreasing blood levels of testosterone

Directions: The group of questions below consists of lettered choices followed by several numbered items. For each numbered item select the **one** lettered choice with which it is **most** closely associated. Each lettered choice may be used once, more than once, or not at all.

Questions 8 and 9

For each of the following clinical presentations, select the laboratory test that would be most helpful in making a clinical diagnosis.

(A) Serum luteinizing hormone and follicle-stimulating hormone
(B) Total testosterone
(C) Serum dehydroepiandrosterone sulfate
(D) Serum 17-hydroxyprogesterone
(E) Serum cortisol

8. A 23-year-old woman gives a history of gradually increasing hair growth accompanied by an increasingly irregular menstrual pattern. In addition, she is concerned that she has not conceived over the last 18 months.

9. A 25-year-old woman gives a history of an abrupt onset of increased hair growth and amenorrhea. In addition, she complains of significant acne and a marked decrease in her breast size.

ANSWERS AND EXPLANATIONS

1. The answer is C. *(I B 1)* Hirsutism initially depends on the number of hair follicles present. One rarely sees hirsutism in Asian women because of the low concentration of hair follicles on their skin.

2. The answer is A. *(II A, B; IV B 1–4)* Elevated levels of dehydroepiandrosterone and dehydroepiandrosterone sulfate suggest adrenal disease. Elevation of 17-hydroxyprogesterone levels suggest adrenal hyperplasia due to a 21-hydroxylase deficiency. Androstenedione is a preandrogen that is secreted chiefly by the ovary; thus, measurement of androstenedione levels is a good screening test when the ovary is suspected of being the source of the excess androgens. Total testosterone is not specific enough to pinpoint the ovary as the source of excess androgen.

3. The answer is C. *(II C 1–3)* Sex hormone binding globulin (SHBG) is a key factor in determining androgen activity. As SHBG increases, there is an increased binding of testosterone and, thus, less free testosterone to exert biologic activity; with a decrease in SHBG, there is an increase in free testosterone. Those conditions, which decrease SHBG are increased androgen production, obesity, hypothyroidism, acromegaly, and corticosteroid therapy, while estrogen therapy, pregnancy and hyperthyroidism tend to increase SHBG.

4. The answer is D. *(V C 1, 2 a–d, E 1–8)* The main goal in treating hirsutism is the elimination of the source of the excess androgens. All of the answers listed in the question (i.e., chemical depilatories, plucking, electrolysis, and bleaching) except the birth control pills are local treatments for hirsutism that do not affect the source of the androgens and, thus, the virilizing process. In a young woman with hirsutism and irregular cycles, the most likely source of the androgens is the ovary. By suppressing ovarian activity with the birth control pills, ovarian steroidogenesis is decreased, and the secretion of the preandrogens is markedly reduced.

5. The answer is B (1, 3). *(II A–C)* In women, androgens are derived from three major sources—the ovary, the adrenal gland, and the peripheral transformation of preandrogens, such as dehydroepiandrosterone (DHEA) and androstenedione, to testosterone. Most testosterone comes from the peripheral transformation in the liver and the skin.

6. The answer is B (1, 3). *(III A 2 b (1); V D 1–3)* In the treatment of hirsutism in which there is no specific cause, an androgen antagonist is often the only therapy that can be offered. Cyproterone acetate is a progestogen that blocks androgen receptors at the cellular level. Cimetidine is a histamine receptor antagonist that also blocks androgen at the receptor level. Spironolactone inhibits the enzyme 5α-reductase, lowering the conversion of testosterone to dihydrotestosterone. Prednisone, a corticosteroid, stimulates hair growth.

7. The answer is E (all). *(V C 2 a–d)* Oral contraceptives cause a decrease in gonadotropin secretion with a consequent decrease in ovarian steroidogenesis and a decrease in secretion of ovarian preandrogens, such as androstenedione. As a consequence of the decreased ovarian steroidogenesis, there is decreased blood testosterone. The estrogen stimulates production of binding globulin from the liver, and the progestogen displaces active androgens at the hair follicle level.

8 and 9. The answers are: 8-A, 9-B. *(IV A 1, B 1–6)* The clinical picture of the 23-year-old woman with a history of gradually increasing hair growth is characteristic of polycystic ovary disease. Measurement of serum dehydroepiandrosterone sulfate, 17-hydroxyprogesterone, and cortisol would indicate adrenal disease. Total testosterone levels may be elevated, but the serum luteinizing hormone (LH) and follicle-stimulating hormone (FSH) would be more specific than total testosterone. In polycystic ovary disease, LH levels are constantly elevated over FSH. With ovulation, LH is only momentarily elevated over FSH.

The abrupt onset of both hirsutism and defeminizing signs (amenorrhea and decreased breast size) is suggestive of an androgen-producing tumor, such as an arrhenoblastoma. In this case, the most definitive test would be measurement of total testosterone because testosterone would be the chief secretory product of the tumor, and levels would be markedly elevated.

36
Menopause
William W. Beck, Jr.

I. PHYSIOLOGY OF THE PERIMENOPAUSE AND MENOPAUSE

A. Menstrual cycle changes

1. Changes in menstrual cycle regularity occur as women progress through their forties.

2. The remaining follicles in both ovaries become less sensitive to gonadotropin stimulation. There is a resultant:
   a. Increase in follicle-stimulating hormone (FSH).
   b. Reduction in estrogen concentration.

   FSH ↑ estrogen ↓

3. The limited follicle maturation leads to either a decreased cycle interval or lapses of cycles with oligomenorrhea.

B. Cessation of menses

1. The menses usually cease between the ages of 50 and 52 years. The reduced level of estrogen from the remaining follicles is no longer sufficient to induce endometrial proliferative changes capable of producing visible menstruation.

2. FSH levels rise 10- to 20-fold above usual cycle levels.

C. Circulating estrogen in postmenopausal women

1. Estrogenic activity is evident for many years after the menopause but at much reduced levels.

2. Estrone, the principal estrogen in a postmenopausal woman, is produced from the androgen precursor, androstenedione, via extraglandular and extrahepatic aromatization.
   a. Most of the androstenedione comes from the adrenal gland.
   b. Ovarian stroma secretes androstenedione for a short time before that tissue becomes quiescent.

3. Obesity is a factor in postmenopausal estrogen levels.
   a. In obese women, there is an increased conversion of androstenedione to estrone.
   b. The conversion reflects the ability of fat cells to aromatize androgens.

4. The extraglandular source of estrogen is sustained for several years and maintains reasonably normal function of such estrogen-dependent tissues as breasts, urethra, vagina, and vulva.

D. Premature menopause is manifested by permanent amenorrhea before 35 years of age. Investigators have suggested that:

1. This phenomenon may be due to a genetic predilection.

2. The ovarian failure may be due to an autoimmune reaction secondary to rheumatoid arthritis or an inflammatory reaction of a mumps infection, which affects the ovaries.

II. TARGET ORGAN RESPONSE TO DECREASED ESTROGEN

A. Vagina

1. The vagina becomes smaller with a diminution in the size of the upper vagina.

2. The vaginal epithelium becomes pale, thin, and dry.
   a. Because proliferation of the vaginal epithelium is estrogen-dependent, there is a decrease in the intermediate and superficial cells in the squamous epithelium.

    b. There is an increase in the parabasal cells, which signifies a shift (regression) in the maturation index.

  3. The labia minora has a pale, dry appearance, and there is a reduction of the fat content of the labia majora.

  4. The pelvic tissues and ligaments that support the uterus and the vagina lose their tone, predisposing to prolapse of the uterus.

B. Uterus

  1. The endometrial tissue becomes sparse with numerous small petechial hemorrhages. The endometrium has an atrophic appearance with scattered endometrial glands.

  2. The myometrium atrophies, and the uterus decreases in size. Fibroids, if present, reduce in size but do not disappear.

C. Breasts. There is a general loss of turgor, form, and fullness of the breasts.

D. Bones. There is a gradual loss of calcium, leading to osteoporosis, which is characterized by a reduction in bone density and fractures. Osteoporosis is often accompanied by pain and deformities, such as a loss of stature.

E. Hair. With the loss of estrogen, there is a relative increase in circulating androgens with a tendency towards an increased quantity of body hair with a male pattern distribution.

III. SEQUELAE OF REDUCED ESTROGEN

A. Vasomotor symptoms

  1. The hot flash or flush is the hallmark of the menopausal woman.
    a. The flush is characterized by the sudden onset of reddening of the skin over the head, neck, and chest, accompanied by a feeling of intense body heat and perspiration.
    b. The flush may last a few seconds or several minutes.
    c. Flushes appear to be more frequent and severe at night or during times of stress.
    d. The vasomotor instability lasts for 1–2 years in most women but may last for as long as 5 years.

  2. The flush appears to coincide with a surge of luteinizing hormone (LH), not FSH, and is preceded by a subjective awareness that a flush is beginning.

  3. Estrogen therapy decreases the frequency and sensitivity of the flushes.
    a. The onset of the flushes initially depends on a reduction of previously established estrogen levels.
    b. Flushes do not occur in hypoestrogenic states, such as gonadal dysgenesis.

B. Altered menstrual function

  1. Oligomenorrhea is followed by amenorrhea.

  2. Menopause is defined as amenorrhea for 6–12 months in women 45 years of age and older.

  3. If vaginal bleeding occurs after 12 months of amenorrhea, endometrial pathology (i.e., polyps, hyperplasia, or neoplasia) must be ruled out.

C. Osteoporosis

  1. Osteoporosis—the main health hazard associated with the menopause—describes the increased porosity (rarefaction) of bone. It is a disease of the axial skeleton with most of the loss occurring to trabecular bone with thinning of the cortex.

  2. Osteoporosis has been associated with decreased estrone and androstenedione levels. Bone loss is most rapid:
    a. After oophorectomy, resulting in castration, in women younger than 45 years of age
    b. In women with gonadal dysgenesis

  3. The consequences of osteoporosis include fractures of the vertebral body (compression fractures), humerus, upper femur, and distal forearm and ribs.

  4. Osteoporosis is more common in white women than in black women.
    a. Approximately 25% of white women over 60 years of age have spinal compression fractures.

b. Approximately 32% of white American women can expect to have one or more hip fractures at some time in their lives if current inadequate methods of prevention and treatment are maintained.

c. An average of 16% of women with hip fractures have died within 4 months of the fracture.

5. Exercise and proper diet have a beneficial effect on bone integrity, and estrogen therapy can retard the process of osteoporosis.

D. The menopausal syndrome includes a variety of symptoms, such as fatigue, headache, nervousness, loss of libido, insomnia, depression, irritability, palpitations, and joint and muscle pain. There is progressive improvement of some of these symptoms with estrogen replacement.

E. Atrophic changes

1. Atrophy of the vaginal mucosa leads to atrophic vaginitis, pruritus of the vulvovaginal area, dyspareunia, and stenosis.

2. Urethral changes with mucosal thinning lead to dysuria, frequency and urgency of urination, and incontinence.

3. There is an increased frequency of cystitis.

4. Vaginal, urethral, and bladder symptoms improve with estrogen therapy.

IV. SEQUELAE OF EXCESS ENDOGENOUS ESTROGEN

A. Dysfunctional uterine bleeding. During the perimenopause (between 40 and 55 years of age), some women manifest estrogen excess, rather than deficiency, by dysfunctional uterine bleeding—that is, irregular and abnormal bleeding. The estrogen excess is not associated with ovulation and, thus, is unopposed by progesterone. Increased endogenous estrogen can result from:

1. Increased levels of precursor androgens in functional and nonfunctional endocrine tumors, liver disease, and stress.

2. Increased aromatization of androgenic precursors associated with obesity, hyperthyroidism, and liver disease.

3. Increased direct secretion of estrogen from ovarian tumors.

B. Endometrial neoplasia

1. Unopposed estrogen that results in endometrial pathology may manifest as dysfunctional uterine bleeding or abnormal bleeding.

2. With any abnormal bleeding over the age of 35 years, there must be an evaluation of the endometrium by dilatation and curettage or endometrial biopsy to rule out organic disease, specifically:
 a. Adenomatous hyperplasia
 b. Carcinoma of the endometrium

C. Therapy. The abnormal bleeding of the perimenopause and the menopause is an entity that is not treated by estrogen replacement therapy because additional estrogen just compounds the problem.

V. ESTROGEN REPLACEMENT THERAPY

{ relief of menopausal symptoms
prevention & treatment of osteoporosis
prevention of vascular disease
Retension of youthful skin }

A. Advantages

1. Relief of menopausal symptoms
 a. Hormone replacement usually eliminates hot flashes and night sweats.
  (1) Progesterone alone is less effective than estrone or estradiol.
  (2) Progestins are not the treatment of choice because they have antiestrogenic properties.
 b. Estrogen replacement provides good prophylaxis against and reversal of atrophic vaginitis, dyspareunia, and degenerative changes in the urethra and urinary bladder. Affective symptoms—depression, insomnia, irritability, and loss of concentration—generally are improved with estrogen therapy.
  (1) Atrophic vaginitis requires continuous therapy.
  (2) Vaginal relaxation is not responsive to estrogen therapy.

2. Prevention and treatment of osteoporosis
 a. Osteoporosis can be prevented with early estrogen replacement therapy.

(1) There is no bone loss, and there is actually new bone formation if therapy is started within 3 years of the last menstrual period.

(2) There is no bone loss but also no new bone formation if therapy is started more than 3 years after the last menstrual period.

(3) Estrogen dosages are as follows:
   (a) Conjugated equine estrogen daily: 0.625–1.25 mg
   (b) Ethinyl estradiol daily: 0.025–0.05 mg
   (c) Estrone sulfate daily: 1–2 mg

(4) Supplemental calcium of 1000–1500 mg/day may also be prescribed.

b. Estrogens are effective in treating osteoporosis and help to eliminate low back pain.

(1) Estrogen replacement therapy at the same doses given above is very effective at reducing the bone density loss per month.

(2) Calcium carbonate (1000–1500 mg daily) alone is effective in reducing bone density loss but less so than estrogen alone.

(3) The combination of estrogen and calcium is most effective in treating osteoporosis.

(4) Vitamin D (400 IU per day) increases calcium resorption from the intestine and has a homeostatic effect on plasma calcium levels.

(5) A regular program of exercise is necessary to assure maintenance of muscle tone.

c. Oophorectomized women appear to be at much greater risk for a rapid onset of osteoporosis than women whose menopause occurs naturally. Preventive estrogen therapy should begin immediately after surgery in these patients.

3. Prevention of cardiovascular disease. Menopausal women who use estrogen show significant reductions in levels of low-density lipoprotein in serum cholesterol and significant increases in levels of high-density lipoprotein (HDL) when compared with nonusers. These are thought to be protective changes in the prevention of cardiovascular disease.

4. Retention of youthful skin. Estrogen replacement therapy induces a series of changes, which help to retain a youthful appearance to the skin.

B. Disadvantages

1. Conditions that could worsen under the influence of estrogen or that could potentiate the effects of the estrogen cannot be treated with estrogen replacement therapy.

a. Metabolic contraindications include:
   (1) Acute liver disease
   (2) Chronically impaired liver function
   (3) Acute vascular thrombosis
   (4) Neuro-ophthalmologic vascular disease

b. Relative contraindications include:
   (1) Seizure disorders
   (2) Hypertension
   (3) Familial hyperlipidemia
   (4) Migraine headaches

2. Cancer

a. Breast cancer. Some studies have suggested a relationship between unopposed estrogen and breast cancer. Risk factors include:
   (1) Late onset of menopause
   (2) Sterility
   (3) Dose and duration of estrogen replacement in women with benign breast disease and intact ovaries
   (4) A positive family history of breast cancer in women with a history of infertility or chronic cystic mastitis

b. Endometrial cancer. The abnormal growth seen with hyperplasia, adenomatous hyperplasia, atypia, and early carcinoma has been associated with unopposed estrogen activity. Retrospective studies have estimated the risk of endometrial cancer in women on estrogen replacement therapy to be increased by four- to eightfold over women not on replacement therapy.
   (1) The risk of endometrial cancer appears to:
      (a) Increase with the duration of exposure and dose of estrogen
      (b) Decrease after the estrogen is stopped
      (c) Be related to continuous versus cyclic therapy
      (d) Be reduced by the addition of a progestin
   (2) Estrogen promotes growth of the endometrium and progestin inhibits that growth. The addition of progestin in sequence with estrogen replacement therapy leads to a reversal of the hyperplasia and a diminished incidence of endometrial cancer.

          (a) Progestin reduces cytoplasmic receptors for estrogen.

          (b) Progestin induces the enzyme (17β-ol-dehydrogenase) that converts estradiol to estrone, thus decreasing the overall intracellular availability of the powerful estradiol.

      (3) It is wise to avoid estrogen replacement therapy in women who are obese, hypertensive, or diabetic and in women with dysfunctional uterine bleeding or high endogenous estrogen levels.

          (a) Before estrogen replacement is given to such women, a pretreatment endometrial biopsy is recommended to ascertain normality of the endometrium.

          (b) Subsequent biopsies every 1–3 years are recommended to insure endometrial stability.

C. Recommendations for replacement therapy

1. Women under 40 who have been castrated and women with gonadal dysgenesis

    a. Cyclic and long-term low-dose (0.625 mg of conjugated estrogen daily from days 1–25 of each calendar month) therapy is recommended for prevention of osteoporosis and target organ atrophy.

    b. Progestin [medroxyprogesterone (Provera), 10 mg daily] is recommended from days 16–25 of each calendar month.

    c. Endometrial biopsy is recommended periodically throughout the therapy.

2. Women with dysfunctional bleeding in the perimenopause

    a. Cyclic progestin therapy is recommended to break up the ongoing effect of the unopposed estrogen on the endometrium; in addition, there should be periodic endometrial biopsies.

    b. Vasomotor reactions in women still menstruating are treated by nonhormonal methods because additional estrogen might worsen the endometrial picture.

3. Menopausal women

    a. Sequential use of estrogen and progestin (as with women under 40 years of age) is recommended starting with a dose of 0.625 of conjugated estrogen and increasing the dose as dictated by the need for symptomatic relief; Provera, 10 mg daily, is used from days 16–25 of the calendar month.

    b. A combined schedule (0.625 or 1.25 mg of conjugated estrogen and 2.5 mg of progestin daily from days 1–25) is an alternative form of therapy and actually supplies less total progestin.

      (1) Estrogen therapy stimulates increased levels of HDL.

      (2) Progestin therapy effectively lowers the level of HDL.

    c. There should be periodic (every 1–3 years) biopsy surveillance.

    d. Atrophic conditions of the vulva, vagina, and urethra found in late menopause can be treated effectively with local (estrogen cream) or low-dose oral therapy. There is substantial absorption of estrogen from the local vaginal application.

4. Alternatives to estrogen therapy.
Medroxyprogesterone (daily Provera or monthly Depo-Provera) is effective for symptomatic relief of hot flashes in women in whom estrogen is contraindicated.

STUDY QUESTIONS

Directions: Each question below contains five suggested answers. Choose the **one best** response to each question.

1. Physiologic characteristics of the perimenopause include all of the following EXCEPT

(A) reduction in the number of ovarian follicles
(B) decreased menstrual cycle length
(C) reduction in the estrogen concentration
(D) decreased secretion of follicle-stimulating hormone (FSH)
(E) reduction in follicle sensitivity to FSH

2. Which of the following menopausal symptoms is not responsive to estrogen replacement therapy?

(A) Vaginal relaxation
(B) Depression
(C) Atrophic vaginitis
(D) Insomnia
(E) Dyspareunia

3. The main health hazard of the menopause is

(A) cardiovascular disease
(B) pelvic relaxation
(C) endometrial cancer
(D) depression
(E) osteoporosis

4. Recommended treatment for osteoporosis includes all of the following EXCEPT

(A) estrogen
(B) progestin
(C) exercise
(D) calcium
(E) vitamin D

Directions: Each question below contains four suggested answers of which **one or more** is correct. Choose the answer

A   if **1, 2, and 3** are correct
B   if **1 and 3** are correct
C   if **2 and 4** are correct
D   if **4** is correct
E   if **1, 2, 3, and 4** are correct

5. Dysfunctional uterine bleeding during the perimenopausal period can be associated with

(1) exogenous estrogen therapy
(2) anovulation
(3) estrogen/progesterone imbalance
(4) increased aromatization of androgenic precursors

6. Increased endogenous estrogen levels during the menopause arise from

(1) peripheral conversion of preandrogens in fatty tissue
(2) secretion of estrogens from the ovarian stroma
(3) secretion of estrogen from a granulosa cell tumor
(4) decreased aromatization of preandrogens in hypothyroidism

7. Contraindications to postmenopausal estrogen replacement therapy include which of the following?

(1) Hypertension
(2) Acute liver disease
(3) Familial hyperlipidemia
(4) Diabetes

8. Positive features of estrogen replacement therapy include

(1) prevention of osteoporosis
(2) a lowering of high-density lipoprotein levels
(3) improvement of urinary frequency and stress incontinence
(4) prevention of endometrial hyperplasia

ANSWERS AND EXPLANATIONS

1. The answer is D. (*I A 1–3*) As women near the menopause, their cycles begin to change. There is a reduction in the number of ovarian follicles, and these follicles become less sensitive to follicle-stimulating hormone (FSH). With a reduced concentration of estrogen from the ovaries, there is less of a negative feedback effect, and the FSH level *rises*. The limited follicle maturation often leads to either a decreased cycle interval or lapses of cycles with oligomenorrhea.

2. The answer is A. [*II A 4, B 1, 2; V A 1 b (1), (2)*] Estrogen replacement therapy has good results in atrophic vaginal conditions, such as atrophic vaginitis and dyspareunia. It is also helpful in improving the affective symptoms associated with the menopause—depression, insomnia, irritability, and loss of concentration. Pelvic tissues and ligaments that support the uterus and the vagina lose their tone in response to decreased estrogen; however, vaginal relaxation is not responsive to estrogen therapy.

3. The answer is E. (*III C 1–5*) Because of the consequences of bone rarefaction, osteoporosis is the main health hazard associated with the menopause. Compression fractures of the vertebrae and fractures of the upper femur demand bed rest and inactivity. An average of 16% of women with hip fractures have died within 4 months of the injury. Osteoporosis is a more widespread problem than either endometrial cancer or cardiovascular disease during the menopause.

4. The answer is B. (*V A 2 a, b*) A coordinated program of estrogen replacement (0.625–1.25 mg of conjugated equine estrogen daily), calcium (1–1.5 g daily), vitamin D (400 IU daily), and exercise is thought to be the best approach to both the prevention and treatment of osteoporosis. Progestin, such as medroxyprogesterone (Provera), may be effective for symptomatic relief during the menopause but does nothing to correct the osteoporosis.

5. The answer is C (2, 4). (*IV A 1, 2, C*) The basic feature of the perimenopausal period is anovulatory bleeding. This irregular, often heavy bleeding, is associated with excess endogenous estrogen that is unopposed by progesterone. There is no imbalance because ovulation does not occur and progesterone is not present. In a situation in which there is increased endogenous estrogen, there would be no reason to add any exogenous estrogen. An additional source of estrogen during the perimenopause is the increased aromatization of androgenic precursors, especially in obese women.

6. The answer is B (1, 3). (*IV A 1–3*) When excess estrogen is found in premenopausal or menopausal women, it can occur from a number of sources. There is an *increased* aromatization of preandrogens to estrogens in obesity, liver disease, and *hyper*thyroidism. The main product of the ovarian stroma is androstenedione and not estrogen. Increased direct secretion of endogenous estrogen is seen with functional ovarian tumors, such as granulosa cell tumors.

7. The answer is A (1, 2, 3). (*V B 1 a, b*) There are clinical conditions that are worsened by exogenous estrogen, such as familial hyperlipidemia and hypertension; both would be reasons for withholding estrogen therapy. In conditions that involve the liver, such as acute disease or cirrhosis, the circulating estrogen is not metabolized as rapidly and, thus, a given dose of replacement estrogen can have a sustained and prolonged effect on target tissues. Diabetes is not worsened by estrogen replacement.

8. The answer is B (1, 3). [*V A 1 b, 2 a, 3, B 2 b (2)*] One of the most important features of estrogen replacement therapy in the postmenopausal woman is the prevention of osteoporosis. In addition, estrogen provides good prophylaxis against the degenerative changes in the urethra and the bladder and can improve urinary frequency and stress incontinence when present. Estrogen causes increases in the level of high-density lipoproteins, not decreases. Unopposed estrogen can cause endometrial hyperplasia; it is progestin that inhibits endometrial growth and prevents the hyperplasia.

37
Pelvic Malignancies
John M. Riva

I. INTRODUCTION. Although cell biology and biochemistry of normal cells and cancer cells are very similar, cancer cells differ from their normal counterparts in that they are aberrantly regulated. Alterations in growth constraints and cellular differentiation frequently lead to autonomous proliferation of abnormal cells to the detriment of the host. Factors responsible for initiating aberrant cellular expression are complex and poorly understood.

II. CERVICAL CANCER

   A. Epidemiology. Epidemiologic factors point to associations between early age of coitus and sexual promiscuity (male and female) and the development of precancerous and cancerous lesions of the cervix.

   1. Increased incidence is related to:
   a. Coitarche (age of first intercourse) during adolescent years
   b. Marriage or conception at an early age
   c. Multiple sexual partners
   d. Cigarette smoking
   e. High-risk male consort (i.e., one whose previous sexual partners developed precancerous or cancerous conditions of the cervix)
   f. Immunosuppression

   2. Viral transmission. Sexually transmitted viruses, such as herpes simplex virus (HSV-2) and human papillomavirus (HPV), have been examined as potential causal agents. Although absolute proof of the human oncogenicity of these viruses is lacking, there is sufficient evidence to implicate them as causal agents.
   a. HSV-2
      (1) There is an increased incidence of Pap (Papanicolaou) smears suggestive of herpes viral infection in women with cervical dysplasia.
      (2) There is a high incidence of positive antibody titers to HSV-2 and AG4, an HSV-2 viral protein, in women with cervical cancer.
      (3) HSV-2 DNA and messenger RNA sequences are present in cervical cancer cells.
   b. HPV
      (1) There is a high incidence of latent (clinically inapparent) papillomavirus infection in women with cervical dysplasia and invasive cancer.
      (2) There is a high incidence of cervical dysplasia and invasive cancers in women with histories of overt genital condyloma acuminatum.
      (3) There is an association with high-risk oncogenic HPV viral types 16 and 18 and high-grade cervical dysplasias and cervical cancers.

   B. Cervical transformation zone (TZ). The region on the ectocervix between the original squamous epithelium and glandular epithelium of the endocervical canal is the site of most squamous preinvasive and invasive neoplasms.

   1. This zone undergoes a transformation from mucus-secreting glandular cells to nonmucus-secreting squamous cells in a process called metaplasia (a change in growth).
   a. Metaplastic change is most active during adolescence and pregnancy where elevated estrogen levels may be the stimulating impetus.
   b. Active metaplasia is most susceptable to viral infection and integration of viral DNA (particularly HPV) into the host's DNA, presumably altering the controls on cellular differentiation.

   2. By-products of cigarette smoke are concentrated in cervical mucus and have been associated with a depletion of the cells of Langerhans, which are macrophages that assist in cell-mediated immunity in the TZ.

C. Evaluation of the abnormal Pap smear

1. **Efficacy of cytologic screening programs**
   a. Invasive carcinoma of the cervix is preceded by a spectrum of preinvasive disease, which can be detected cytologically. Detection and simple local treatments of preinvasive cervical disease can prevent invasive cancer.
   b. Regular cervical cancer screening programs have demonstrated a significant decrease in mortality from cervical cancer. Unscreened populations can have as high as a 10-fold or more increase in mortality from cervical cancer.

2. **Frequency of cervical cytologic screening**
   a. Screening should be initiated at the onset of sexual activity.
   b. Women with high-risk factors should be screened annually.
   c. Women with low-risk factors and two consecutive negative annual Pap smears can be screened every other year.

3. **Management of the abnormal Pap smear**
   a. **Classification.** There has been a recent trend to provide descriptive terminology to abnormal cervical cytology. Descriptive terminology varies from laboratory to laboratory. A simple summary is provided below.
      (1) **Class I:** Normal
      (2) **Class II:** Atypical benign. No dysplastic cells are appreciated. This group includes:
         (a) Squamous atypia
         (b) Atypical squamous metaplasia
         (c) Koilocytic atypia
         (d) Inflammatory atypia
         (e) Radiation atypia
      (3) **Class III:** Suspicious. This group includes mild, moderate, and severe dysplastic cells. Some laboratories include carcinoma-in-situ in this category, while others include it as **class IV**.
      (4) **Class V:** Positive for malignancy
   b. **Current diagnostic recommendations** suggest that all women with a class II or greater Pap smear undergo colposcopic evaluation unless there is an obvious invasive cancer in which tissue biopsies for diagnosis will suffice. Women with class II Pap smears have 15%–50% risk of having a dysplastic lesion that is not detected cytologically.
   c. **Colposcopy.** This technique involves inspection of the TZ and the squamocolumnar junction under 7.5–30 power magnification, following the application of a 3%–5% acetic acid solution. An endocervical canal curettage (ECC) is performed in conjunction with colposcopy to rule out dysplasia within the canal that is colposcopically inapparent.
   d. **Treatment recommendations** are based on the colposcopic findings as outlined below.
      (1) **Class II Pap/cervical biopsies without dysplasia but with squamous or koilocytic atypia:** Repeat the Pap smear every 6 months, and perform an annual colposcopy. This group has a 9%–33% risk of developing a dysplastic lesion within 2 years.
      (2) **Cervical dysplasia/squamocolumnar junction visualized/ECC negative:** Outpatient local destruction of TZ
      (3) **Cervical dysplasia with either a nonvisualized squamocolumnar junction or a positive ECC:** Outpatient cone biopsy of the cervix
      (4) **Microinvasive carcinoma:** Cone biopsy
      (5) **Class III or greater Pap smear/negative colposcopy and ECC:** Diagnostic cone biopsy

4. **Treatment of cervical preinvasive disease.** Preinvasive cervical disease is a spectrum of lesions of increasing severity: mild dysplasia or cervical intraepithelial neoplasia (CIN I), moderate dysplasia (CIN II), and severe dysplasia/carcinoma-in-situ (CIN III). These dysplasias have the potential for progression to invasive cervical cancer in up to 33% of women within a 2–15-year period if left untreated.
   a. **Locally destructive treatment modalities** for cervical dysplasias/carcinoma-in-situ include:
      (1) Electrocautery
      (2) Cryotherapy
      (3) Cold coagulation
      (4) Diathermy loop
      (5) Laser vaporization
   b. **The goal of treatment** is to incorporate the entire TZ within the treatment field and create a thermal injury to a sufficient depth (5–7 mm) to include potentially dysplastic epithelium underlying the TZ.

(1) Cure rates for one treatment range from 85%–96%.
(2) Repeat treatment of the adequately evaluated persistent lesion effects a cure rate of 95%.
  c. Post-treatment follow-up. The risk of persistent or recurrent lesions is 5%–15%. Of these lesions, 85% are detected within 2 years of the initial treatment. Follow-up of the treated patient should include:
    (1) An initial Pap and colposcopy at 3 months
    (2) A Pap smear every 6 months
    (3) An annual colposcopy for at least 2 years
    (4) Hysterectomy for those patients who have persistent severe lesions despite repeated conservative local destructive techniques

D. Invasive cervical cancer

1. Microinvasive carcinoma of the cervix. Much controversy surrounds the exact definition of this "early" invasive cancer of the cervix. A commonly adopted definition in the United States is a depth of invasion of less than 3 mm with no lymphovascular space involvement and no confluent tongues of tissue.
  a. The diagnosis can only be made on a thoroughly examined cone biopsy.
  b. The incidence of pelvic lymph node metastases is less than 1%.
  c. Total abdominal hysterectony is the preferred treatment of choice although cervical conization with negative margins can be used in women wishing to preserve fertility.
  d. Cure rates are 95%.

2. Invasive carcinoma of the cervix. These invasive lesions are either clinically inapparent and found on histologic inspection of a cone biopsy (depth of invasion more than 3 mm, lymphovascular space involvement, or both) or are clinically obvious in which case a simple biopsy confirms the diagnosis.
  a. Symptoms
    (1) Postcoital or irregular bleeding are the most common symptoms.
    (2) Malodors, bloody discharge, and deep pelvic pain are seen in locally advanced disease.
  b. Age. Mean age of diagnosis is aproximately 45 years. Primary cervical cancers diagnosed before age 30 or after the age of 70 occur in about 7% and 16% of women, respectively.
  c. Histology. Squamous carcinomas (85%) and adenocarcinoma (13%) account for most invasive cervical disease. There appears to be no difference in survival between these two groups when matched for grade, size of lesion, or stage. Rare tumors of the cervix include small cell carcinomas, verrucous carcinomas, sarcomas, and lymphomas.
  d. Staging. Clinical assessment of the extent of disease includes the following:
    (1) Stage I: Carcinoma is confined to the cervix (extension to uterine corpus should be disregarded).
      (a) Stage IA: Microinvasive carcinoma
      (b) Stage IB: All other cases of stage I
    (2) Stage II: Carcinoma extends beyond the cervix but not onto the pelvic sidewall. The cancer extends into the vagina but not the lower third.
      (a) Stage IIA: No obvious parametrial involvement
      (b) Stage IIB: Obvious parametrial involvement
    (3) Stage III. Carcinoma extends onto the pelvic sidewall. On rectal examination, there is no cancer-free space between the tumor and the pelvic sidewall. The tumor extends to the lower third of the vagina. All cases of hydronephrosis or nonfunctioning kidney should be included in stage III diagnoses unless another cause for these conditions can be found.
      (a) Stage IIIA: No extension to pelvic sidewall
      (b) Stage IIIB: Extension to pelvic sidewall, hydronephrosis, or nonfunctioning kidney
    (4) Stage IV: Carcinoma extends beyond the true pelvis or clinically involves the mucosa of the bladder or rectum.
      (a) Stage IVA: Spread to adjacent organs
      (b) Stage IVB: Spread to distant organs
  e. Pretreatment staging evaluations. The diagnostic workup of a women with histologically confirmed invasive cervical cancer is designed to examine the known patterns of spread, such as direct extension, lymphatic involvement, or hematogenous spread.
    (1) Mandatory tests
      (a) Chest x-ray
      (b) Intravenous pyelogram
      (c) Barium enema
      (d) Cystoscopy and proctosigmoidoscopy under anesthesia

   (2) Optional tests
      (a) CAT scan
      (b) Nuclear magnetic resonance (NMR) imaging
      (c) Lymphangiography
      (d) Fine needle aspiration radiologically guided
f. Treatment. Therapeutic measures are governed by the patient's clinical stage, age, and general health. Primary modalities include surgery, and radiotherapy. Chemotherapy can be used as an adjunct to radiotherapy as radiation sensitizers or for control of locally recurrent or distant metastatic disease.
   (1) Surgery involves radical hysterectomy with periaortic and pelvic lymphadenectomy. This procedure involves the en bloc removal of the uterus, cervix, upper third of the vagina, the parametrium, and the uterosacral and uterovesical ligaments. In addition, the lymphatics of the lower periaortic, common iliac, and pelvic regions are removed en bloc.
      (a) The best results are achieved in patients with a tumor volume of 3 cm or less with no lymph node metastasis.
      (b) Comparable cure rates between surgery and radiotherapy are the rule in the treatment of early stage (IB and IIA) disease.
      (c) Surgery alone is generally reserved for patients with low volume local disease who are reasonably young and medically sound. Ovarian preservation is an important component of these operations.
      (d) Five-year survival with surgery
         (i) Stage IB: 84%
         (ii) Stage IIA: 52%
   (2) Radiotherapy. This treatment modality can be used for all stages of cervical cancer either for curative or palliative intent.
      (a) It can be used in conjunction with surgery for bulky (4 cm or more) stage IB and IIA tumors and with chemotherapy (i.e., hydroxyurea, cisplatin, and 5-fluorouracil) for locally advanced stage IIB–IVA tumors to improve survival.
      (b) Tumor cells appear more sensitive to the effects of ionizing irradiation and are less capable of repair of lethal damage than normal tissue.
      (c) Five-year survival with radiotherapy
         (i) Stage IB: 85%
         (ii) Stage IIA: 80%
         (iii) Stage IIB: 67%
         (iv) Stage IIIA: 45%
         (v) Stage IIIB: 33%
         (vi) Stage IVA: 14%
g. Follow-up evaluation. It is estimated that approximately 35% of patients with invasive cervical cancer have persistent or recurrent disease. Most of these (85%) have a recurrence of disease within 3 years of the initial treatment. Thus, frequent checkups are mandatory in the first 3 years.
   (1) Evaluations include:
      (a) Pelvic examinations
      (b) Pap smears
      (c) Periodic chest x-rays
      (d) Intravenous pyelograms
   (2) Suspicious signs or symptoms include:
      (a) Persistent cervical lesion
      (b) Unexplained weight loss
      (c) Unilateral leg edema
      (d) Pelvic or sciatic pain
      (e) Serosanguineous vaginal discharge
      (f) Progressive ureteral obstruction
      (g) Supraclavicular node enlargement
      (h) Persistent cough or hemoptysis
h. Treatment of recurrent disease. Treatment rests with determining whether or not recurrent disease is locally confined or metastatic.
   (1) Locally confined
      (a) In patients treated primarily with surgery, pelvic radiotherapy can salvage about 25%.
      (b) In patients treated primarily by radiotherapy and in whom extensive presurgical and intraoperative evaluations reveal no evidence of metastatic tumor, partial or total pelvic exenteration (i.e., en bloc removal of the uterus, cervix, vagina, parametrium, bladder, or rectum) can be curative in as many as 70% of cases.
   (2) Metastatic recurrence. These patients are generally treated with chemotherapy. Cure

rates are exceedingly rare, and response rates are variable and of limited duration. Radiotherapy can be used in the palliation of troublesome painful metastases.

III. ENDOMETRIAL CANCER

A. Epidemiology

1. Incidence. There are approximately 37,000 new cases of endometrial cancers per year in the United States and 2900 deaths. The incidence of this malignancy appears to be decreasing.

2. Increased risk of endometrial cancer has been associated with:
   a. **Obesity.** Women who are 20–50 lbs over their ideal body weight have a 3-fold increased risk of endometrial cancer. Women who are more than 50 lbs over their ideal body weight have a 9-fold increased risk.
   b. **Chronic anovulation/polycystic ovary disease.** The increased risk seen in patients with chronic anovulation has been attributed to unopposed estrogen stimulation of the endometrium.
   c. **Granulosa–theca cell ovarian tumors.** A hormonally active estrogen-producing stromal tumor of the ovary has been associated with a 25% incidence of a concurrent endometrial cancer.
   d. **Exogenous unopposed estrogen.** There is a significant correlation between exogenous oral estrogen usage and endometrial cancer when estrogen therapy is administered without the protective effects of a cyclic progestational agent.

B. Pathophysiology. Conversion of adrenal or ovarian androstenedione (an androgenic precursor to estrogens) in the peripheral adipose tissue to estrone (a weak estrogen) shuts off the normal cyclic function of the hypothalamic–pituitary–ovarian axis. As a result, ovulation and the subsequent production of progesterone, a potent "antiestrogenic" hormone, ceases. **There is then a chronic, unabated stimulation of the endometrium by estrone, leading to endometrial hyperplasia (a premalignant lesion) and endometrial carcinoma.** Unopposed exogenous estrogen or estrogen-producing ovarian tumors stimulate the endometrium in a similar fashion.

C. Endometrial hyperplasia is thought to be a precursor to endometrial carcinoma. There is a spectrum of glandular proliferation with varying degrees of architectural disarray, that is, epithelial stratification with or without cytologic atypia. No invasion can be demonstrated. The risk of progression to endometrial carcinoma is 1%–14% in untreated hyperplasias. This risk is greatest in postmenopausal women and in women with atypical adenomatous hyperplasias.

1. Types of endometrial hyperplasia
   a. **Adenomatous hyperplasia.** This entity is manifested by proliferation of glands at the expense of the stroma. Glands are hyperchromatic and are separated by strands of stroma. There is no invasion or cytologic atypia.
   b. **Atypical adenomatous hyperplasia.** This hyperplasia is considered carcinoma-in-situ of the endometrium. It is manifested histologically by glandular proliferation with intense hyperchromatism and nuclear atypia. There is little intervening stroma but no invasion.

2. Treatment of endometrial hyperplasias
   a. **The teenager** invariably responds to cyclic estrogen/progestin for 6 months at which time endometrial sampling should be repeated. If the patient continues to be anovulatory after medical treatment, oral estrogen/progestin or cyclic medroxyprogesterone (10 mg for 10 days every other month) should be continued to induce stabilization of the endometrium and to control withdrawal bleeding.
   b. **Women of childbearing age** can be treated with three courses of cyclic estrogen/progestin followed by a repeat endometrial sampling.
      (1) If pregnancy is desired, ovulation can be induced with clomiphene citrate.
      (2) If pregnancy is not desired, the woman should be evaluated as to the cause of anovulation and treated with either cyclic estrogen/progestin or cyclic medroxyprogesterone (see above).
   c. **Perimenopausal and postmenopausal women.** Treatment is predominantly medical by:
      (1) Three to six months of cyclic medroxyprogesterone (10–20 mg for 10–12 days every month) or an intramuscular depot of injections of medroxyprogesterone acetate (200 mg intramuscularly every 2 months for three courses).
         (a) Intramuscular injections are beneficial in women with symptomatic vasomotor flushes.
         (b) Repeat sampling at 3–6 months is mandatory.
      (2) Persistent endometrial hyperplasia following progestational therapy is associated with

a subsequent risk of developing endometrial carcinoma in 40%–80% of cases. This occurs in approximately 3% of treated patients.

(3) Hysterectomy is warranted in women with either persistent hyperplasia following progestational agents or in women with severe atypical adenomatous hyperplasia.

3. **Prevention of endometrial hyperplasias.** In women on estrogen replacement therapy, the addition of a cyclic progestational agent (i.e., medroxyprogesterone, 5–10 mg for the first 12 days of each monthly cycle) has dramatically reduced the risk of endometrial hyperplasia and carcinoma.

D. Endometrial carcinoma

1. **Symptoms.** The most common symptom is irregular menses or postmenopausal bleeding. The chance of detecting an occult endometrial carcinoma in an asymptomatic postmenopausal woman is exceedingly low.

2. **Age.** The median age for endometrial cancer is 61 years.

3. **Histology.** The principle histologic subtypes of endometrial carcinoma are adenocarcinoma (60%) and adenoacanthoma (22%). The remaining subtypes are papillary serous carcinoma, clear cell adenocarcinoma, and adenosquamous carcinoma. The latter subtypes are associated with a poorer 5-year survival for stage I disease than the more common endometrial carcinomas. Histologic differentiation correlates with depth of myometrial penetration, pelvic and periaortic lymphatic metastases, and overall 5-year survival.
   a. **Grade 1:** Well-differentiated adenocarcinoma
   b. **Grade 2:** Moderately differentiated carcinoma with partly solid components
   c. **Grade 3:** Poorly differentiated carcinoma with predominantly solid sheets of tumor cells of undifferentiated carcinoma

4. **Staging**
   a. **Stage I:** Confined to the corpus
      (1) **Stage IA:** Length of uterine cavity 8 cm or less
      (2) **Stage IB:** Length of uterine cavity more than 8 cm
      (3) Each stage I tumor is also described according to the grade of the tumor; for example, stage IB3 describes a carcinoma in which the uterine cavity is more than 8 cm in depth and the tumor is poorly differentiated.
   b. **Stage II:** Involvement of the corpus and cervix
   c. **Stage III:** Extension outside of the corpus but not outside the true pelvis
   d. **Stage IV:** Mucosal involvement of the bladder or rectum or extension beyond the true pelvis

5. **Diagnosis and staging evaluation**
   a. **Fractional dilatation and curettage.** This procedure is the formal method of diagnosis. It entails:
      (1) Curetting the endocervical canal to detect occult disease
      (2) Measuring the depth of the uterine cavity
      (3) Dilating the cervix
      (4) Curetting the contents of the endometrial cavity
   b. **Alternative diagnostic tests.** This group includes endometrial biopsy and endoscopically directed biopsies of the endometrium by means of hysteroscopy.
   c. **Staging workup following diagnosis**
      (1) Chest x-ray
      (2) Intravenous pyelogram or CAT scan
      (3) Barium enema or proctosigmoidoscopy
      (4) Cystoscopy

6. **Treatment.** Trends in the United States are changing from preoperative radiotherapy for early stage disease (stage I and II carcinomas with occult endocervical involvement) to a surgical staging evaluation that includes total abdominal hysterectomy and a bilateral salpingo-oophorectomy and periaortic lymph node sampling, peritoneal cytology, assessment of estrogen and progesterone receptor status, and a pathologic evaluation of the depth of myometrial penetration. The need for subsequent postoperative radiotherapy can be made for those patients at high risk for local recurrence.
   a. **Stage I, grade 1 carcinomas.** This group of tumors has a low incidence of poor prognostic features. Surgery (total abdominal hysterectomy and bilateral salpingo-oophorectomy) alone is the treatment of choice. In the event of deep myometrial penetration, adjuvant pelvic radiotherapy can be administered.
   b. **Stage IA or IB, grade 2–3 carcinomas.** The surgical staging evaluation is as outlined above

(see section III D 6). Adjuvant postoperative pelvic radiotherapy is used for:
  (1) Myometrial invasion of more than half of the myometrium
  (2) Involvement of pelvic lymph nodes

  c. Stage II carcinomas with occult disease on ECC
  (1) False-positive ECCs occur in more than 60% of cases. It has a similar prognosis to stage I tumors.
  (2) The surgical staging evaluation is as outlined above (see section III D 6).
  (3) Adjuvant postoperative pelvic radiotherapy is used for:
    (a) Extensive cervical involvement
    (b) Penetration of more than half of the myometrium
    (c) Involvement of the pelvic lymph nodes

  d. Stage II carcinomas with obvious cervical extension
  (1) Grade 3 tumors are associated with a high incidence of pelvic lymph node metastases, distant metastases, and a poor prognosis.
  (2) There are two approaches to treatment. The first approach entails radical hysterectomy, bilateral salpingo-oophorectomy, and periaortic and pelvic lymphadenectomy; the second approach entails pelvic radiotherapy and intracavitary radium followed in 4 weeks by a total abdominal hysterectomy and bilateral salpingo-oophorectomy.
    (a) Radical hysterectomy should be reserved for those patients with low-grade tumors, who are otherwise medically healthy and preferably young. In patients with a prior history of extensive abdominopelvic surgery or chronic pelvic inflammatory disease (PID) where intra-abdominal adhesions are expected, this treatment modality may be preferred because of the increased risk of radiation-induced small bowel injury in patients treated by radiotherapy.
    (b) Combined radiotherapy and surgery. This approach is less morbid than radical hysterectomy. Given the fact that many patients with endometrial carcinoma are older; obese; and suffer from hypertension, adult onset diabetes, or both, the combined approach is preferred in patients with stage II tumors with obvious cervical extension.

  e. Stage III and IV adenocarcinoma. Treatment in these patients must be individualized. In most instances, treatment programs that involve surgery with chemotherapy, hormonal therapy, and radiation therapy can be devised.

  f. Recurrent disease. Treatment for recurrent disease must be individualized, depending upon the extent and site of recurrence, hormonal receptor status, and the patient's health. Treatment programs can include exenterative procedures, radiotherapy, chemotherapy, and hormonal therapy.

IV. OVARIAN CANCER

A. Incidence

1. Ovarian cancer is the leading cause of death attributable to gynecologic cancers in the United States. Approximately 12 out of every 1000 women will develop the disease, but only 2–3 of the 12 will be cured.

2. The incidence starts to rise in the fifth decade and continues to rise until the eighth decade. The postmenopausal patient is at high risk for developing ovarian cancer.

3. Ovarian cancer is silent in its early development.
   a. In over 70% of cases, the ovarian disease has spread beyond the pelvis before the diagnosis is made.
   b. There is no dependable serodiagnostic screening test other than periodic pelvic examinations.
      (1) No cytologic sampling from the cervix, vaginal pool, or cul-de-sac washing has been useful as a screening tool.
      (2) It is the combined responsibility of the physician and the patient to ensure that a pelvic examination occurs every 6 months during the postmenopausal years in order that ovarian enlargement, or the "postmenopausal palpable ovary" can be detected.

B. Pathophysiology

1. Ovarian neoplasias are categorized according to the site of origin, including the following:
   a. Epithelial
   b. Sex cord stromal
   c. Germ cell
   d. Nonspecialized stromal
   e. Metastatic

2. The initial spread is to adjacent peritoneal surfaces and retroperitoneal lymph nodes; however, spread may be to any surface and to the omentum.
   a. Extra-abdominal and intrahepatic metastases occur late in the course of the disease and only in a small percentage of cases.
   b. As a terminal event, bowel obstruction caused by massive serosal involvement is common.

C. **Staging**

1. **Stage I:** Limited to the ovaries
   a. **Stage IA:** Limited to one ovary; no ascites
      (1) No tumor on the external surface; capsule intact
      (2) Tumor present on the external surface or capsule ruptured or both
   b. **Stage IB:** Limited to both ovaries; no ascites
      (1) No tumor on the external surface; capsule intact
      (2) Tumor present on the external surface or capsule ruptured or both
   c. **Stage IC:** Tumor either stage IA or IB but with ascites present or with positive peritoneal washings

2. **Stage II:** Involvement of one or both ovaries with pelvic extension
   a. **Stage IIA:** Extension or metastases to the uterus or tubes or both
   b. **Stage IIB:** Extension to other pelvic tissues
   c. **Stage IIC:** Tumor either stage IIA or IIB but with ascites present or with positive peritoneal washings

3. **Stage III:** Involvement of one or both ovaries with intraperitoneal metastases outside the pelvis or positive retroperitoneal nodes or both

4. **Stage IV:** Involvement of one or both ovaries with distant metastases

D. **Categories of tumors**

1. **Epithelial tumors.** These tumors arise from the coelomic mesothelium, which is capable of differentiating into both benign and malignant tumors. The transition from benign to malignant is not abrupt; there is an intermediate or borderline category. Distinguishing benign, borderline, or malignant tumors is important in terms of treatment and prognosis. Epithelial malignancies represent 82% of all ovarian malignancies.
   a. The predominant cell types are:
      (1) **Serous**
         (a) One out of three serous tumors is malignant.
         (b) Serous cancers are more than three times as common as the mucinous variety and seven times as common as the endometrioid variety.
         (c) Serous cystadenoma carcinoma, the most common type of ovarian cancer, tends to be bilateral in 35%–50% of cases.
      (2) **Mucinous**
         (a) One out of five mucinous tumors are malignant.
         (b) Mucinous tumors are bilateral in 10%–20% of cases.
      (3) **Endometrioid**
         (a) The microscopic pattern is similar to primary carcinoma of the endometrium.
         (b) Areas of endometriosis in the ovary may be present.
         (c) The prognosis is much better than that of the serous and mucinous carcinomas.
   b. The prognosis for each stage of epithelial ovarian tumors is linked to the grade of the tumor; poorly differentiated tumors have a poor prognosis. Long-term survival of patients with borderline or well-differentiated cancers after primary surgery is common.

2. **Sex cord stromal neoplasms.** Granulosa–theca cell tumors, granulosa cell tumors, and Sertoli-Leydig cell tumors, which comprise 3% of all ovarian neoplasms, are derived from mesenchymal stem cells in the ovarian cortex. These tumors have the potential to secrete estrogen. Endometrial hyperplasia has been reported with more than 50% of these tumors, and cancer in 5%–10%.
   a. **Granulosa–theca cell tumors** occur both in premenarchal, menopausal, and postmenopausal women and induce abnormal bleeding and breast development.
   b. **Granulosa cell tumors** have the following characteristics:
      (1) They are bilateral only 10% of the time.
      (2) They vary in size from microscopic to tumors that fill the abdomen.
      (3) They are characterized histologically by Call-Exner bodies—that is, rosettes or follicles of granulosa cells often with a central cavity.
      (4) Approximately 30% of these tumors recur, usually more than 5 years after removal of the primary tumor with occasional recurrences after 30 years.

    c. Sertoli-Leydig cell tumors (e.g., androblastoma and arrhenoblastoma) are rare tumors of mesenchymal origin.

      (1) Their usual endocrine activity is androgenic.

      (2) Defeminization is the classic feature of the androgen-secreting tumors, including breast and uterine atrophy, which is followed by masculinization, including hirsutism, acne, receding hairline, clitorimegaly, and voice changes.

3. Germ cell tumors. Malignant germ cell tumors are believed to arise from primitive germ cells in the ovary, which give rise to either dysgerminoma or tumors of totipotential cells. The latter tumors can differentiate into either embryonal carcinoma, which, in turn, can be differentiated into extraembryonic structures, such as endodermal sinus or choriocarcinoma, or embryonal structures, such as the malignant teratomas. These tumors represent 5% of all ovarian malignancies but account for over two-thirds of all malignant ovarian neoplasms in women under the age of 20 years.

    a. Dysgerminoma. The histologic appearance demonstrates sheets of round to oval cells with clear cytoplasm and a centrally placed nucleus with prominent nucleoli. There is a characteristic lymphocytic infiltrate within fibrous septae. Occasionally there are syncytiotrophoblastic giant cells. Other characteristics of dysgerminomas include the following:

      (1) They are the most common germ cell tumor, accounting for approximately 50% of cases.

      (2) Ninety percent of dysgerminomas are found in women under the age of 30.

      (3) The propensity for lymphatic invasion is great.

      (4) Tumors can secrete detectable amounts of human chorionic gonadotropin (HCG).

      (5) Bilateral tumors occur in more than 20% of cases.

      (6) Tumors are exquisitely radiosensitive.

    b. Embryonal carcinoma. The histologic appearance demonstrates solid sheets of anaplastic cells with abundant clear cytoplasm, hyperchromatic nuclei, and numerous mitotic figures. Embryonal carcinoma is further characterized by the following:

      (1) The median age of patients with embryonal carcinoma is 15 years.

      (2) The tumor elaborates both α-fetoprotein and HCG; the latter trophic hormone levels may be responsible for precocious puberty in the prepubertal girl.

      (3) Most often, the tumor is unilateral with explosive growth tendencies, leading to large tumor masses and acute abdominal pain.

    c. Endodermal sinus tumor. The histologic appearance consists of a glomerulus-like structure resembling the papillae of the endodermal sinus in the rat's placenta. This pathognomonic structure is known as the Schiller-Duval body. This tumor is further characterized by the following:

      (1) The median age of patients with endodermal sinus tumors is 19 years.

      (2) A primary tumor is unilateral 95% of the time; the right ovary is most commonly affected.

      (3) α-Fetoprotein is a tumor marker.

      (4) There is a tendency toward rapid expansion.

    d. Choriocarcinoma. This primary tumor must be distinguished from metastatic disease to the ovary from a gestational choriocarcinoma. The histologic appearance is that of atypical to highly anaplastic cyto- and syncytiotrophoblastic elements. This tumor is further characterized by the following:

      (1) It commonly occurs in young women.

      (2) It is rarely bilateral.

      (3) It elaborates HCG.

      (4) It can present as a pelvic mass and precocious puberty in prepubertal girls.

    e. Malignant teratomas. This broad spectrum of tumors arise from embryonal elements, which have differentiated into the embryonal somatic structures of the ectoderm, mesoderm, and entoderm. These tumors can be either solid or cystic and can give rise to:

      (1) Immature malignant teratoma. The principle tumor element is atypical neural epithelial elements.

      (2) Monodermal tumors. These tumors involve highly specialized tumors of thyroid tissue (struma ovarii) or neurosecretory tissue (carcinoid).

      (3) Mature teratoma with malignant transformation. The principle tumor type that undergoes malignant transformation in the mature teratoma is squamous elements.

4. Gonadoblastoma. This is a rare ovarian tumor found in patients with dysgenetic gonads and a karyotype that includes a Y chromosome.

    a. They are composed of granulosa, theca, Sertoli, and Leydig cells.

    b. They frequently contain calcifications.

    c. They have a tendency to develop dysgerminomatous overgrowth; therefore, in the presence of a Y chromosome, all dysgenetic gonads should be removed as soon as they are diagnosed.

E. Diagnosis

1. **Signs and symptoms.** Ovarian cancers usually produce few symptoms until the disease is advanced.
   a. Abdominal distension caused by ascites is often the presenting complaint.
   b. Lower abdominal pain, a pelvic mass, and weight loss are additional features.

2. **Early detection** of ovarian cancer depends on periodic pelvic examinations, especially after 40 years of age.

3. **Pelvic ultrasound** is helpful in characterizing the size and architecture of the adnexal mass. Approximately 95% of ovarian cancers are greater than 5 cm. Multicystic and solid components and free fluid in the cul-de-sac are ultrasonic features suggestive of ovarian carcinoma.

4. **CA 125**, an ovarian cancer antigen, is elevated above the normal range in greater than 85% of patients with ovarian cancer.

5. **Abdominopelvic CAT scan, barium enema, and chest x-ray** are helpful in the evaluation of the extent of disease in women suspected of having an ovarian cancer.

6. **Surgical staging evaluation**
   a. Exploratory laparotomy through a vertical abdominal incision, allowing a thorough evaluation of the upper abdomen
   b. Peritoneal washings from the pelvis and upper abdomen
   c. Inspection of all peritoneal and diaphragmatic surfaces
   d. Sampling of pelvic and para-aortic lymph nodes
   e. Omentectomy
   f. A wedge biopsy of the contralateral ovary to exclude occult disease in young women who wish to preserve fertility and who have an ovarian cancer apparently confined to one ovary

F. Treatment

1. **Epithelial tumors**
   a. In patients with stage IA well-differentiated tumors confirmed on staging laparotomy, surgery alone is sufficient therapy.
   b. In all other patients with early stage (I and II) cancers with no residual tumor apparent, either intraperitoneal instillation of ^{32}P, a radioactive colloidal isotope, which emits β-radiation up to a depth of 7 mm, or whole abdominopelvic radiotherapy have been associated with an improved survival.
   c. In patients with stage III and IV cancers, complete surgical excision in the form of a tumor debulking procedure is the desired initial treatment approach. Adjuvant combination chemotherapy with cisplatin and cyclophosphamide for 6–9 courses is recommended to treat residual disease.
   d. Second-look laparotomy following the completion of chemotherapy in patients with no clinically detectable disease is recommended to tailor subsequent treatment recommendations.
   e. Five-year survival rates
      (1) **Stage I:** 66.4%
      (2) **Stage II:** 45.0%
      (3) **Stage III:** 13.3%
      (4) **Stage IV:** 4.1%

2. **Sex cord stromal tumors**
   a. Total abdominal hysterectomy and bilateral salpingo-oophorectomy following adequate surgical staging constitute definitive therapy in most patients.
   b. In young women with stage IA disease who desire fertility, a conservative approach with uterine and contralateral adnexal preservation is indicated.
   c. Patients with advanced or recurrent disease should be surgically debulked. If residual tumor is less than 2 cm, abdominopelvic radiotherapy may be beneficial. Chemotherapy is used in bulky residual or recurrent disease. Vincristine, actinomycin D, and cyclophosphamide are active agents.

3. **Germ cell tumors**
   a. **Dysgerminoma**
      (1) **Stage IA:** Conservative surgery
      (2) **Greater than stage IA.** Therapy consists of either:
         (a) Radiotherapy to the whole abdomen and pelvis with a boost to the para-aortic region

      (b) Chemotherapy. This involves 3–4 intensive courses with vinblastine, cisplatin, and bleomycin.

  b. Nondysgerminomatous germ cell tumors
    (1) Stage IA. Conservative surgery
    (2) All other cases. Aggressive chemotherapy as outlined for dysgerminoma

V. VAGINAL CANCER

A. Squamous cell carcinoma is usually located in the upper half of the vagina.

  1. Symptoms
    a. The most frequent symptom is a vaginal discharge, which is often bloody.
    b. Urinary symptoms occur because of the close proximity of the upper vagina to the vesicle neck with resulting compression of the bladder.
    c. The elasticity of the posterior vaginal fornix allows lesions in that area to become quite large, especially in sexually inactive women, before they are detected.

  2. Age. This rare malignant cancer occurs in women between 35 and 70 years of age.

  3. Lymphatic spread. The upper vagina is drained by the common iliac and hypogastric nodes while the lower vagina is drained by the regional lymph nodes of the femoral triangle.

  4. Staging
    a. Stage I: Limited to the vaginal mucosa
    b. Stage II: Involvement of the subvaginal tissue but no extension onto the pelvic sidewall
    c. Stage III: Extension onto the pelvic sidewall
    d. Stage IV: Extension beyond the true pelvis or involvement of the mucosa of the bladder or rectum

  5. Treatment. Treatment of squamous cell carcinoma is primarily by radiotherapy. Large carcinomas of the vault or vaginal walls are treated initially with external radiation; this shrinks the neoplasm so that local radiation therapy will be more effective.

  6. Five-year survival rates
    a. Stage I: 65%
    b. Stage II: 60%
    c. Stage III: 35%
    d. Stage IV: 9%

B. Diethylstilbestrol (DES)-related adenocarcinoma. DES was used in the 1940s and 1950s in high-risk pregnancies—diabetes, habitual abortion, threatened abortion, and other obstetric risk situations—to prevent pregnancy wastage. In all documented cases, DES was begun before the eighteenth week of pregnancy.

  1. Age
    a. There is a peak frequency of 19.5 years for patients with a history of DES exposure and clear cell adenocarcinoma of the vagina.
    b. The risk of development of these carcinomas through the age of 24 years in DES-exposed females has been calculated at 0.14 to 1.4/1000.

  2. Characteristics of clear cell carcinoma
    a. Approximately 40% of the cases occur in the cervix, and the other 60% primarily in the upper half of the vagina.
    b. The incidence of lymph node metastases is high; about 18% in stage I and 30% or more in stage II.

  3. Treatment
    a. If the cancer is confined to the cervix and the upper vagina, radical hysterectomy and upper vaginectomy with pelvic lymphadenectomy and ovarian preservation is recommended.
    b. Advanced tumors and lesions involving the lower vagina are more suitable for irradiation, which should include treatment of the pelvic nodes and parametrial tissues.

  4. Five-year survival rates are comparable to those for the squamous tumors of the cervix and upper vagina.

VI. VULVAR CARCINOMA

A. Epidemiology. Factors associated with vulvar carcinoma include:

  1. A history of vulvar condylomata or granulomatous venereal disease is common.

2. Vulvar carcinomas occasionally arise from areas of carcinoma-in-situ.

3. They occur more frequently in women who have been treated for invasive squamous carcinomas of the cervix or vagina.

4. More than half of the patients are between the age of 60 and 79 years of age.

5. Less than 15% are under the age of 40.

B. Etiology. Little is known about causal factors in this disease. Recently, human papillomavirus types 16 and 18 have been detected in squamous cancer of the vulva.

C. Symptoms. Recognition of a lesion is often accompanied by a delay in diagnosis because of either self-treatment by the patient or lack of recognition by the treating physician. Vulvar cancer usually presents with:

1. A history of chronic vulvar irritation or soreness

2. A visible lesion on the labia, which is often sore

D. Histology. Squamous carcinoma comprises 90% of these tumors. The remaining 10% are comprised of adenosquamous carcinoma, adenocarcinoma, malignant melanoma, verrucous carcinoma, and sarcomas.

E. Patterns of spread

1. Local expansion involves the contiguous structures of the urethra, vagina, perineum, anus, rectum, and pubic bone.

2. Lymphatic spread. Metastases follow the lymphatic drainage pattern of the vulva, which includes superficial inguinal groups, deep femoral groups, and pelvic nodes.

3. Hematogenous spread occurs in the advanced or recurrent cases.

F. Diagnosis. Incisional or excisional biopsy of the suspicious lesion under local or general anesthesia confirms the diagnosis.

G. Pretreatment evaluation includes a clinical assessment of:

1. Tumor size (T)
   a. T_1: Tumor confined to the vulva that is 2 cm or less in size
   b. T_2: Tumor confined to the vulva that is greater than 2 cm in size
   c. T_3: Tumor of any size that spreads to the urethra, vagina, perineum, or anus
   d. T_4: Tumor of any size that infiltrates the bladder and rectal mucosa

2. Node assessment (N)
   a. N_0: No regional nodes palpable
   b. N_1: Nodes palpable in either groin but not enlarged or mobile (not clinically suspicious)
   c. N_2: Nodes palpable in either groin and enlarged and mobile (are clinically suspicious)
   d. N_3: Fixed or ulcerative nodes

3. Metastases (M)
   a. M_0: No metastases
   b. M_1: Palpable pelvic nodes
   c. M_2: Other distant metastases

H. Staging

1. Stage I: $T_1N_0M_0$ and $T_1N_1M_0$

2. Stage II: $T_2N_0M_0$ and $T_2N_1M_0$

3. Stage III: $T_3N_0M_0$, $T_1N_2M_0$, $T_2N_2M_0$, and $T_3N_2M_0$

4. Stage IV: $T_4N_0M_0$, $T_4N_1M_0$, $T_4N_2M_0$, or any N_3, M_{1a}, or M_{1b} tumors

I. Treatment

1. Microinvasive carcinoma. There is no uniform acceptance as to the exact definition, but a commonly accepted definition includes the factors listed below. Treatment includes wide (3 cm) local excision and sampling of the ipsilateral superficial inguinal nodes.
   a. The lesion is less than or equal to 1 cm in size.

        b. Focal invasion is no greater than 5 mm in depth.

        c. There is no lymphovascular space involvement.

    2. Invasive squamous carcinoma. Therapy includes:

        a. Stage I and II disease. Radical vulvectomy with inguinal and deep femoral adenopathy. Pelvic radiotherapy is recommended for patients with involved nodes.

        b. Stage III and IV disease. Therapy is tailored to the exact extent of the disease and the patient's general health. Therapy includes either radical or exenterative surgery alone or in combination with radiotherapy.

        c. Metastatic or recurrent disease. Therapy is tailored to the clinical situation.

J. Five-year survival rates

    1. Stage I: 71.4%

    2. Stage II: 47.2%

    3. Stage III: 32.0%

    4. Stage IV: 10.5%

STUDY QUESTIONS

Directions: Each question below contains five suggested answers. Choose the **one best** response to each question.

1. Colposcopic examination of the cervix of a 38-year-old woman yields a negative biopsy and a positive endocervical curettage. Which of the following is appropriate follow-up?

(A) Repeat the Pap smear in 3 months
(B) Repeat the colposcopic examination in 3 months
(C) Perform conization of the cervix
(D) Perform a vaginal hysterectomy
(E) No follow-up required

2. A patient presents with a gross lesion on her cervix, which appears to involve a small portion of the adjacent vagina. Biopsy of the lesion reveals invasive squamous cell carcinoma. Pelvic examination reveals thickening of the right parametrium but not out to the pelvic sidewall. What is the stage of this cancer?

(A) Stage IA
(B) Stage IB
(C) Stage IIA
(D) Stage IIB
(E) Stage III

3. The correct stage for a $T_2N_1M_0$ carcinoma of the vulva is

(A) stage I
(B) stage II
(C) stage III
(D) stage IV
(E) none of the above

4. Which of the following tumors is most sensitive to radiation therapy?

(A) Serous cystadenocarcinoma
(B) Endometrioid cancer
(C) Gonadoblastoma
(D) Arrhenoblastoma
(E) Dysgerminoma

5. A woman with stage I, grade I adenocarcinoma of the endometrium is treated with a total abdominal hysterectomy and a bilateral salpingo-oophorectomy. Examination of the uterine pathology reveals myometrial invasion to a depth of 3 mm. Follow-up should involve

(A) no further therapy
(B) local vaginal cuff radiation
(C) external pelvic radiation
(D) para-aortic lymph node biopsy
(E) medroxyprogesterone therapy

Directions: Each question below contains four suggested answers of which **one or more** is correct. Choose the answer

A   if **1, 2, and 3** are correct
B   if **1 and 3** are correct
C   if **2 and 4** are correct
D   if **4** is correct
E   if **1, 2, 3, and 4** are correct

6.   Epidemiologic factors that are associated with cervical cancer include which of the following?

(1) Early age of coitarche
(2) Sexual promiscuity
(3) Latent human papillomavirus infection of the cervix
(4) High-risk male consort

7.   Endometrial hyperplasia could be expected in which of the following conditions?

(1) Polycystic ovary disease
(2) Cystic teratoma
(3) Granulosa–theca cell tumor
(4) Sertoli-Leydig cell tumor

8.   Correct statements concerning ovarian dysgerminoma include which of the following?

(1) It is a germ cell tumor
(2) The median age of women with this tumor is 45 years
(3) It is bilateral in about 20% of cases
(4) It is a radioresistant tumor

9.   Procedures that are helpful in the surgical staging of ovarian cancer include which of the following?

(1) Peritoneal cytology
(2) Pelvic and para-aortic lymph node sampling
(3) Omentectomy
(4) Transverse lower abdominal incision

ANSWERS AND EXPLANATIONS

1. The answer is C. [*II C 3 c, d (3), 4 b*] An endocervical canal curettage (ECC) is performed with a colposcopy to rule out dysplasia within the canal that is colposcopically inapparent. With a negative colposcopic examination and a positive ECC, cervical dysplasia can only be adequately assessed by a cone biopsy and histologic inspection of the endocervical glands, which contain the abnormal epithelium. A repeat Pap smear or colposcopic examination in 3 months leaves known disease in the canal unevaluated or untreated. Conization of the cervix is not only a diagnostic procedure, it is also a minor procedure, which is therapeutic in 85% of cases.

2. The answer is D. [*II D 2 d (1), (2)*] Stage II cervical cancers involve the cervix and the vagina or the parametrium. Stage IIA involves the vagina without evidence of parametrial involvement. Stage IIB involves infiltration of the parametrium but not out to the pelvic sidewall.

3. The answer is B. (*VI G 1–3, H*) Vulvar staging is based on the tumor size (T), regional nodal assessment (N), and metastatic assessment (M) system. A $T_2N_1M_0$ tumor is a stage II tumor in which a tumor of 2 cm or more is confined to the vulva and is accompanied by papable nodes that are not enlarged or mobile. There is no metastasis present.

4. The answer is E. (*IV D 3 a (6), F 3 a*) The dysgerminoma is the most common form of germ cell tumor. It has a favorable prognosis because of its radiosensitivity. Even though there is a 25% recurrence rate following conservative surgical treatment, most of these recurrent cases will have a complete remission after radiation therapy.

5. The answer is A. (*III D 6 a*) The patient described in the question has a low-grade endometrial cancer that is limited to the inner one-third of the myometrium. Therefore, no further therapy other than the hysterectomy and bilateral salpingo-oophorectomy is indicated, and a very high cure rate can be expected. If the tumor was of a higher grade or involved the outer one-third of the myometrium, external pelvic radiation following the hysterectomy would be indicated.

6. The answer is E (all). (*II A 1 a–f*) Epidemiologic studies associate an early age of first intercourse (coitarche) and sexual promiscuity with an increased incidence of cervical cancer. Cigarette smoking, a high-risk male consort (i.e., one whose previous sexual partners developed precancerous or cancerous conditions of the cervix), and marriage or conception at an early age are additional risk factors. Sexually transmitted viruses, such as herpes simplex virus and human papillomavirus, have also been implicated as causal agents.

7. The answer is B (1, 3). (*III A 2 b, B, C*) The etiology of endometrial hyperplasia appears to involve the secretion of estrogen that is unopposed by progesterone. Unopposed estrogen is characteristic of chronic anovulatory states, such as polycystic ovary disease, and estrogen-secreting tumors, such as the granulosa–theca cell tumor. The cystic teratoma is not characterized by estrogen secretion, and the Sertoli–Leydig cell tumor secretes an androgen that would not produce endometrial hyperplasia.

8. The answer is B (1, 3). (*IV D 3 a*) Dysgerminoma is a tumor of germ cell origin. Over 90% of these tumors are found in women under the age of 30. They are bilateral in 20% of cases and are exquisitely radiosensitive.

9. The answer is A (1, 2, 3). (*IV E 6 a–f*) A staging laparotomy for ovarian cancer involves a generous vertical abdominal incision to enable the surgeon to assess adequately the upper abdomen for occult metastatic disease. A transverse lower abdominal incision limits the surgeon's ability to adequately visualize, palpate, or sample the upper abdomen for occult disease. Peritoneal cytology, pelvic and para-aortic lymph node sampling, and omentectomy are also performed to detect occult metastatic disease.

38
Medicolegal Considerations in Obstetrics and Gynecology
Luciano Lizzi

I. INTRODUCTION. Law defines the set of agreements made among the members and groups in a society. Medicine is one such group in which law permeates, defining and regulating the relationship between the physician and patient, the physician and hospital, and the physician and society at large. Moreover, legal issues dealing with access to medical care and consumer demands regarding health care are dominant in public policy discussions. Obstetrics and gynecology exists at the cutting edge of these matters because it involves the most critical aspects of life, such as conception, reproduction, and abortion. Thus, it is important for the student of medicine to understand, at least in a preliminary fashion, the legal issues that involve the practice of obstetrics and gynecology.

II. MALPRACTICE

A. Definition. Malpractice is professional misconduct that indicates an unreasonable lack of skill in carrying out one's professional duties. Thus, a professional is accused of acting in a negligent manner.

B. Elements of negligence

1. **Duty.** A physician has a particular duty or obligation to the patient. A physician–patient relationship exists when a patient presents to a physician who agrees to undertake her care in a fiduciary manner. It is a form of implied contract. In this relationship, a physician must act:
   a. In accordance with specific standards established or accepted by the profession
   b. As a reasonable physician, taking reasonable care of a patient and not taking unreasonable risks

2. **Breach of duty.** When a physician fails to act in accordance with professional norms, thus violating a standard of care, he or she has committed a breach of duty. This breach must be substantiated by the testimony of an expert.

3. **Causation.** A reasonable connection between an act or a failure to act by a physician and a patient's injury (i.e., causation) must be established.

4. **Damages.** Actual loss, injury, or damage must have occurred.

C. Recovery. The patient/plaintiff must prove that it is more probable than not that the elements of negligence are satisfied (**preponderance of the evidence**) in order to recover damages.

III. PRECONCEPTION ISSUES. A constitutional right of privacy protects an individual's procreative choice from government intrusion. The right to use contraception was the earliest right to reproductive freedom (*Griswold v. Connecticut*, 1965).

A. Oral contraceptives

1. Most lawsuits regarding oral contraceptives are product liability cases against the manufacturer.
   a. The general rule is that a manufacturer must provide patients with a written warning of all untoward side effects.
   b. A physician must inform patients of the possible side effects and explain the alternative methods of contraception. All of these discussions must be documented.

2. **A physician has a duty to:**
   a. Perform a thorough physical examination.
   b. Perform relevant laboratory examinations.
   c. Warn patients of possible adverse side effects.

WAIT 2-3 mos
I pills to be preg.
to be preg.

    d. Monitor closely patients who develop side effects.

    e. Advise patients to use an alternative form of contraception for 2–3 months before attempting to conceive since there is evidence of aneuploidy among abortuses of women who recently stopped oral contraceptives (*Jorgensen v. Meade Johnson Labs*, 1973).

B. Intrauterine devices (IUDs) have been the center of legal and medical controversy regarding contraceptives ever since the Dalkon shield was recalled in 1984 and $500 million was paid in damages to 9500 women.

  1. All IUDs except for the Progestasert and the recently released Paragard have been withdrawn by the manufacturers because of litigation costs. Most lawsuits have been product liability cases, which state that the IUD is unreasonably dangerous because of defective design and caused:

    a. Uterine and pelvic infections

    b. Infertility

    c. Perforation

    d. Ectopic pregnancy

  2. A physician has a duty to:

    a. Inform patients of the risk of an IUD insertion and use.

    b. Explain alternative methods of contraception and their risks.

    c. Perform a physical examination.

    d. Perform a Pap test and cervical cultures.

    e. Examine patients in 3 months after insertion of an IUD and then yearly thereafter.

C. Sterilization

  1. Definition. Sterilization is a surgical procedure undertaken for the express purpose of eliminating reproductive capacity.

  2. Voluntary sterilization

    a. Public hospitals cannot refuse to perform sterilization procedures since it would abridge a woman's reproductive right of privacy.

    b. Private physicians and hospitals may, however, decline to perform this procedure on moral grounds.

    c. Federal funding regulations require that a Department of Health and Human Services consent form be signed between 30 and 180 days prior to surgery. Consent cannot be obtained if the patient is:

      (1) Less than 21 years of age

      (2) In labor

      (3) Under the influence of alcohol or drugs

      (4) Mentally incompetent

      (5) Having an abortion

  3. A physician has a duty to inform patients that:

    a. The operation will result in sterility.

    b. The procedure is permanent.

    c. There are alternative forms of contraception.

    d. There is no guarantee of sterility, and thus, an intrauterine or an ectopic pregnancy can occur.

  4. Involuntary sterilization. Twenty states authorize involuntary sterilization of genetically retarded wards of the state. However, it is generally required that patients:

    a. Have permanent medical conditions

    b. Have adequate sexual capacity

    c. Have a high probability of transmitting a genetic disease

    d. Are unable to care for children

    e. Are unable to use alternative methods of contraception

    f. Will suffer minimal risk of personal injury from the procedure

IV. GENETIC COUNSELING. Five percent of all newborns are born with a congenital disorder.

A. Routine genetic screening

  1. Legislation requires phenylketonuria testing in newborns.

  2. Voluntary sickle cell screening centers are available.

  3. Prenatal maternal serum α-fetoprotein testing to determine the risk for neural tube defects or Down's syndrome is routinely recommended.

   4. Semen donors are routinely screened.

B. A physician involved in prenatal care has a duty to:

   1. Test for rubella exposure.

   2. Offer maternal serum α-fetoprotein testing.

   3. Obtain a genetic history.

   4. Recognize a genetic disease in the parents or siblings of the conceptus.

   5. Offer pregnant women referral to a genetic counselor if there is:
      a. A genetic or congenital abnormality in a family member
      b. A family history of a genetic problem
      c. Abnormal development in a previous child
      d. Mental retardation in a previous child
      e. Maternal age greater than or equal to 35 years
      f. Specific ethnic background suggestive of a genetic abnormality (e.g., Tay-Sachs disease)
      g. Exposure to drugs or teratogens
      h. A history of three or more spontaneous abortions
      i. A history of infertility
      j. A desire on the patient's part

C. Particular genetic problems of which a physician must be aware

   1. Teratogens
      a. Rubella
      b. Dilantin
      c. Alcohol
      d. Nicotine
      e. Illicit drugs

   2. Autosomal dominant disorders
      a. Neurofibromatosis
      b. Hereditary familial polyposis

   3. Autosomal recessive disorders
      a. Cystic fibrosis
      b. Infantile polycystic kidneys
      c. Congenital deafness
      d. Tay-Sachs disease
      e. Thalessemia

   4. X-linked disorders
      a. Duchenne muscular dystrophy
      b. Hemophilia

D. Amniocentesis must be offered to pregnant women with:

   1. Age of 35 years or greater

   2. A history of multiple miscarriages

   3. A family history of genetic disease

   4. An abnormal maternal serum α-fetoprotein

V. TERMINATION OF PREGNANCY

A. Right of privacy. A woman's right to abortion falls within a right of privacy interpreted by the Supreme Court to exist within the constitution. This right was upheld in *Roe v. Wade, 1973.*

B. Trimester model

   1. During the first trimester, the decision to abort is a decision that is strictly between a woman and her physician.

   2. During the second trimester, the state may impose regulations reasonably related to a woman's health.

   3. After the second trimester or after the fetus is viable, the state may regulate or proscribe abortion, except when necessary to preserve a woman's health, in order to advance its interest in potential life.

C. **State restrictions.** Since 1973, the time of the abortion decision, states have formulated many laws to limit a woman's access to abortion. The Supreme Court has allowed or disallowed these restrictions on access to abortions, depending on whether the law intended to limit a woman's right of reproductive privacy or if the legislators had a woman's health in mind.

1. **Allow restrictions** on access to abortion in laws requiring:
   a. Parental consent of minors as long as the minor can seek permission from a court in the event of parental disapproval
   b. Licensing of medical facilities where abortions are performed
   c. The presence of a second physician

2. **Disallow restrictions** on access to abortion in laws requiring:
   a. A waiting period
   b. Lengthy information describing the details of the abortion process to women seeking an abortion
   c. Humane disposition of abortuses

D. **Federal financing.** In *Harris v. McCrae* (1980), the Supreme Court upheld the Hyde amendment, which prohibits the use of federal Medicaid funds for abortion unless the woman's life is in danger. It stated that although a state is free to fund abortion and childbirth expenses, it may deny public funds for elective abortions in order to express its preference for normal childbirth.

VI. **NEW REPRODUCTIVE TECHNOLOGIES.** New techniques, such as artificial insemination by husband or donor, in vitro fertilization, embryo transfer, and embryo freezing have created a change in society's concept of the family. A child may be born with as many as five parents: a genetic father, a social father, a genetic mother, a gestational mother, and a social mother. These technologies create legal issues of linkage, inheritance, legitimacy, adultery, confidentiality, the legal status of residual embryos, the particular "parent" responsibilities for a child's diseases and defects, and the legal status and rights of each "parent."

A. **Artifical insemination**

1. **Definition.** Inoculation of a husband's (AIH)* or a donor's (AID) semen into the female genital tract is called artifical insemination.

2. **Consent of the husband.** When the husband of a child's mother consents to artificial insemination, he obtains the same legal right and obligations as a natural parent, including:
   a. The duty to support the child
   b. The right to visitation in case of divorce

3. **Right to privacy.** Given the Supreme Court's enshrinement of a right to privacy, when a single woman requests AID, a public institution providing these services cannot abridge this woman's right to privacy and, thus, would logically have to provide this service; however, a private practitioner could choose not to provide this service. To date, there has not been a case about this issue.

4. *The Model Uniform Parentage Act* states that records pertaining to AID shall be kept confidential in a sealed file and are not subject to inspection except upon order of the court for good cause.

5. **A physician has a duty to explain that there is:**
   a. No guarantee of pregnancy
   b. A possibility of birth defects
   c. A possibility of acquiring a sexually transmitted disease despite screening

6. **Liability** may arise when:
   a. A physician has not adequately screened a donor for genetic defects or venereal diseases.
   b. A husband's consent has not been obtained.

B. **In vitro fertilization**

1. **Definition.** In in vitro fertilization, sperm and ova are obtained, incubated outside the body, and then the blastocyst is implanted into a uterus.

2. **Legal concepts**
   a. When a husband provides sperm and a wife provides an ovum, traditional family principles apply. This is similar to AIH.

---

*AIH = artificial insemination by husband; AID = artificial insemination by donor.

b. When a donor provides sperm and a wife provides an ovum, legal concepts of AID and adoption apply.

c. When the ovum comes from a female donor and is fertilized and then transferred into another woman's uterus, the legal relationships arising are complex and not clearly formulated. The essential question is whether genetic material, a contractual relationship, or carrying and giving birth determine the claim of motherhood.

C. Surrogate motherhood

1. **Definition.** When a wife is incapable of bearing a child, a couple enters into a contract with another woman (a surrogate mother) who agrees to be artificially inseminated with the husband's semen, to carry and bear a child, and to relinquish her rights to the child. In exchange, she receives payment for medical care, lost wages, clothing, and hospitalization.

2. **Legitimacy and paternity**
   a. Both common law and statutory enactments presume that a child born to a married woman is the legitimate child of that woman and her husband.
   b. Criminal sanctions against the sale of infants pose problems for a couple entering into a contract with a surrogate mother.
   c. Other laws prohibit paying or offering to pay in order to obtain a parent's consent for adoption.
   d. Arguments against surrogate motherhood include the following:
      (1) It undermines the traditional family model.
      (2) It threatens the institution of marriage.
      (3) It cheapens and destroys maternal bonding.
      (4) It treats children as commodities.
      (5) It exploits poor women as vehicles to fulfill the dreams of the rich.
   e. Both Great Britain (*Warnock Report*) and Australia (*Waller Report*) have outlawed surrogate motherhood.
   f. Problems arising in the surrogate contract include the following:
      (1) Surrogate mothers develop maternal feelings toward their infants and refuse to give them to the husband and his wife (e.g., *re Baby M,* 1987).
      (2) Surrogate mothers decide not to honor the contract and terminate the pregnancy.
      (3) Surrogate mothers expose the fetus to teratogens or addicting drugs.
      (4) The infant is defective, and the contractive couple decides not to accept it.
      (5) There is a multiple gestation.

D. Embryo freezing

1. **Definition.** Embryo freezing entails the freezing of unused fertilized ova for future implantation.

2. **Problems**
   a. Concerns have been raised as to the propriety of eugenic considerations and commercialism.
   b. The disposition of unused embryos has been deemed unethical by some critics.
   c. If the parents die, the rights and obligations of frozen embryos has yet to be decided.

VII. BIRTH-RELATED SUITS

A. Wrongful conception

1. **Definition.** Conception is deemed wrongful if it arises after:
   a. Failed sterilization
   b. Ineffective prescription of contraception
   c. Failure to diagnose pregnancy in a timely fashion
   d. An unsuccessful abortion

2. **Liability** arises secondary to a physician's negligence, resulting in the birth of an unplanned child. Negligence is based on:
   a. The improper performance of a sterilization procedure or an abortion
   b. The failure to ascertain the success of the procedure
   c. The failure to inform the woman about the possibility of procedural failures

B. Wrongful birth and wrongful life

1. **Definition**
   a. Wrongful birth is an action brought by parents of a child, alleging that a child with a con-

genital defect was born due to negligent genetic counseling. Thus, a physician has failed to:
  (1) Recognize a genetic problem
  (2) Recognize a condition that places a fetus at risk for a genetic problem
  (3) Inform the mother of the ability to detect genetic problems and to offer termination
  b. **Wrongful life** is an action similar to wrongful birth; however, the child brings suit against the physician, alleging that no life at all would have been preferable to life with a congenital defect.

2. The physician should perform a genetic evaluation as outlined in section IV to minimize liability.

VIII. BIRTH INJURY

A. **Definition.** A birth injury results when an obstetrician's neglect results in injury to a child, such as birth trauma or brain damage.

B. **Negligence** may arise from a failure to:

1. Monitor fetal heart rate adequately

2. Assess the degree of risk of a pregnancy

3. Perform expedient delivery, resulting in perinatal asphyxia that leads to brain damage

4. Monitor a pregnancy adequately

5. Use obstetric forceps properly

C. **Brain damage.** Current studies indicate that it is impossible to isolate a single cause of brain dysfunction. The National Institutes of Health have stated that:

1. Mental retardation is multifactorial, resulting from a combination of genetic, biochemical, viral, and developmental factors and is not necessarily related to birth trauma.

2. Severe mental retardation and epilepsy are possibly associated with birth asphyxia but only when accompanied by cerebral palsy, which is associated with birth asphyxia, prematurity and intrauterine growth retardation.

IX. INFORMED CONSENT

A. **General definition.** "Every human being of adult years and sound mind has a right to determine what shall be done with his own body" (*Schloendorff v. Society of New York Hospital*, 1914).

B. **Negligence theory of consent.** To sue successfully under this theory, the patient/plaintiff must show that:

1. A physician disclosed an inadequate amount of significant information.

2. The patient agreed to therapy based on this inadequate information.

3. The patient was harmed.

4. If the significant information had been given, the suggested therapy would have been refuted.

C. **Disclosure rules** establish the appropriate standard of care in obtaining informed consent. States differ as to which standard is applicable.

1. **Majority rule** is the objective view of consent where a physician needs to disclose only information that a reasonable physician would disclose and need not disclose information that would not customarily be disclosed. This rule operates from the physician's point of view.

2. **Minority rule** is the subjective view of consent where a physician needs only to disclose information that a reasonable patient in similar circumstances would wish to know to make a reasonable decision.

D. **General guidelines in obtaining informed consent**

1. A physician must obtain a patient's informed consent prior to treating her.

2. A physician must provide information concerning the probable benefits, risks, and nature of the suggested diagnostic or therapeutic interventions.

3. A physician must provide an explanation of reasonable alternatives to the recommended intervention and consequences of no intervention.

4. Information must be:
   a. What a reasonable practitioner would reveal under similar circumstances
   b. What a reasonable patient would consider significant under similar circumstances

5. Exceptions to informed consent include the following:
   a. If a risk is not reasonably foreseeable, it need not be disclosed.
   b. Disclosure may be partial if full disclosure would be detrimental to a patient's best interest.
   c. If the danger is commonly known, it can be assumed that the patient knows of the danger.
   d. The patient may request not be told of risks.
   e. If the risk concerns the improper performance of an appropriate procedure, it need not be disclosed.
   f. In an emergency requiring prompt attention without which death or serious injury would result and where a patient is in a condition in which reflection is impossible, informed consent is not required.
   g. If a patient is declared either generally or specifically incompetent, informed consent cannot be legitimately obtained.

E. Procedure for obtaining informed consent. Informed consent is a process by which a physician imparts information to a patient who by virtue of this information may intelligently decide whether to submit to and participate in the physician's proposed intervention. Thus, the physician must do the following:

1. Discuss the intervention honestly and explain it in layman's terms along with the reason for its necessity.

2. Explain the risks inherent in the procedure.

3. Explain alternatives and the probable result of no intervention.

4. Allow the patient to ask questions.

5. Document the conversation, listing the major risks and alternatives presented.

6. Explain that it is the patient's right to know a reasonable amount about the proposed intervention and that this right is being forfeited if she refuses to discuss the intervention. Document this.

7. Inform the patient about the risks and the recovery time.

8. Do not alter records.

9. Obtain the consent in person.

X. RISK MANAGEMENT

A. Definition. The systematic process of identifying, evaluating, and addressing malpractice risk defines risk management.

B. Methods to decrease liability risk in an obstetrics practice

1. Treat all pregnancies with concern, and consider none routine.

2. Evaluate past obstetric, genetic, medical, and family histories.

3. Look for a family history of growth retardation, developmental delay, mental retardation, and cerebral palsy.

4. Ask about drugs or toxic exposures.

5. Recognize diabetes mellitus, hypertension, previous stillbirth, advanced maternal age, and postdates pregnancy.

6. Realize that 30% of high-risk intrapartum patients were low-risk patients antepartum.

7. Consider fetal heart rate monitoring.

8. Make frequent visits when the patient is in labor, and stay with her if anything unusual occurs.

9. Obtain umbilical arterial blood gas values at delivery.

10. Obtain a scalp pH in labor with poor variability or with severe variables on fetal monitor tracing.

11. Use oxytocin with caution.

12. Evaluate the progress of labor closely.

C. Education. A physician's role is one of educator, and thus, he or she must educate the public about the realities of what medicine can offer. Expectations of outcomes are difficult to dispel and are reinforced by paternalistic physicians who are hesitant to inform their patients of realistic medical capabilities.

D. Medical records. The medical record is an account of the events that have occurred in the care of a patient. It should reveal a timely analysis of those events, the thoughts of a physician about the patient, and a plan to handle possible occurrences. It should include:

1. The patient's name

2. The date and time

3. Appropriate signature and title

4. Explanations of unusual events or therapies

5. Documentation of procedures

6. Documentation of discharge instructions

7. No arguments, criticisms, contradictions, or illegible entries

8. A single line through any error initialed by the author of the statement

E. Operative notes should not be procedural instructions. It should include:

1. The indications for surgery

2. The type of procedure performed

3. Departures from the routine procedure

4. Unusual findings

5. Difficulties encountered

F. Discharge summary should simply and clearly state:

1. Dates of hospitalization

2. The reason for hospitalization

3. Procedures performed

4. The events of the hospital stay

G. Patient communications. A breakdown in communication is the leading cause of malpractice litigation. Therefore, a physician should do the following:

1. Communicate information in a way that demonstrates concern.

2. Avoid criticism that would adversely affect a patient's self-image.

3. Communicate frequently with a patient's family.

4. Increase the amount of time spent with the patient, especially when modern technologies, which tend to be depersonalizing, are used.

COURT CASES

In re Baby M, 525 A 2a 1128 (New Jersey Superior Court, 1987)

Griswold v. Connecticut, 381 US 479 (US Supreme Court, 1965)

Harris v. McCrae, 448 US 297, (US Supreme Court, 1980)

Jorgensen v. Meade Johnson Laboratories, 483 F 2nd 277 (US Court of Appeals, Tenth Circuit, 1973)

Roe v. Wade, 410 US 113 (US Supreme Court, 1973)

Schloendorff v. Society of New York Hospital, 211 NY 125, 105 NE 92 (New York, 1914)

STUDY QUESTIONS

Directions: Each question below contains five suggested answers. Choose the **one best** response to each question.

1. An obstetrician is called at home by a woman who is in labor. Although she has never been to see the obstetrician for a prenatal visit, she would like him to deliver her infant. The obstetrician refuses to attend to her since he is in the middle of dinner. She subsequently delivers a healthy infant at home. If this woman sues the physician for negligence, his best defense would be which of the following?

(A) Labor is not a disease, so it was not necessary to attend to this pregnant woman
(B) Since the woman did not come for prenatal visits, she is not entitled to a physician
(C) Since the woman gave birth to a healthy infant, no harm was done
(D) Since the physician never accepted the woman as a patient, no physician–patient relationship existed
(E) The physician does not take care of patients who call him at home.

2. Most intrauterine devices have been unavailable recently because of which of the following reasons?

(A) The materials used to manufacture them have become extraordinarily expensive
(B) They have been found to be unreasonably dangerous and cause multiple pelvic problems
(C) The cost of litigation is well above the time, expense, and profit needed by manufacturers to produce them
(D) The demand for this form of contraceptive has fallen
(E) This statement is false; many intrauterine devices are still available

3. When obtaining consent for a laparoscopic tubal ligation the physician must do all of the following EXCEPT

(A) explain that the operation will result in an inability to have children
(B) call the patient's husband to be certain he is aware of his wife's desire for sterility
(C) explain that there is no guarantee of sterility
(D) ask the patient to call if she should miss her menses or develop any pain after the procedure
(E) explain other forms of contraception, including a vasectomy

4. A 32-year-old woman is 12 weeks pregnant. She has no history of Down's syndrome in her family, but she has decided that she could not live with an infant with Down's syndrome. She requests an interview with a genetic counselor to talk about amniocentesis. The physician should do which of the following?

(A) Explain that you understand her concerns and will set up an appointment for her
(B) Explain that she has only a small risk of having a child with Down's syndrome and she should not be concerned
(C) Tell her that it is too risky to subject her infant to an amniocentesis given the small risk of having an infant with Down's syndrome
(D) Explain that although you understand her concerns, you cannot ethically use up a genetic counselor's time simply for reassurance
(E) Refer her to another physician since she is trying to tell you how to practice obstetrics

5. In 1973, the Supreme Court upheld the right to obtain an abortion. In doing so, it established a trimester model. In this model, the Supreme Court explained all of the following concepts EXCEPT

(A) the right to abortion is unqualified, and the decision to obtain an abortion should be strictly between a woman and her physician
(B) during the third trimester, the state may proscribe abortion in order to further its interest in fetal life
(C) during the first trimester, a woman's right to abortion is absolute
(D) during the second trimester, the state may impose regulations on facilities that provide abortions
(E) during the third trimester, a physician may perform an abortion as a lifesaving measure

Directions: Each question below contains four suggested answers of which **one or more** is correct. Choose the answer

A   if **1, 2, and 3** are correct
B   if **1 and 3** are correct
C   if **2 and 4** are correct
D   if **4** is correct
E   if **1, 2, 3, and 4** are correct

6.   In counseling a couple who wishes artificial insemination by donor, a physician should

(1) obtain consent from both husband and wife
(2) explain that there is no guarantee of pregnancy
(3) explain that despite screening, birth defects are possible
(4) explain that despite screening, sexually transmitted diseases can be transmitted

ANSWERS AND EXPLANATIONS

1. The answer is D. (*II B 1–4*) In order for a physician to be sued for negligence, the plaintiff must clear four hurdles. These are that a duty existed, the duty was breached, that because of the breach of duty, harm was directly caused, and real damage occurred. In this case no physician–patient relationship existed, since the physician refused to help a person who was not his patient. Although it might be argued that it would have been morally correct for the physician to attend to this woman, the law does not recognize a duty to rescue. A physician–patient relationship must be entered into voluntarily and not coerced on either part.

2. The answer is C. (*III B 1*) Although the Dalkon shield was responsible for many cases of pelvic infection, the risk for this is only slightly higher than normal with other IUDs, such as the Copper-7 and Lippe's Loop. Because of defending challenges to the safety of IUDs, manufacturers have found it less costly simply to stop manufacturing these devices. The IUDs now on the market are available at high cost to the consumer and are inserted only after extensive explanations are given to the patient of the possible risks involved.

3. The answer is B. (*III C 3*) When obtaining consent for sterilization, the physician must explain that the procedure is permanent, but failures do occur, and these failures may result in pregnancy. Thus, if a woman misses her menses after a tubal ligation, the physician must rule out pregnancy. If she complains of pelvic pain, it is imperative to rule out ectopic pregnancy. In addition, prior to a sterilization procedure, a patient must be informed about all of the possible contraceptive alternatives.

4. The answer is A. (*IV B 5 j*) All obstetricians must realize that the physician–patient relationship in this field is one of collaboration. Thus, situations where a reasonable request on the part of a concerned patient should be denied are rare. All women are at risk for having an infant with Down's syndrome; 35 years of age is the age at which this risk approximates the risk of fetal loss secondary to amniocentesis. An individual, however, may not want to take *any* risk of having an infant with Down's syndrome, and prenatal testing grants her some security. Denying a woman access to this type of testing is not only cruel but may be later challenged as breaching a duty to provide access to prenatal testing and infringing on a right to procreative privacy.

5. The answer is A. (*V A, B*) In *Roe v. Wade* (1973), the Supreme Court extended the right to privacy to encompass a woman's right to obtain an abortion. In doing so, it explained that this right is not absolute except for the first trimester. In the second trimester, the state may limit this right by imposing regulations in order to preserve a woman's health. In the third trimester, the state may limit this right to the extent that abortion may be performed *only* to preserve maternal health.

6. The answer is E (all). (*VI A 2, 5, 6*) The couple who wishes artificial insemination by donor (AID) must be told of the risks of acquiring birth defects and sexually transmitted diseases. There are some sexually transmitted diseases for which screening is not routine (e.g., human papillomavirus) or about which there is no information (e.g., no screening was available for the human immunodeficiency virus 5 years ago). In this process, it is essential that the husband give his consent, because in so doing he is accepting all responsibility for the child born from this AID process.